SCREENING FOR DOWN SYNDROME
IN THE FIRST TRIMESTER

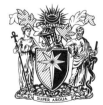

RCOG Press

Since 1973 the Royal College of Obstetricians and Gynaecologists has regularly convened Study Groups to address important growth areas within obstetrics and gynaecology. An international group of eminent scientists and clinicians from various disciplines is invited to present the results of recent research and to take part in in-depth discussions. The resulting volume, containing the papers presented and also edited transcripts of the discussions, is published within a few months of the meeting and provides a summary of the subject that is both authoritative and up to date.

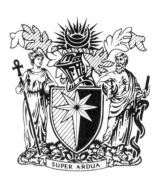

Previous Study Group publications available

Hypertension in Pregnancy
Edited by F. Sharp and
E. M. Symonds

Early Pregnancy Loss
Edited by R.W. Beard and F. Sharp

AIDS in Obstetrics and Gynaecology
Edited by C.N. Hudson and
F. Sharp

Fetal Growth
Edited by F. Sharp, R.B. Fraser
and R.D.G. Milner

Micturition
Edited by J.O. Drife, P. Hilton
and S.L. Stanton

HRT and Osteoporosis
Edited by J.O. Drife and
J.W.W. Studd

Antenatal Diagnosis of Fetal Abnormalities
Edited by J.O. Drife and D. Donnai

Prostaglandins and the Uterus
Edited by J.O. Drife and
A.A. Calder

Infertility
Edited by A.A. Templeton and
J.O. Drife

Intrapartum Fetal Surveillance
Edited by J.A.D. Spencer and
R.H.T. Ward

Early Fetal Growth and Development
Edited by R.H.T. Ward, S.K. Smith
and D. Donnai

Ethics in Obstetrics and Gynaecology
Edited by S. Bewley and R.H.T. Ward

The Biology of Gynaecological Cancer
Edited by R. Leake, M. Gore
and R.H.T. Ward

Multiple Pregnancy
Edited by R.H.T. Ward and
M. Whittle

The Prevention of Pelvic Infection
Edited by A.A. Templeton

Screening for Down Syndrome in the First Trimester

Edited by

J.G. Grudzinskas and R.H.T. Ward

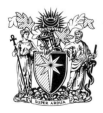

RCOG Press

It was not possible to refer all the material back to the authors or discussants, but it is hoped that the proceedings have been reported fairly and accurately.

The Royal College of Obstetricians and Gynaecologists gratefully acknowledges the support of the 32nd Study Group by Johnson & Johnson Clinical Diagnostics.

J. G. Grudzinskas MB, BS, MD, FRACOG, FRCOG
Academic Unit of Obstetrics, Gynaecology and Reproductive Physiology, St Bartholomew's and the Royal London School of Medicine and Dentistry, Holland Wing, The Royal London Hospital, Whitechapel Road, London E1 1BB, UK

R. H.T. Ward MA, MB, BChir, FRCOG
Consultant Obstetrician and Gynaecologist, University College Hospital Medical School, London WC1E 6HX, UK

First published 1997

The use of registered names, trademarks, etc. in this publication does not imply, even in the absence of a specific statement, that such names are exempt from the relevant laws and regulations and therefore free for general use.

Product liability: the publisher can give no guarantee for information about drug dosage and application thereof contained in this book. In every individual case the respective user must check its accuracy by consulting other pharmaceutical literature.

ISBN 0 902331 98 1

DECLARATION OF INTEREST

All contributors to the Study Group were invited to make a specific Declaration of Interest in relation to the subject of the Study Group. This was undertaken and all contributors complied with this request.

Published by the **RCOG Press** at the
Royal College of Obstetricians and Gynaecologists
27 Sussex Place, Regent's Park
London NW1 4RG

Registered Charity No. 213280

Cover designed by Geoffrey Wadsley

Printed by Henry Ling, The Dorset Press, Dorchester DT1 1HD

Contents

SECTION 9: PRACTICAL ISSUES OF SCREENING PROGRAMMES

SECTION 10: RECOMMENDATIONS

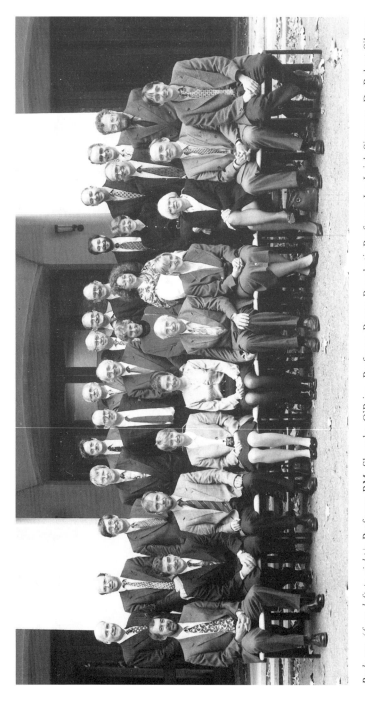

Back row (from left to right): Professor P.M. Shaughn O'Brien, Professor Bruno Brambati, Professor Joe Leigh Simpson, Dr Robert Silman, Professor Timothy Chard, Professor Kypros H. Nicolaides, Dr James N. Macri, Professor Bent Norgaard-Pedersen.

Middle row (from left to right): Mr R. Humphry Ward, Dr Nicholas R. Hicks, Professor Nicholas J. Wald, Dr Timothy M. Reynolds, Dr David J. Torgerson, Mr Kevin Spencer, Professor Eva D. Alberman, Dr Françoise Muller, Professor Theresa M. Marteau, Professor Martin J. Whittle, Professor Howard S. Cuckle.

Front row (from left to right): Dr David A. Aitken, Dr Chris Davies, Dr Roland Zimmermann, Dr M. Ann Harper, Dr Mary C.M. Macintosh, Professor Matteo Adinolfi, Dr Carole A. Barry-Kinsella, Dr Lucia Tului, Professor J. Gedis Grudzinskas, Mr Eric Jauniaux.

Participants

Professor Matteo Adinolfi
The Galton Laboratory, University College London, Wolfson House, 4 Stephenson Way, London NW1 2HE and the Department of Obstetrics and Gynaecology, University College Hospital, University College London, 86–96 Chenies Mews, London WC1E 6HX, UK

Dr David A. Aitken
Top Grade Scientist, Duncan Guthrie Institute of Medical Genetics, Yorkhill NHS Trust, Glasgow G3 8SJ, UK

Professor Eva D. Alberman
Emeritus Professor, Department of Environmental and Preventive Medicine, Wolfson Institute, The Medical College of St Bartholomew's Hospital, Charterhouse Square, London EC1M 6BG, UK

Professor Bruno Brambati
Head of Prenatal Diagnosis Unit, First Institute of Obstetrics and Gynaecology, University of Milan, Via Commenda 12, 20122 Milan, Italy

Professor Timothy Chard
Department of Obstetrics and Gynaecology, St Bartholomew's and the Royal London School of Medicine and Dentistry, West Smithfield, London EC1A 7BE, UK

Professor Howard S. Cuckle
Professor of Reproductive Epidemiology, Centre for Reproduction Growth and Development, Research School of Medicine, 34 Hyde Terrace, Leeds LS2 9LN, UK

Professor J. Gedis Grudzinskas
Academic Unit of Obstetrics, Gynaecology and Reproductive Physiology, St Bartholomew's and the Royal London School of Medicine and Dentistry, 4th Floor, Holland Wing, The Royal London Hospital, Whitechapel Road, London E1 1BB, UK

Dr Nicholas R. Hicks
Consultant Public Health Physician, Department of Public Health and Health Policy, Oxfordshire Health Authority, Old Road, Headington, Oxford OX3 7LG, UK

Mr Eric Jauniaux
Senior Lecturer in Fetal Medicine/Honorary Consultant in Obstetrics and Gynaecology, Academic Department of Obstetrics and Gynaecology, 86–96 Chenies Mews, London WC1E 6HX, UK

Dr Mary C.M. Macintosh
Consultant Obstetrician and Medical Care Epidemiologist, Institute of Epidemiology, 34 Hyde Terrace, Leeds LS2 9LN, UK

Professor Theresa M. Marteau
Professor of Health Psychology, Psychology and Genetics Research Group, UMDS, Old
Medical School Building, London SE1 9RT, UK

Dr Françoise Muller
Laboratoire de Biochimie, Hôpital Ambroise Paré, 9 Avenue Charles de Gaulle, 92104
Boulogne, France

Professor Kypros H. Nicolaides
Harris Birthright Research Centre for Fetal Medicine, King's College Hospital School of
Medicine, Denmark Hill, London SE5 8RX, UK

Professor Bent Nørgaard-Pedersen
Professor and Head of Department, Department of Clinical Biochemistry, Statens Serum
Institut, Artillerivej 5, DK-2300, Copenhagen S, Denmark

Dr Timothy M. Reynolds
Consultant Chemical Pathologist, Clinical Chemistry Department, Burton Hospitals NHS
Trust, Burton Hospital, Belvedere Road, Burton upon Trent, Staffordshire DE13 0RB, UK

Dr Robert Silman
Senior Lecturer in Reproductive Physiology and Honorary Consultant, Academic
Department of Obstetrics and Gynaecology, St Bartholomew's and the Royal London
School of Medicine and Dentistry, The Royal London Hospital, Whitechapel Road,
London E1 1BB, UK

Professor Joe Leigh Simpson
Ernst W. Bertner Chairman and Professor, Department of Obstetrics and Gynecology;
Professor, Department of Molecular and Human Genetics, Baylor College of Medicine,
One Baylor Plaza, Houston, Texas 77030-3498, USA

Mr Kevin Spencer
Consultant Biochemist, Endocrine Unit, Clinical Biochemistry Department, Harold Wood
Hospital, Gubbins Lane, Romford, Essex RM3 0BE, UK

Dr David J. Torgerson
Research Fellow, National Primary Care Research and Development Centre, Centre for
Health Economics, The University of York, York YO1 5DD, UK

Dr Jan M. M. Van Lith
Department of Obstetrics and Gynaecology, Academic Medical Centre, Meibergdreef 9,
1105 AZ Amsterdam, The Netherlands

Professor Nicholas J. Wald
Department of Enviromental and Preventive Medicine, Wolfson Institute, The Medical
College of St Bartholomew's Hospital, Charterhouse Square, London EC1M 6BG, UK

Mr R. Humphry T. Ward
Consultant Obstetrician and Gynaecologist, University College Hospital, 86–96 Chenies
Mews, London WC1E 6HX, UK

Dr Roland Zimmermann
Department of Obstetrics, University Hospital, CH-8091 Zurich, Switzerland

Discussants and observers

Dr Carole A. Barry-Kinsella
Academic Department of Obstetrics and Gynaecology, Rotunda Hospital, Parnell Square,
Dublin 1, Republic of Ireland

Dr Chris Davies
Scientific Adviser, Johnson & Johnson Clinical Diagnostics, Forest Farm Estate,
Whitchurch, Cardiff CF4 7YT, UK

Dr M. Ann Harper
Consultant/Senior Lecturer, Royal Maternity Hospital, Grosvenor Road, Belfast BT12
6BB, Northern Ireland

Dr James N. Macri
Director, NTD Laboratories Inc., 403 Oakwood Road, Huntington Station, New York
11746, USA

Professor P.M. Shaughn O'Brien
Professor and Head of Department, School of Postgraduate Medicine, Thornburrow
Drive, Hartshill, Stoke-on-Trent ST4 7QB, UK

Professor Martin J. Whittle
Department of Fetal Medicine, Birmingham Women's Hospital, Metchley Park Road,
Birmingham B15 2TG, UK

Additional contributors

Dr Josef Achermann
Department of Obstetrics, University Hospital, CH-8091 Zurich, Switzerland

Dr Ezio Alberti
First Institute of Obstetrics and Gynaecology, University of Milan, Via Commenda 12,
20122 Milan, Italy

Dr Hans Baumann
Department of Obstetrics, University Hospital, CH-8091 Zurich, Switzerland

Dr Franz Binkert
Department of Obstetrics, University Hospital, CH-8091 Zurich, Switzerland

Dr Farideh Z. Bischoff
Department of Obstetrics and Gynecology, Baylor College of Medicine, One Baylor Plaza,
Houston, Texas 77030-3498, USA

Dr Maria Brizot, Research Fellow, Harris Birthright Research Centre for Fetal Medicine,
King's College Hospital School of Medicine, Denmark Hill, London SE5 8RX, UK

Dr Luico Bronz
Department of Obstetrics, University Hospital, CH-8091 Zurich, Switzerland

Dr Michael Christiansen
Department of Clinical Biochemistry, Statens Serum Institut, Artillerivej 5, DK-2300,
Copenhagen S, Denmark

Dr Hans Conzin
Department of Obstetrics, University Hospital, CH-8091 Zurich, Switzerland

Dr Jennifer A. Crossley
Principal Scientist, Duncan Guthrie Institute of Medical Genetics, Yorkhill, Glasgow G3 8SJ, UK

Dr Sherman Elias
Department of Obstetrics and Gynecology, Department of Molecular and Human Genetics, Baylor College of Medicine, One Baylor Plaza, Houston, Texas 77030-3498, USA

Dr John Fletcher
Directorate of Public Health and Health Policy, Oxfordshire Health Authority, Old Road, Headington, Oxford OX3 7LG, UK

Dr Verena Geissbühler
Department of Obstetrics, University Hospital, CH-8091 Zurich, Switzerland

Dr Allan Hackshaw, Research Fellow, Department of Enviromental and Preventive Medicine, Wolfson Institute, The Medical College of St Bartholomew's Hospital, Charterhouse Square, London EC1M 6BG, UK

Dr Terrence W. Hallahan
Research Division, NTD Laboratories Inc., 403 Oakwood Road, Huntington Station, New York 11746, USA

Dr Ray Iles, Department of Obstetrics and Gynaecology, St Bartholomew's and the Royal London School of Medicine and Dentistry, West Smithfield, London EC1A 7BE, UK

Dr David A. Krantz
Research Division, NTD Laboratories Inc., 403 Oakwood Road, Huntington Station, New York 11746, USA

Dr Dorothy E. Lewis
Department of Microbiology and Immunology, Baylor College of Medicine, One Baylor Plaza, Houston, Texas 77030-3498, USA

Dr Penelope L. Noble, Research Fellow, Harris Birthright Research Centre for Fetal Medicine, King's College Hospital School of Medicine, Denmark Hill, London SE5 8RX, UK

Dr Jürg Obwegeser
Department of Obstetrics, University Hospital, CH-8091 Zurich, Switzerland

Professor Charles Rodeck
Department of Obstetrics and Gynaecology, University College Hospital, University College London, 86–96 Chenies Mews, London WC1E 6HX, UK

Ms Sarah Rutter
Information Officer, Down's Syndrome Association, 155 Mitcham Road, London SW17 9PG, UK

Dr Guido Savoldelli
Department of Obstetrics, University Hospital, CH-8091 Zurich, Switzerland

Dr Neil J. Sebire, Research Fellow, Harris Birthright Research Centre for Fetal Medicine, King's College Hospital School of Medicine, Denmark Hill, London SE5 8RX, UK

Dr Jon Sherlock
The Galton Laboratory, University College London, Wolfson House, 4 Stephenson Way, London NW1 2HE and the Department of Obstetrics and Gynaecology, University College Hospital, University College London, 86–96 Chenies Mews, London WC1E 6HX, UK

Dr Rosalinde J.M. Snijders, Research Fellow, Harris Birthright Research Centre for Fetal Medicine, King's College Hospital School of Medicine, Denmark Hill, London SE5 8RX, UK

Dr Lucia Tului
First Institute of Obstetrics and Gynaecology, University of Milan, Via Commenda 12, 20122 Milan, Italy

Preface

For some years, there have been indications that ultrasound and biochemical serum markers applicable in the first trimester could provide information about the risk of having a pregnancy affected by Down syndrome (DS). Many have argued that this information, if available earlier in pregnancy, would constitute a significant advance in that women would be reassured by having been advised about low risk or diagnostic tests could be performed sooner if a high-risk status was assigned. Others have argued that the introduction of screening in the first trimester would be ineffective because of the substantial changes required in provision of antenatal care, the identification of pregnancies which would spontaneously abort and the cost implications. Concern has also been expressed about the anticipated increased demand for invasive tests such as chorionic villus sampling, health education for general practitioners and midwives and counselling services. For these reasons, the 32nd RCOG Study Group met to discuss issues surrounding Screening for Down Syndrome in the First Trimester.

Cuckle's chapter on the epidemiology of DS addresses many issues surrounding what is and is not known about the occurrence of screening for this condition with particular respect to ethnic and life-style aspects. The endocrine and metabolic events of early pregnancy are reviewed to provide the reader with a basis for why certain serum markers have been evaluated as risk indicators.

Silman reviews the ethical and social issues surrounding screening for DS. Chapters by Wald, Reynolds and Aitken provide an authoritative basis for a better understanding of the mathematical models used to identify women at risk.

The British and American experience in second trimester screening has been reviewed by Chard and Simpson respectively outlining the historical basis of existing strategies in the second trimester and emphasising the speed with which some centres have already embraced first trimester screening, possibly rendering the use of randomised controlled trials for the validation of first trimester screening inappropriate.

Serum markers have been extensively reviewed, emphasising the simplicity of new techniques for handling samples, the prominent place of serum measurements, in particular of pregnancy associated plasma protein-A and free β-human chorionic gonadotrophin in the first trimester and other markers possibly applicable in the middle rather than at the end of the first trimester.

Ultrasonic markers for fetal aneuploidy have been extensively reviewed. The central place of nuchal translucency screening at 10–13 weeks' gestation is described in detail by Nicolaides, emphasising the effectiveness of this screening test at the District General Hospital level if supported by an active external quality-control service, the use of ultrasound equipment of a particular specification and cost and staff training. Zimmermann and Muller describe their early experience in the combined use of serum and ultrasound markers. Alternatives to biochemical screening such as the identification of fetal cells in the maternal circulation and cervical canal are reviewed.

Jauniaux has reviewed the need for expansion of CVS and amniocentesis of high quality, emphasising the possible need for centralisation of these invasive tests to reduce the risk of complications.

Macintosh, Marteau and Rutter critically address the issues surrounding the communication of tests results, counselling and the views of women who have had screening procedures. The effectiveness of screening for DS is presented in financial terms by Torgerson and Hicks asking whether screening for DS should be offered at all.

These chapters and the discussions which followed formed the basis of the final session of the meeting from which the editors have attempted to distil a series of recommendations for clinical practice, future research and health education and policy.

June 1997

J.G. Grudzinskas
R.H.T. Ward

SECTION 1
GENERAL ASPECTS

Chapter 1

Epidemiology of Down syndrome

Howard S. Cuckle

Many reviews have been published on the epidemiology of Down syndrome but they are too general to provide for the needs of those engaged in antenatal screening for the disorder. In this paper the focus is specifically on screening issues.

The assessment of screening for any disorder begins with the epidemiological considerations of prevalence and natural history; generally screening is only worthwhile for common, serious conditions. Once this basic requirement has been established attention usually turns to the screening test itself. However, unlike most tests, multi-marker screening for Down syndrome uses epidemiology for the interpretation of the test result, in the allowance for covariables when calculating marker levels and in monitoring the entire screening programme. Increasingly the screening programme is being extended to include other types of aneuploidy with similar epidemiological considerations to Down syndrome.

Prevalence and natural history

With the recent decline in birth prevalence of neural tube defects, Down syndrome is the most common serious abnormality found at birth in the UK. The expected birth prevalence, in the absence of antenatal diagnosis and therapeutic abortion, is currently about 1.4 per 1000; almost one thousand affected births a year.

Although there is a high infant mortality rate, life-expectancy for those born in the 1990s is probably in excess of 60 years (Baird and Sadovnick 1988). Improved survival, more effective treatment of associated malformations particularly of the heart and digestive system, together with specific educational programmes means that affected individuals can have a higher quality of life than in the past.

However, not all are capable of benefiting from these developments. Down syndrome remains the most common known cause of severe mental handicap. For example, a survey in the late 1970s among handicapped young adults in three London boroughs found that 20% had Down syndrome (Mitchell and Woodthorpe 1981); the second largest group with a known cause were the 4% who had cerebral palsy. In addition to the congenital mental handicap it is likely that many affected adults will suffer cognitive deficits from pathological changes in the brain normally associated with Alzheimer's disease.

There is a high intrauterine lethality for fetuses with Down syndrome. Much of this occurs in the early weeks of pregnancy but the survival rate is low even for affected fetuses that have not miscarried by the late first trimester and remains considerably reduced for those alive in the middle of the second trimester. The best evidence for this comes from follow-up studies of women who had invasive prenatal diagnosis but refused an offer of termination when Down syndrome was found. The combined results from three studies including a total of 110 pregnancies diagnosed after mid-trimester amniocentesis found a 29% fetal loss rate (Hook *et al.* 1989). A larger series of 168 cases from the National Down Syndrome Cytogenetic Register for England and Wales found an overall loss rate of 35% and this could be broken down further according to gestation (Hook *et al.* 1995). Less than a half of those known to be alive at 14–16 weeks survived to term and by 25–27 weeks four-fifths survived. A further eight pregnancies included in the Register were diagnosed after first trimester chorionic villus sampling and six of them miscarried.

Test interpretation

It can be shown statistically that the optimal way of interpreting the multi-marker profile is to estimate the risk of Down syndrome from the marker levels (Royston and Thompson 1992). This is done by modifying the prior risk, that attained before testing, by a factor known as the 'likelihood ratio' derived from the marker profile and comparing the posterior risk with a fixed cut-off risk. If the risk is greater than the cut-off the result is regarded as 'screen positive', otherwise it is 'screen negative'. This approach will yield a higher detection rate for a given false-positive rate than any other method of test interpretation. It also provides a way of encapsulating the result for the purposes of counselling. The method is optimal even if a single marker is used and whether the marker is physical or biochemical.

The prior risk of Down syndrome can be expressed as a probability, say p, or a rate of 1 in $1/p$ and needs to be converted into an odds of $p:(1-p)$. The posterior risk is calculated by multiplying the left hand side of the odds by the likelihood ratio (x) from the marker profile and the result re-expressed as the rate of 1 in $1+(1-p)/px$ or the probability $px/(1+p(x-1))$. The prior risk can be related to the chance of having a term pregnancy with the disorder or the chance of the fetus being affected at the time of testing. In so far as the aim of screening is to reduce birth prevalence the former is the most appropriate. But screening is also about providing women with information on which to base an informed choice about prenatal diagnosis and to some the risk of an affected fetus is more relevant than an affected birth. The most robust estimates of likelihood ratio are derived from statistical models of marker frequency distributions in affected and unaffected pregnancies.

Two major risk factors are used to derive the prior risk, namely maternal age and family history. Other risk factors can be incorporated but this is not widespread practice at present.

Maternal age

The risk of having a term pregnancy with Down syndrome increases rapidly with maternal age, particularly after age 30. The best available estimate of risk is obtained from combining the results of published population studies of birth prevalence for individual years of age which were carried out before prenatal diagnosis became common. The most widely cited meta-analysis combined all eight published studies, including a total of 4000–5000 Down syndrome and more than 5 million unaffected births, and curve fitted a three parameter additive-exponential curve to overcome statistical fluctuation (Cuckle et al. 1987). In a recent meta-analysis Hecht and Hook (1994) reviewed the eight studies and fitted a series of different curves: using five instead of three parameters, restricting the studies to those thought most likely to be complete and restricting the age range used for parameter calculation. There is little practical difference between the results of the two meta-analyses over the 15–45 year age range but the five parameter curve of Hecht and Hook yields much lower risks for women aged over 45. Even with the combined published series there are relatively few cases at these advanced ages to judge the goodness of fit. However, in women aged over 45 the Down syndrome detection rate is extremely high for all the common marker combinations (Cuckle et al. 1996) and it is unlikely to be greatly affected by the choice of risk curve.

Information on the maternal age-specific risk of Down syndrome in the mid-trimester of pregnancy is available from studies of amniocentesis carried out for reasons other than a family history. A large multicentre European collaborative study has published results on nearly 53 000 amniocenteses in women aged 35 or older including over 600 resulting in a diagnosis of Down syndrome (Ferguson-Smith and Yates 1984). A logistic regression curve was fitted to the data but it would be invalid to extrapolate this curve to young women.

The best estimate of mid-trimester risk across all ages is to apply the known fetal survival rate of affected pregnancies in women who refused termination following amniocentesis to the age-specific term risk. This has been shown to be reasonably consistent with the observed rates at amniocentesis for women aged over 35 (Cuckle and Wald 1990) and it is assumed that it also applies to younger women.

Several large studies of maternal age-specific Down syndrome rates have been published for older women having first trimester chorionic villus sampling. Two recent meta-analyses have been carried out using overlapping subsets of the studies (Snijders et al. 1994; Macintosh et al. 1995). Both fitted curves to the combined data, compared the age-specific rates with the expected term risk from Cuckle et al. (1987) and found that there was an estimated 54% fetal loss rate. In the absence of a large number of women diagnosed in the first trimester and followed up to term, the best estimate of late first trimester risk for all ages is to apply this factor to the term risk.

Previous Down syndrome

If a woman has had a previous pregnancy with Down syndrome and the additional chromosome 21 was *non-inherited* there is an increased risk of recurrence. Three studies have been published with data that can be used to derive a maternal age-specific risk. In a meta-analysis of the total data from 3983 pregnancies including 28 with Down syndrome it appears that the recurrence risk is additive (Cuckle and Wald 1990). A similar excess compared with the age-specific risk from Cuckle *et al.* (1987) was found in each of three age bands. The average excess was equivalent to 0.42% at mid-trimester and 0.34% at term. The best estimate of prior risk in such women is to add this excess to the age-specific probability before converting it into an odds. This results in a relatively large risk for young women but by the age of about 35–40 the risk is not markedly increased above that for women without a family history.

If the previously affected pregnancy was an *inherited* case of Down syndrome the recurrence risk is high enough to dwarf the age-specific risk at most ages. On average the resultant risk can be approximated by adding 10% risk to the age-specific probability but expert genetic advice will be needed in individual cases.

Other factors

Many studies have been reported on whether or not Down syndrome risk is related to paternal age. No clear consensus has emerged principally because of the high correlation between maternal and paternal ages. The ideal study would be based on couples with highly discordant ages, but they are rare. Now, such a series is available from the central register of the French national programme for artificial insemination by donors. This programme provides a natural experiment with no correlation between the ages of the sperm donor and recipient. Preliminary results from nearly 12 000 pregnancies including 25 with Down syndrome show a clear trend in prevalence with paternal age of 1.4, 2.3 and 4.1 per 1000 for fathers aged under 35, 35–9 and 40 or more, respectively (Jalbert 1996). If these results are confirmed as the series expands it may be worthwhile incorporating paternal age into the prior risk calculation.

Several other factors have been associated with Down syndrome risk including maternal thyroid disease, excess exposure to ionising radiation, infrequent intercourse and grand multiparity. However, they are either difficult to quantify or there are insufficient data to estimate a precise risk. For example grand multiparity has recently received attention following a presentation at the 14th European Congress of Perinatal Medicine in 1994. In an orthodox Jewish population with a high rate of grand multiparity a high Down syndrome risk was reported even after allowing for maternal age. Some excess might be expected from women having multiple miscarriages because of undiagnosed aneuploidy and a balanced parental translocation. The phenomenon remains to be confirmed and it will take an extremely large study to do so.

Covariables

The marker levels themselves are calculated after allowing for one or more covariables. Allowance for gestational age and the presence of twins are mandatory whereas other covariables are optional. None of the optional co-variables will have a major impact on the discriminatory power of the test but all of them can markedly change the risk for the individual woman. Hence the allowance for covariables can be seen as a way of improving the information on which a woman makes an informed choice about prenatal diagnosis.

The calculations used to allow for each of the covariables are usually made with the implicit assumption that there is no confounding covariable. They assume that the covariable is not *per se* related to the risk of Down syndrome. Epidemiological data are needed to establish whether or not this assumption is valid.

Gestational dating

Nearly all the Down syndrome screening markers which are currently being used or planned for the near future vary with gestational age. This is allowed for either by the use of multiples of the gestation specific median (MoMs), deviations from the median or by taking the ratio between more than one gestation dependent marker. However, none of these methods of adjustment avoid the effect of errors in gestational assessment. Small errors can have a disproportionate effect on the estimated Down syndrome risk. In practice there are several strategies to minimise this effect with the intention of increasing the detection rate, reducing the false-positive rate or both. Some centres can organise services so that all women have an ultrasound dating scan prior to screening. Others can only ensure that this is done for those with uncertain dates, pill withdrawal periods and irregular or long cycles. Some centres use only dates to calculate marker levels but reinterpret the result when a scan is eventually done. However, in practice those with positive screening results are more likely to have a reinterpretation than if the result was negative. Because of 'regression to the mean' this leads to a large reduction in the false-positive rate but it also means a reduction in detection. One way of avoiding this bias is to ensure that borderline negative results are also reinterpreted. Another approach, adopted by many centres, is to only reclassify a positive result as negative if the gestational correction is large (say 2–3 weeks or more).

All of these strategies assume that the ultrasound result is unbiased. This would not be the case if in pregnancies with Down syndrome the average gestational age based on the scan differed from the dates gestation. A bias could be beneficial or detrimental depending on the direction of bias and the markers used. With the current most commonly used marker combinations a negative bias will reduce detection.

The short stature associated with children with Down syndrome is reflected *in utero* by short femur lengths measured by ultrasound. Thus if these biometric measurements were to be used to estimate gestation there would be negative bias. Infants with Down syndrome are growth retarded at term (Khoury *et al.* 1988) and it is therefore possible that biometric measures in early pregnancy may be reduced. An international multicentre collaborative study has investigated possible bias in the two main biometric measures of gestation, crown–rump length and biparietal diameter (Wald *et al.* 1993). In 55 case-control sets using the former and 146 for the latter the median difference in measurements was zero for both measures. Therefore provided femur length is avoided ultrasound should not seriously bias screening results.

Maternal weight

All the maternal serum marker levels investigated so far have shown a tendency to decrease with increasing maternal weight. This is presumably due to a fixed mass of fetal product being diluted in a heavy woman and concentrated in a small one. The relationship is weakest for unconjugated oestriol (uE$_3$) probably reflecting the fact that some of the circulating hormone is maternal in origin. To allow for the negative associations it is standard practice for levels to be divided by the expected value for the weight based on a regression curve. Since the average weight is likely to differ between populations unless a centre produces its own curve or ensures that the average weight is similar to that where the regression was originally done adjustment may introduce inaccuracy. If the maternal weight differed in affected pregnancies there would also be bias. However, in one study of 51 pregnancies with Down syndrome the median weight did not differ from that in over 3000 unaffected controls (Wald and Cuckle 1987).

Twins

For all the maternal serum marker found so far the median level in unaffected twin pregnancies is close to double that of singletons. In discordant twins the average maternal marker level is almost equivalent to the sum of the average for an affected and an unaffected singleton pregnancy. There is no need to adjust marker levels in twins to allow for these increases but the parameters of the statistical models used to calculate likelihood ratios must be altered accordingly.

On theoretical grounds the prior risk of Down syndrome per twin pregnancy should be greater than the risk in singleton pregnancies. Since there are two fetuses, if the probability of the second being affected is independent of the first, the risk that at least one twin is affected would be double that of singletons. In fact the risk will be somewhat less than double because monozygous twins will be concordant for Down syndrome so reducing the overall risk. Theoretical age-specific risks have been published based on 20% monozygosity (Rodis *et al.* 1990) although they incorrectly assume that the monozygosity rate is unaffected by age.

However, the observed prevalence of Down syndrome in twin pregnancies is much less than the theoretical calculations predict. A meta-analysis of four cohort studies including a total of 64 twins with Down syndrome yielded a birth preva- lence only 18% higher in twin pregnancies than in singletons (Wald and Cuckle 1987). When this is extended to include a more recent large study based on notifications to the Office of Populations Censuses and Surveys (Doyle *et al.* 1990) taking the combined total of twins with Down syndrome to 106 the prevalence was only 3% greater than for singletons.

None of the five studies was stratified for maternal age and the chance of having a twin increases with age. Therefore, the observed small increase in the crude Down syndrome prevalence rate among twins implies a reduction in the age-specific prevalence rate. Until there is a more precise estimate of these rates it is probably best to assume that the prior term risk for twins does not differ from that of singletons. The prior risk during pregnancy is even more problematic. The discrepancy between the observed crude rate and that expected from theoretical calculations may be accounted for by a particularly high intrauterine lethality for affected twins. If so the prior risk for a twin during pregnancy may be much higher than for singletons. There are insufficient published data on which to judge this at present.

Smoking

Most of the biochemical markers are influenced by maternal smoking but the biggest effect is in the reduction of human chorionic gonadotrophin (hCG). The extent of this reduction is large enough for some centres to consider routinely adjusting levels for smoking in a similar way to maternal weight. However, there is a large body of evidence which suggests that smoking is less common in the mother's of infants with Down syndrome than in women of comparable age with unaffected pregnancies. If so adjustment would lead to a reduction in the estimated risk of Down syndrome in affected pregnancies unless different prior risks were used for smokers and non-smokers.

There are seven published series with adequate maternal age matching or adjustment reporting smoking rates in Down syndrome and unaffected pregnancies. The relative risks of Down syndrome given maternal smoking were 0.34 (Shiono *et al.* 1986; Hook and Cross 1988), 0.51 (Palomaki *et al.* 1993), 0.56 (Hook and Cross 1985), 0.63 (Cuckle *et al.* 1990), 0.66 (Kline *et al.* 1981; Hook and Cross 1988), 0.88 (Stoll *et al.* 1990) and 1.03 (Cuckle *et al.* 1990). Meta-analysis could be used to calculate likelihood ratios for adjusting the prior age-specific risk according to smoking habit.

Ethnic origin

Several investigators have reported that the average level of one or more maternal serum markers of Down syndrome was different in an ethnic subgroup compared with the general screened population. Thus it is well established for women of Afro-Caribbean ancestry and many screening programmes adjust levels accordingly. There is also interest in making adjustments for women whose origins are in the Indian subcontinent, the Far East and for Arabs.

Although all the published studies used to estimate maternal age-specific risk of Down syndrome were largely based on Caucasian populations there is no reason to believe the risk curves cannot be applied generally. There have been several reports of relatively high or low birth prevalence figures in different ethnic groups. However, none of them was carried out in a population with reliable parental dates of birth. Unless proper age standardisation can be carried out these studies must be considered unproven.

Vaginal bleeding

The presence of vaginal bleeding in early pregnancy is associated with an increase in maternal serum α-fetoprotein (AFP) level and could mask the relatively low level expected in a pregnancy affected by Down syndrome. This is probably not a sufficiently large effect to consider routine adjustment, particularly since AFP is a weak marker of Down syndrome. None the less, some would want to reinterpret tests in which the other maternal serum markers would indicate a high risk if considered alone but the inclusion of AFP yields a low risk.

There are five published studies giving the rate of vaginal bleeding in pregnancies with Down syndrome compared with an unaffected control group of comparable maternal age and in which information on vaginal bleeding had been collected before the outcome of pregnancy was known (Cuckle *et al*. 1994). In the combined data including over 300 affected pregnancies the rate of vaginal bleeding was 1.7-fold higher in those with Down syndrome compared with unaffected pregnancies. Since vaginal bleeding is associated with spontaneous abortion it is possible that the excess relates to non-viable pregnancies. However, in the three studies restricted to term pregnancies the effect was still present and in a large study of pregnancies ending in second trimester spontaneous abortion the rate of first trimester bleeding was no higher in chromosomally abnormal fetuses than in those with a normal karyotype (Strobino and Pantel-Silverman 1987).

To fully account for vaginal bleeding when calculating Down syndrome risk requires adjustment of AFP, adjustment of the prior risk and allowance for the fact that bleeding is more common in older women. A method for doing this has been published by Cuckle and colleagues (1994).

Reproductive factors

A negative association between maternal serum hCG level and gravidity or parity has now been found in several studies. Some centres may want to make allowance for this in calculating hCG levels. Correlations with other markers have also been reported but not as consistently. If markers are adjusted, with the possible exception of grand multiparity, there is no reason why prior risks should be altered.

Abnormal marker levels have been reported in women who have achieved pregnancy following assisted conception although there is no consistency between studies. More work is needed to clarify the matter and if a clearer effect emerges this would be of importance to those women with positive test results who are reluctant to consider amniocentesis. There are insufficient data to judge whether the prior risk of Down syndrome in those undergoing assisted reproduction differs from spontaneous pregnancies. However, despite the lack of concrete information when there is *in vitro* fertilisation of a donor egg the age of the donor should be used to estimate prior risk rather than the mother.

Epidemiological monitoring

The ongoing quality assessment of a multi-marker screening programme should not rest simply on a standard laboratory-based approach. A tolerably small degree of inaccuracy in one marker may lead to serious error if compounded by a similarly small inaccuracy in another marker. Moreover the overall performance of the screening programme will be dependent on factors outside the direct control of the laboratory such as the accuracy of gestational dating. For these reasons laboratory quality assessment needs to be supplemented with the epidemiological monitoring of performance.

There are several possible performance indices of performance but the most useful in day-to-day monitoring are the overall median of the gestation adjusted values (e.g. MoMs) and the overall positive rate. A sudden and consistent change in these indices is an important early sign of a problem. The effect on the positive rate of screening quality will not be uniform across all ages: a greater effect will be seen in younger women than in those who are older. This is because at young ages the cut-off is in the upper tail of risks for Down syndrome pregnancies.

The Down syndrome detection rate is the ultimate measure of performance but care is needed in interpreting the observed rate. First, the confidence interval around a given rate is great and in a small centre it may take years to derive a reliable estimate. Secondly, the observed rate is biased upwards since most non-viable true-positives are terminated whereas the corresponding non-viable false-negatives will go undiagnosed. Furthermore it is possible that the test detects affected fetuses with a different survival rate *in utero* than those it misses. One way of overcoming these problems is to derive the detection rate from the false-negative rate estimated by the number of affected births divided by the number expected from the maternal age distribution.

Other aneuploidy

Many cases of other types of aneuploidy are discovered as a result of antenatal screening for Down syndrome. Some of these are incidental findings of an abnormal fetal karyotype when prenatal diagnosis is performed because of a positive test and would not have been discovered otherwise. Hence the literature on the distribution of marker levels in these disorders is biased. None the less there are strong underlying associations and some centres now routinely interpret the Down syndrome screening result at least for Edwards' syndrome risk.

Edwards' syndrome is a lethal condition with about one-third dying in the neonatal period, one-half by two months and only a few per cent surviving the first year as severely mentally handicapped individuals (Goldstein and Nielsen 1988). In the rare cases of mosaicism or partial trisomy 18 the survival is more favourable as is the phenotype. There are insufficient data to indicate whether the marker levels are different in the more viable cases, or in the rarer genotypes. In 10–20% of cases of Edwards' syndrome there is an associated neural tube or abdominal wall defect. The distribution of maternal serum AFP levels in such cases may not be as high as expected for the physical defect and not as low as expected for the chromosomal anomaly (Barkai *et al.* 1993).

The maternal age-specific risk of Edwards' syndrome can be taken to be a fixed fraction of the corresponding risk for Down syndrome. The relative frequency of the disorders are 1/10, 1/4.5 and 1/3 at term, mid-trimester and in late first trimester, respectively. These relative frequencies are derived from the ratio of Edwards' and Down syndrome cases in neonates, at amniocentesis and at chorionic villus biopsy. When six series of routinely karyotyped neonates were combined (Hook and Hammerton 1977), there was a total of seven cases of Edwards' syndrome and 71 of Down syndrome (a relative frequency of 1/10). In five large amniocentesis series combined (Hook *et al.* 1984) together with the multicentre European study (Ferguson-Smith and Yates 1984) there was a total of 241 cases of Edwards' syndrome and 1086 of Down syndrome in women age 35 or more (a relative frequency of 1/4.5). This is consistent with a 1/10 relative frequency at term. The fetal loss rate for Edwards' syndrome is higher than for Down syndrome, 68% compared with 29% (Hook *et al.* 1989), so the expected relative frequency at birth for the pregnancies in the amniocentesis series would have been 70/738 or 1/11. Moreover, the combined results from the amniotic fluid studies showed no significant differences in the relative frequency according to maternal age.

References

Baird, P. and Sadovnick, A.D. (1988) Life expectancy in Down Syndrome adults. *Lancet* **ii**, 1354–6

Barkai, G., Goldman, B., Ries, L., Chaki, R., Zer, T. and Cuckle, H. (1993) Expanding multiple marker screening for Down's syndrome to include Edwards' syndrome. *Prenat Diagn* **13**, 843–50

Cuckle, H.S. and Wald, N.J. (1987) Vaginal bleeding in pregnancies associated with fetal Down syndrome. *Prenat Diagn* **7**, 619–22

Cuckle, H.S. and Wald, N.J. (1990) 'Screening for Down syndrome' in R.J. Lilford (Ed.) *Prenatal Diagnosis and Prognosis*, pp.67–92. London: Butterworth

Cuckle, H.S., Wald, N.J. and Thompson, S.C. (1987) Estimating a woman's risk of having a pregnancy associated with Down's syndrome using her age and serum alpha-fetoprotein level. *Br J Obstet Gynaecol* **94**, 387–402

Cuckle, H.S., Wald, N.J., Densem, J. *et al.* (1990) The effect of smoking in pregnancy on maternal serum alpha-fetoprotein, unconjugated oestriol, human chorionic gonadotrophin, progesterone and dehydroepiandrosterone sulphate levels. *Br J Obstet Gynaecol* **97**, 272–6

Cuckle, H., van Oudgaarden, E.D., Mason, G. and Holding, S. (1994) Taking account of vaginal bleeding in screening for Down's syndrome. *Br J Obstet Gynaecol* **101**, 948–53

Cuckle, H., Sehmi, I. and Holding, S. (1996) Nomograms to help inform women considering Down's syndrome screening. *Eur J Obstet Gynaecol Reprod Biol* **69**, 69–72

Doyle, P.E., Beral, V., Botting, B. and Wale, C.J. (1990) Congenital malformations in twins in England and Wales. *J Epidemiol Community Health* **45**, 43–8

Ferguson-Smith, M.A. and Yates, J.R.W. (1984) Maternal age specific rates for chromosome aberrations and factors influencing them: Report of a collaborative European study on 52,965 amniocenteses. *Prenat Diagn* **4**, 5–44

Goldstein, H. and Nielsen, K.G. (1988) Rates and survival of individuals with trisomy 13 and 18. Data from a 10-year period in Denmark. *Clin Genet* **34**, 366–72

Hecht, C.A. and Hook, E.B. (1994) The imprecision in rates of Down syndrome by 1-year maternal age intervals: a critical analysis of rates used in biochemical screening. *Prenat Diagn* **14**, 729–38

Hook, E.B. and Cross, P.K. (1985) Cigarette smoking and Down Syndrome. *Am J Hum Genet* **37**, 1216–24

Hook, E.B. and Cross, P.K. (1988) Maternal cigarette smoking, Down Syndrome in live births, and infant race. *Am J Hum Genet* **42**, 482–9

Hook, E.B. and Hammerton, J.L. (1977) 'The frequency of chromosome abnormalities detected in consecutive newborn studies; differences between studies; results by sex and severity of phenotypic involvement' in E.B. Hook and I.H. Porter (Eds) *Population Cytogenetics: Studies in Humans*, pp. 63–79. New York: Academic Press

Hook, E.B., Cross, P.K. and Regal, R.R. (1984) The frequency of 47,+21, 47,+18, and 47+13 at the uppermost extremes of maternal ages: results on 56,094 fetuses studied prenatally and comparisons with data on livebirths. *Hum Genet* **68**, 211–20

Hook, E.B., Topol, B.B. and Cross, P.K. (1989) The natural history of cytogenetically abnormal fetuses detected at midtrimester amniocentesis which are not terminated electively: New data and estimates of the excess and relative risk of late fetal death associated with 47,+21 and some other abnormal karyotypes. *Am J Hum Genet* **45**, 855–61

Hook, E.B., Mutton, D.E., Ide, R., Alberman, E. and Bobrow, M. (1995) The natural history of Down Syndrome conceptuses diagnosed prenatally that are not electively terminated. *Am J Hum Genet* **57**, 875–81

Jalbert, P.M. (1996) Down's syndrome incidence and paternal age. *Screening News* **3**, 5

Khoury, M.J., Erickson, J.D., Cordero, J.F. *et al.* (1988) Congenital malformations and intrauterine growth retardation: a population study. *Pediatrics* **82**, 83–90

Kline, J., Stein, Z., Susser, M. and Warburton, D. (1981) 'New insights into epidemiology of chromosomal disorders: their relevance to the prevention of Down's syndrome' in P. Mitler (Ed.) *Frontiers in Knowledge in Mental Retardation, Vol. II. Biochemical Aspects,* pp. 131–41, Baltimore: University Park Press

Macintosh, M.C.M., Wald, N.J., Chard, T. *et al.* (1995) Selective miscarriage of Down's syndrome fetuses in women aged 35 years and older. *Br J Obstet Gynaecol* **102**, 798–801

Mitchell, S.J.F. and Woodthorpe, J. (1981) Young mentally handicapped adults in three London boroughs: prevalence and degree of disability. *J Epidemiol Community Health* **35**, 59–64

Palomaki, G.E., Knight, G.J., Haddow, J.E. *et al.* (1993) Cigarette smoking and levels of maternal serum alpha-fetoprotein, unconjugated estriol, and hCG: impact on Down syndrome screening. *Obstet Gynecol* **81**, 675–8

Rodis, J.F., Egan, J.F.X., Craffey, A. *et al.* (1990) Calculated risk of chromosomal abnormalities in twin gestations. *Obstet Gynecol* **76**, 1037–41

Royston, P. and Thompson, S.G. (1992) Model-based screening by risk with application to Down's syndrome. *Stat Med* **11**, 257–68

Shiono, P.H., Klebanoff, M.A. and Berendes, H.W. (1986) Congenital malformations and maternal smoking during pregnancy. *Teratology* **34**, 65–71

Snijders, R.J.M., Holzgreve, W., Cuckle, H. and Nicolaides, K.H. (1994) Maternal age-specific risks for Trisomies at 9–14 weeks' gestation. *Prenat Diagn* **14**, 543–52

Stoll, C., Alembik, Y., Dott, B. and Roth, M.P. (1990) Epidemiology of Down syndrome in 118,265 consecutive births. *Am J Med Genet Suppl* **7**, 79–83

Strobino, B.A. and Pantel-Silverman, J. (1987) First-trimester vaginal bleeding and the loss of chromosomally normal and abnormal conceptions. *Am J Obstet Gynecol* **157**, 1150–4

Wald, N.J. and Cuckle, H.S. (1987) 'Recent advances in screening for neural tube defects and Down's syndrome' in C.H. Rodeck (Ed.) *Fetal Diagnosis of Genetic Defects. Baillière's Clin Obstet Gynaecol* **1**, 649–76

Wald, N.J., Smith, D., Kennard, A. *et al.* (1993) Biparietal diameter and crown–rump length in fetuses with Down's syndrome: implications for antenatal serum screening for Down's syndrome. *Br J Obstet Gynaecol* **100**, 430–5

Chapter 2

Endocrinology and metabolism in early pregnancy

J. Gedis Grudzinskas

Introduction

Complications in pregnancy are common in particular in the first trimester, at least 10–15% of all recognised pregnancies failing to proceed beyond 12 weeks' gestation (for review, see Stabile *et al.* 1992). The most common complication is spontaneous miscarriage, and it is notable that the most frequent abnormality observed in this condition is aneuploidy. The most eloquent theoretical explanation for these events has been proposed by Roberts and Lowe (1975). Scientists and clinicians have nevertheless searched for markers to try to determine whether there are any biochemical hormonal or ultrasonic events which may be exploited either to provide reassurance to the woman that her pregnancy is proceeding normally or identify women at risk of spontaneous miscarriage or abnormalities of embryonic/fetal development. It is not surprising that proteins and hormones of fetal or trophoblastic origin have been studied extensively in this light in particular in the first trimester (for review see Grudzinskas *et al.* 1985). This chapter reviews some of the molecular aspects of fetal and trophoblastic hormones and proteins as well as fetal and maternal factors (Table 2.1) which may influence serum measurements of these substances.

Trophoblast proteins and hormones

Human chorionic gonadotrophin (hCG)

Human chorionic gonadotrophin has close structural similarities to pituitary luteinising hormone (LH), follicle-stimulating hormone (FSH), and thyroid-stimulating hormone (TSH), consisting of two protein chains, the α and β

Table 2.1. Principal fetal, trophoblast and maternal hormones and proteins in human pregnancy

	Gene location
Fetal	
Alphafetoprotein (AFP)	chromosome 4
Fetal antigen 1 (FA1)	not known
Fetal antigen 2 (FA2)	not known
Trophoblast	
Human chorionic gonadotrophin (hCG)	α chromosome 6
	β chromosome 19
Human placental lactogen (hPL)	chromosome 17
Schwangerschafts/protein 1 (SP1)	chromosome 19
Pregnancy-associated plasma protein A (PAPP-A)	chromosome 9
Oestrogen receptor	chromosome 6
Progesterone receptor	chromosome 11
Ovarian	
Inhibin[a]	α chromosome 2
	β-A chromosome 7
	β-B chromosome 2
Endometrial	
Glycodelin	chromosome 9
Insulin like growth	
factor binding protein	chromosome 7
Pituitary	
Luteinising hormone[b]	α chromosome 6
	β chromosome 19
Follicle stimulating hormone[c]	α chromosome 6
	β chromosome 11
Prolactin[d]	chromosome 6
Growth hormone[e]	chromosome 17

[a] Barton *et al.* 1989; [b] Naylor *et al.* 1983; [c] Watkins *et al.* 1987; [d] Owerbach *et al.* 1981; [e] George *et al.* 1981 (For other references, see text.)

subunits. The chains are joined by non-covalent bonds. Both subunits have side chains of carbohydrate residues, principally sialic acid, which constitute some 12% of the molecule. The α subunit has 92 amino acid residues and is almost identical to the α subunits of LH, FSH and TSH. The β subunit has 145 amino acid residues. Thirty of these, at the carboxy terminus of the molecule, are unique to hCG. The remaining 115 residues are very similar to the 115 residues of the β subunit of LH; 80% of the sequence is identical. The molecular weights of the α subunit, the β subunit, and the whole molecule are 14,930, 23,470 and 38,400, respectively (Bahl *et al.* 1972; Morgan *et al.* 1975; Fiddes and Goodman 1981).

Within the trophoblast the synthesis of the α and β subunits of hCG is independent, i.e. the subunit is encoded by a single gene on chromosome 6 (6q 12-21) (Fiddes and Goodman 1981) and the β subunit by a family of six genes on the long arm of chromosome 19 (Graham *et al.* 1987). The two subunits combine in the cell prior to release as intact hCG, and for this reason only small quantities of the free subunits appear in the circulation. The production of β subunit appears to be the rate-limiting factor; the trophoblast can synthesise much greater quantities of α subunit than β subunit, but combination of the two is essential for release from the cell. The β subunit production peaks at 8–10 weeks, declining thereafter, but α subunit levels increase until term (Hoshina *et al.* 1984).

The main proposed function for hCG is maintenance of the corpus luteum in early pregnancy. The mechanisms that control hCG synthesis are still largely unknown. It is suggested that in early pregnancy some factor stimulates trophoblastic hCG synthesis. Later in pregnancy this factor either declines or is replaced by another which actively reduces hCG production. No hypothesis as to what such factors must be has been put forward. There is some evidence that cyclic adenosine monophosphate or luteinising hormone releasing factor will stimulate hCG production in placental explants, but it is difficult to relate this to control *in vivo*.

The measurement of hCG has an established place in the diagnosis of pregnancy, screening for ectopic pregnancy, Down syndrome and other aneuploidies and monitoring trophoblastic disease (see Chapter 12).

Human placental lactogen (hPL)

Placental lactogen (hPL) is a protein with close similarities to pituitary prolactin and growth hormone (96% homology). It consists of a single chain of 191 amino acids without carbohydrate residues. There are two intrachain disulphide (–S–S–) links. The molecular weight is 21 600 (Chard 1982).

In common with many other proteins, hPL is initially synthesised in the form of a larger molecule, having an additional 20 amino acids at the amino terminus. This extra 'signal' sequence is removed as part of the process of secretion. hPL is encoded by a gene cluster on chromosome 17 (George *et al.* 1981).

hPL is produced by syncytiotrophoblast, and fits very well to the model of control by mass of trophoblast, i.e. the concentrations in maternal blood increase slowly and appear to parallel the size of the placental mass. Maximum levels are reached at 32 weeks' gestation. Most investigators agree that hPL levels are related to placental mass, and secondarily to fetal weight. Serum hPL measurements are no longer used in the assessment of fetal well-being, as other biophysical methods of fetal assessment are far superior (Chard 1982).

Schwangerschaftsprotein 1 (SP1)

This protein has a molecular weight of 90 000 and the electrophoretic mobility of a β_1-globulin. A large part (30%) of the molecule consists of carbohydrate containing sialic acid. Its biological activity is unknown, although it forms part of a large family of proteins of which carcinoembryonic antigen (CEA) is the most familiar (Grudzinskas *et al.* 1982). SP1 is coded by a gene on chromosome 19 (19q13.1) (Barnett *et al.* 1989; Niemann *et al.* 1989). SP1 levels are significantly lower in ectopic and failing pregnancies than in pregnancies with good outcome (Seppala *et al.* 1980; Mantzavinos *et al.* 1991; Johnson *et al.* 1993). SP1 measurements in the first and second trimester of pregnancy are currently being evaluated as a secondary screening test for Down syndrome (Macintosh *et al.* 1993; Christiansen and Nørgaard-Pedersen, Chapter 15).

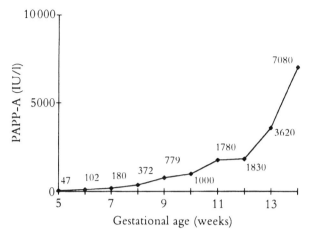

Fig. 2.1. Serum levels of pregnancy-associated plasma protein in seven women during early normal pregnancy (from Chemnitz *et al.* 1986).

Pregnancy associated plasma protein-A (PAPP-A)

PAPP-A is a pregnancy specific glycoprotein produced by trophoblast. It is detectable in maternal serum from 28 days after conception and increases throughout gestation with a doubling time of 4–5 days in the first trimester (Fig. 2.1). PAPP-A is a glycoprotein with α_2 electrophoretic mobility and a molecular weight of 750 000–820 000. Various functions have been proposed, notably as an inhibitor of enzymes such as granulocyte elastase. No specific control mechanisms are known (Stabile *et al.* 1988). The gene for PAPP-A is located on the distal part of the long arm of chromosome 9 (9q33.1) (Silahtoraglu *et al.* 1993). Depressed serum PAPP-A levels are seen in association with early pregnancy failure (spontaneous miscarriage and ectopic pregnancy) and in association with fetal aneuploidy (El-Farra and Grudzinskas 1995). A number of retrospective studies have defined a relationship between low levels of PAPP-A in the first trimester and Down syndrome and other trisomies (Spencer *et al.* 1992; Wald *et al.* 1992; Aitken *et al.* 1993; Brambati *et al.* 1993a, b, 1994). This difference is greatest at the earliest gestations and decreases rapidly towards the second trimester. Serum PAPP-A levels in affected pregnancies at 6–11 weeks are substantially lower (0.27 MoM) than those seen in normal pregnancies (Brambati *et al.* 1993a). By the second trimester the difference is no longer evident (Aitken *et al.* 1993). It has been proposed that using first trimester measurements of maternal serum PAPP-A, serum free βhCG and maternal age to define the 5% of women at highest risk of Down syndrome, and offering karyotyping to this 5% it is possible to detect 70% of cases of Down syndrome. This proposal has been supported recently in a large multicentre study (Wald *et al.* 1996).

Oestriol

The principal oestrogen in human pregnancy is oestriol, which has hydroxyl groups at C-3, C-16 and C-17. The first step of synthesis involves the removal of six carbon atoms from the side chain of cholesterol leaving the 21-carbon steroid pregnenolone. In the fetal adrenal gland pregnenolone is converted into the C_{19} steroid dehydroepiandrosterone (DHEA) which passes to the fetal liver where it is hydroxylated to 16-OH-DHEA and in turn to the placenta where an aromatase confers the characteristic oestrogen A-ring to produce oestriol. In the fetal circulation the majority of these steroids exist as sulphate conjugates. The placenta has a high content of a sulphatase enzyme which is essential for the conversion of 16-OH-DHEA-SO_4 in the trophoblast prior to aromatisation (Siiteri and MacDonald 1966; France and Liggins 1969; Shearman 1979). In cases of sulphatase deficiency little or no oestriol is secreted into the mother. In maternal blood, half or more of the oestriol circulates in the form of 16-glucosiduronate conjugates which is also the principal form in urine. Around one-half of oestrogens are directed through the enterohepatic circulation. In the bile the main form is oestriol-3-sulphate-16-glucosiduronate.

There is no information on the function of oestriol in pregnancy; an almost complete deficiency, in the absence of placental sulphatase, seems to have no effect on maternal or fetal well-being. Similarly, there is little information on control mechanisms, other than the general mechanisms already proposed. Certain specific factors affect oestriol synthesis. It is deficient in the absence of placental sulphatase, in adrenal hypoplasia, in anencephaly and following administration of corticosteroids. The last three situations all have in common a reduction in the synthesis of the main precursor, DHEA. The oestrogen receptor is coded on the long arm of chromosome 6 (Gosden *et al.* 1986). Depressed serum levels are also seen in association with trisomy 21 (Canick *et al.* 1988). The measurement of oestriol in maternal blood was introduced to assess fetal well-being in the third trimester. Currently, serum oestriol measurements in the second trimester are used in conjunction with hCG and AFP to identify women at increased risk of having a Down syndrome baby (Spencer 1994).

Progesterone

This trophoblast steroid does not depend on fetal precursors. After six weeks of pregnancy the placental secretion of progesterone takes over from that of the corpus luteum. The major excretion product in urine is pregnanediol. Progesterone is believed to play a major role in the maintenance of early pregnancy, especially in the transformation of the endometrium to the decidua. The progesterone receptor is coded on the long arm of chromosome 11 (Law *et al.* 1987). Progesterone concentrations are depressed in women with spontaneous miscarriages and ectopic pregnancy and this, in conjunction with hCG levels, may be useful in the diagnosis of this condition (Stabile and Grudzinskas 1994), but not fetal aneuploidy.

Fetal proteins

Alpha fetoprotein (AFP)

AFP is a protein synthesised by the fetal liver and yolk sac, which is believed to serve an oncotic function in the fetus similar to that of albumin in the adult. AFP is a glycoprotein in which more than 39% of the amino acid sequence resembles albumin. The gene for AFP is coded on the long arm of chromosome 4 (4q 11-22) (Harper and Dugaiczyk 1983). Serum AFP levels in ectopic pregnancy tend to be higher than in intrauterine pregnancies (Grosskinsky *et al.* 1993). Serum AFP levels are measured in screening for open neural tube defects (elevated levels) and Down syndrome (depressed levels). Maternal serum levels of AFP (MSAFP) in the second trimester tend to be lower in pregnancies affected by Down syndrome, the median level in an affected pregnancy is 0.75 multiples of the normal median (MoM) of normal pregnancies. In the first trimester, the situation is very similar: a number of studies report MSAFP in Down syndrome as 0.7–0.8 MoM of normal pregnancies (Brambati *et al.* 1986; Crandall *et al.* 1993; Casals *et al.* 1996). Current research is addressing whether MSAFP in first trimester serum will be as useful as it is in the second trimester.

Fetal antigen 1 (FA1)

Fetal antigen 1, like its partner FA2, was first identified in second trimester amniotic fluid and the fetal origin was suggested by its distribution in fetal and maternal compartments and tissues (Fay *et al.* 1988; Tornehave *et al.* 1989). High concentrations of FA1 were found in second-trimester amniotic fluid and in fetal serum, whereas the concentration in normal human serum was found to be approximately 20 ng/ml, which is 1000 times less than in second-trimester fetal serum (Fay *et al.* 1988). Studies on fetal tissues (week 7) have demonstrated FA1 immunoreactivity in the hepatocytes of the fetal liver (Tornehave *et al.* 1989). Subsequently, the presence of FA1 was observed within the cytoplasm of nearly all glandular cells of the first trimester anlage of the fetal pancreas (Tornehave *et al.* 1993), the relative number of FA1-positive glandular cells decreasing as the development of the fetal pancreas progresses. Postnatally the expression of FA1 is restricted to the insulin-producing β cells of the islets of Langerhans (Tornehave *et al.* 1993; Jensen *et al.* 1993). It is suggested that FA1 is synthesised as a membrane-anchored protein and released into the circulation after enzyme cleavage, and that circulating FA1 represents the post-translationally modified gene product of human dlk which, in turn, is identical to human adrenal-specific mRNA pG2 (Jensen *et al.* 1994). FA1 has the potential to be an index of organ specific or general embryonic or fetal development.

Fetal antigen 2 (FA2)

FA2 was first identified in amniotic fluid (Fay *et al.* 1988; Tornehave *et al.* 1989) and has been shown to be identical to the aminopropeptide of the α1 chain of collagen type 1 (Teisner *et al.* 1992). Biochemical characterisation has revealed several molecular forms of the protein which differ in both size (Fay *et al.* 1988; Rasmussen *et al.* 1992a) and charge (Price *et al.* 1995a). An ELISA has been developed and used to demonstrate the presence of FA2 in normal serum (Rasmussen *et al.* 1992b). A radioimmunoassay has also been described (Price *et al.* 1995b) and a standard prepared (Price *et al.* 1994). In amniotic fluid there are two major high-molecular-mass FA2 types and several low-molecular-mass forms

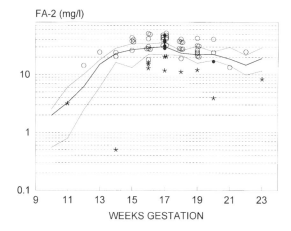

Fig. 2.2. Fetal antigen-2 (FA-2) concentrations in trisomy 21, trisomy 18 and trisomy 13 amniotic fluid quantified using radioimmunoassay. FA-2 concentrations were measured in 47 trisomy 21 cases (○), 12 trisomy 18 (★) and six trisomy 13 (●) amniotic fluid samples, using radioimmunoassay. Values are presented in relation to the median and 95% confidence interval of the normal range.

(Price *et al.* 1995a). Levels rise steeply from 10 to 14 weeks, peak at 17 weeks and then fall slightly by 23 weeks. FA2 holds the promise of being a marker of fetal mesodermal activity, tumour activity or tissue regeneration. A comparison of amniotic fluid FA2 levels between 10 and 23 weeks' gestation in normal pregnancies and pregnancies affected by trisomy, showed significantly higher FA2 levels in trisomy 21 and significantly lower levels in trisomy 18 (Fig. 2.2) (Price *et al.* 1995b).

Decidual-endometrial proteins

Insulin-like growth factor binding protein-1 (IGFBP-1) (also known as PP12, placental protein 12)

The identification of IGFBP-1 as a major secretory product of decidualised endometrium suggests that studies of the IGFs and their binding proteins may contribute to implantation. IGFBP-1 is a 25 kDa growth hormone independent, acid-stable protein found in fetal and adult serum and also in amniotic, follicular and cerebrospinal fluid. IGFBP-3 is the main serum IGFBP with a molecular weight of 29 kDa and is growth hormone dependent. In the peripheral circulation, IGFBP-3 forms a 150 kDa complex and in pregnancy both IGFBP-3 and IGFBP-2 are present in the peripheral circulation but in reduced concentrations. However, IGFBP-1 increases steadily throughout pregnancy (Seppala *et al.* 1992). Maternal serum IGFBP-1 levels greater than those in non-pregnant women are observed from week seven onward. The maximum levels are reached at 22–23 weeks. There is a correlation between endometrial IGFBP-1 and progesterone levels (Rutanen *et al.* 1982, 1984).

The primary stucture of IGFBP-1 has been determined and the single gene encoding IGFBP-1 located on the short arm of chromosome 7 (7 p12-13) (Jalkunen *et al.* 1989). The gene encodes a single 1.6 kb mRNA species expressed in gestational endometrium from the first and third trimesters of pregnancy, secretory endometrium, liver and hepatoma cell lines but not in proliferative endometrium or trophoblastic tissue obtained at term (Julkunen *et al.* 1988). Using *in situ* hybridisation, the mRNA for IGFBP-1 has been identified in a population of stromal cells in late secretory phase endometrium and decidua (Julkunen *et al.* 1990). The production by the decidualised endometrium of a peptide that controls the bioavailability of growth factors suggests that the human endometrium may exert local control on the development and growth of the placenta and influences fetal metabolism, since it is present in the amniotic cavity (Giudice *et al.* 1990; Rutanen *et al.* 1982). Hustin and colleagues (1994) have reported the apparent selective expression of IGFBP-1 at the implantation site in humans in the earliest days of pregnancy.

Glycodelin (also known as placental protein 14 (PP14) and progesterone-dependent endometrial protein)

Biochemical and immunohistochemical observations (Wahlstrom *et al.* 1985) have shown that glycodelin is the most abundant protein derived from glandular epithelium of late secretory endometrium. The protein is actively secreted into the uterine cavity (Bell and Dore-Green 1987). Glycodelin is a glycoprotein which expresses polymorphism, has a molecular weight of 42–43 kDa, contains 17.5% carbohydrate, and the gene is located on chromosome 9 (Van Cong *et al.* 1991).

Circulating levels increase 20-fold from the late secretory phase to the early first trimester whereas tissue levels increase only two-fold, suggesting that much of the rise is due to the increase in the mass of the decidua (Bell 1988). Significant amounts of glycodelin have not been detected in any tissue in the adult or fetus, except the reproductive organs (Tornehave *et al.* 1989; Waites *et al.* 1990; Karmarainen *et al.* 1996).

Serum glycodelin levels are high in the late luteal and menstrual phases of the normal menstrual cycle. A number of observations suggest that progesterone might be an important control factor (Fay *et al.* 1990). Circulating levels of glycodelin start to rise one week after ovulation. In a conceptual cycle, the rise continues with a doubling time of 2.5 days; the levels peak within four weeks (Joshi 1987). The levels remain high for up to 8–10 weeks after which there is a fall, a pattern similar to hCG (Bell *et al.* 1985; Joshi *et al.* 1982; Julkunen *et al.* 1985; Than *et al.* 1987). A similar pattern is observed by quantitative immuno-histochemistry of the endometrium (Bolton *et al.* 1988). The correlation suggests that fetal PP14 originates from the mother, although it is surprising that a protein of this size would cross the placenta. At term, glycodelin levels in the fetus correlate with but are 10-fold less than those in the mother (Bell *et al.* 1985). The glycodelin concentration in amniotic fluid is 100- to 1000-fold higher than that in maternal blood. The highest levels in amniotic fluid are found at 8–10 weeks. Serum glycodelin levels are lower in ectopic pregnancy than in non-complicated intrauterine pregnancies, and when using in combination with hCG concentration, may distinguish between normal and abnormal implantation (Nylund *et al.* 1992; Ruge *et al.* 1992).

Conclusion

The measurement of hormones and proteins in maternal and fetal blood, amniotic and coelomic fluids provides useful information about the intrauterine environment and embryonic and fetal development in addition to that obtained by high resolution ultrasonography. This is certainly the case in relation to subsequent miscarriage of a live fetus and the detection of women at increased risk of trisomy 21 and other aneuploidies. However, the knowledge that the genes for α interferon receptor and superoxidase dismutase are, among others, situated on chromosome 21 has not advanced our ability to screen more effectively for Down syndrome. The further study of metabolic and endocrine events in early pregnancy will permit the development of better screening programmes in early pregnancy.

References

Aitken, D.A., McCaw, G. and Crossley, J.A. (1993) First trimester biochemical screening for fetal chromosome abnormalities and neural tube defects. *Prenat Diagn* **13**, 68–9

Bahl, O.P., Carlson, R.B., Bellisario, R. and Swaminathan, N. (1972) Human chorionic gonadotrophin amino acid sequence of the alpha and beta subunits. *Biochem Biophys Res Commun* **48**, 416–22

Barnett, T.R., Pickle, W., Rae, P.M., Hart, J., Kamarck, M. and Elting, J. (1989) Human pregnancy-specific beta-1-glycoproteins are coded within chromosome 19. *Am J Hum Genet* **44**, 890–3

Barton, D.E., Yang-Feng, T.L., Mason, A.J., Seeburg, P.H. and Francke, U. (1989) Mapping of genes of inhibin subunits, α, βA and βB on human and mouse chromosomes and studies of jsd mice. *Genomics* **5**, 91–9

Bell, S.C. (1986) Secretory endometrial and decidual proteins: studies and clinical significance of a maternally derived group of pregnancy associated serum proteins. *Hum Reprod* **1**, 129–43

Bell, S.C. (1988) Secretory/endometrial decidual proteins and their function in early pregnancy. *J Reprod Fertil Suppl* **36**, 109

Bell, S.C. (1989) Decidualization and insulin-like growth factor (IGF) binding protein: implications for its role in stromal cell differentiation and the decidual cell in haemochorial placentation. *Hum Reprod* **4**, 125–30

Bell, S.C. and Dore-Green, F. (1987) Detection and characterization of human secretory pregnancy-associated and endometrial alpha-2-globulin (α2-PEG) in uterine luminal fluid. *J Reprod Fertil* **11**, 13

Bell, S.C., Hales, M.W., Patel, S.R. *et al.* (1985) Protein synthesis and secretion by the human endometrium and decidua during early pregnancy. *Br J Obstet Gynaecol* **92**, 793

Bolton, A.E., Pockley, A.G., Stoker, R.J. *et al.* (1988) 'Biological activity of placental protein 14' in M. Chapman, J.G. Grudzinskas and T. Chard (Eds) *Implantation: Biological and Clinical Aspects,* pp.135–44. London: Springer-Verlag

Brambati, B., Simoni, G., Bonacchi, I. and Piceni, I. (1986) Fetal chromosomal aneuploidies and maternal serum alphafetoprotein levels in the first trimester. *Lancet* **ii**, 165–6

Brambati, B., Macintosh, M.C.M., Teisner, B. *et al.* (1993a) Low maternal serum levels of pregnancy associated plasma protein A in the first trimester in association with abnormal karyotype. *Br J Obstet Gynaecol* **100**, 324–6

Brambati, B., Tului, L., Bonnachi, I., Shrimanker, K., Suzuki, Y. and Grudzinskas, J.G. (1993b) Serum PAPP-A and free beta hCG are first trimester screening markers for Down syndrome (Abstract). *Hum Reprod* **8**, (Suppl 1), 183

Brambati, B., Tului, L., Bonnachi, I., Suzuki, Y., Shrimanker, K. and Grudzinskas, J.G. (1994) 'Biochemical screening for Down syndrome in the first trimester' in J.G. Grudzinskas, T.

Chard, M. Chapman and T. Cuckle (Eds) *Screening for Down Syndrome* pp. 289–94. Cambridge: Cambridge University Press

Canick, J.A., Knight, G.J., Palomaki, G.E., Haddon, J.E., Cuckle, H. and Wald, N.J. (1988) Low second trimester maternal serum unconjugated oestriol in pregnancies with Down's syndrome. *Br J Obstet Gynaecol* **95**, 330–3

Casals, E., Fortuny, A., Grudzinskas, J.G. *et al.* (1996)First-trimester biochemical screening for Down syndrome with the use of PAPP-A, AFP and β-hCG. *Prenat Diagn* **16**, 405–10

Chard, T. (1982) 'Placental lactogen: biology and clinical applications' in J.G. Grudzinskas, B. Turner and M. Seppala (Eds) *Pregnancy Proteins, Biology, Chemistry and Clinical Applications*, pp.101–18. Sydney: Academic Press

Chemnitz, J., Folkersen, J., Teisner, B. *et al.* (1986) Comparison of different antibody preparations against pregnancy-associated plasma protein-A (PAPP-A) for use in localisation and immunoassay studies. *Br J Obstet Gynaecol* **93**, 916–23

Crandall, B.F., Hanson, F.W., Keener, S., Matsumoto, M. and Miller, W. (1993) Maternal serum screening for alpha-fetoprotein, unconjugated oestriol and human chorionic gonadotrophin between 11 and 15 weeks of pregnancy to detect fetal chromosome abnormalities. *Am J Obstet Gynecol* **168**, 1864–9

El-Farra, K. and Grudzinskas, J.G. (1995) Will PAPP-A be a biochemical marker for screening of Down's syndrome in the first trimester? *Early Pregnancy Biol Med* **1**, 4–12

Fay, T.N., Jacobs, I.J., Teisner, B. *et al.* (1988) Two fetal antigens (FA1 and FA2) and endometrial proteins (PP12 and PP14) isolated from amniotic fluid. Preliminary observations in fetal and maternal tissues. *Eur J Gynaecol Biol* **29**, 73–5

Fay, T.N., Jacobs, I.J., Teisner, B. *et al.* (1990) A biochemical test for the direct assessment of endometrial function: measurement of the major secretory endometrial protein PP14 in serum during menstruation in relation to ovulation and luteal function. *Hum Reprod* **5**, 382

Fiddes, J.C. and Goodman, H.M. (1981) The gene encoding the common alpha-subunit in the four human glycoprotein hormones. *J Mol Appl Genet* **1**, 3–18

France, J.T. and Liggins, G.C. (1969) Placental sulphatase deficiency. *J Clin Endocrinol Metab* **29**, 138–41

George, D.L., Phillips, J.A., Francke, U. and Seeburg, P.H. (1981) The genes of growth hormone and chorionic somatomammotrophin are on the long arm of human chromosome 17 in region q21 to qter. *Hum Genet* **57**, 138–41

Giudice, L.C., Farrell, E.M., Pham, H., Lamson, G. and Rosenfeld, R.G. (1990) Insulin-like growth factor binding proteins in the maternal serum throughout gestation and in the puerperium: effects of a pregnancy-associated serum protease activity. *J Clin Endocrinol Metab* **71**, 806–16

Gosden, J.R., Middleton, P.E. and Rout, D. (1986) Localisation of the human oestrogen receptor gene to chromosome 6q24-q27 by in-situ hybridization. *Cytogenet Cell Genet* **43**, 218–20

Graham, M.Y., Otani, T., Boime, I., Olsen, M.V., Carle, G.F. and Chaplin, D.D. (1987) Cosmid mapping of the human chorionic gonadotrophin beta subunit genes by field-inversion gel electrophoresis. *Nucleic Acids Res* **15**, 443–7

Grosskinsky, C.M., Hage, M.L., Tyrey, L., Christakos, A.C. and Hughes, C.L. (1993) hCG, progesterone, alpha-fetoprotein, and estradiol in the identification of ectopic pregnancy. *Obstet Gynecol* **81**, 705–9

Grudzinskas, J.G. (1995) 'Endocrinological and metabolic assessment of early pregnancy' in G. Chamberlain (Ed.) *Turnbull's Obstetrics* (2nd ed.), pp.185–94. Edinburgh: Churchill Livingstone

Grudzinskas, J.G., Teisner, B. and Seppala, M. (Eds) (1982) 'Pregnancy specific beta glycoprotein' in *Pregnancy Proteins, Biology, Chemistry and Clinical Applications*, pp.179–262. Sydney: Academic Press

Grudzinskas, J.G., Westergaard, J.G. and Teisner, B. (1985) 'Pregnancy-associated plasma protein A in normal and abnormal pregnancies' in P. Bischof and A. Klopper (Eds) *Proteins of the Placenta. Biochemistry, Biology and Clinical Application*, p.184. Basel: Karger

Harper, M.E. and Dugaiczyk, A. (1983) Linkage of evolutionarily related serum albumin and AFP genes within q11-22 of chromosome 4. *Am J Hum Genet* **35**, 565–72

Hoshina, M., Hussa, R., Paltillo, R., Camel, M.H. and Boime, I. (1984) The role of trophoblast differentiation in the control of the hCG and hPL genes. *Adv Exp Med Biol* **176**, 299–311

Hustin, J., Philippe, E., Teisner, B. and Grudzinskas, J.G. (1994) Immunohistochemical localization of two endometrial proteins in the early days of human pregnancy. *Placenta* **7**, 701–8

Jalkunen, M., Suikkari, A.M., Koistinen, R. *et al.* (1989) Regulation of insulin-like growth factor-binding protein 1: production by human granulosa luteal cells. *J Clin Endocrinol Metab* **69**, 1174–9

Jensen, C.H., Teisner, B., Hojrup, P. *et al.* (1993) Studies on the isolation, structural analysis and tissue localisation of fetal antigen 1 and its relation to human adrenal-specific cDNA, pG2. *Hum Reprod* **8**, 635–41

Jensen, C.H., Krogh, T.N., Hojrup, P. *et al.* (1994) Protein structure of fetal antigen 1 (FA1). A novel circulating human epidermal growth factor-like protein expressed in neuroendocrine tumours and its relation to the gene products of dlk and pG2. *Eur J Biochem* **225**, 83–92

Johnson, M.R., Riddle, A.F., Irvine, R. *et al.* (1993) Corpus luteum failure in ectopic pregnancy. *Hum Reprod* **8**, 1491–5

Joshi, S.G. (1987) Progestogen-dependent human endometrial protein: a marker for monitoring human endometrial function. *Adv Exp Med Biol* **230**, 167

Joshi, S.G., Bank, J.G., Henriques, E.S. *et al.* (1982) Serum levels of progestogen-associated endometrial protein during the menstrual cycle and pregnancy. *J Clin Endocrinol Metab* **55**, 642

Julkunen, M., Rutanen, E.M., Koskimies, A. *et al.* (1985) Distribution of placental protein 14 in tissues and body fluids during pregnancy. *Br J Obstet Gynaecol* **92**, 1145

Julkunen, M., Koistinen, R., Aalto-Setala, K., Seppala, M., Janne, O.A. and Kontula, K. (1988) Primary structure of human insulin-like growth factor-binding protein/placental protein 12 and tissue-specific expression of its mRNA. *FEBS Lett* **236**, 295–302

Julkunen, M., Koistinen, R., Suikkari, A.-M., Seppala, M. and Janne, O.A. (1990) Identification by hybridization histochemistry of human endometrial cells expressing mRNAs encoding a uterine betalactoglobulin homologue and insulin-like growth factor-binding protein-1. *Mol Endocrinol* **4**, 700–7

Karmarainen, M., Leivo, I., Koistinen, R. *et al.* (1996) Normal human ovary and ovarian tumours express glycodelin, a glycoprotein with immunosuppressive and contraceptive properties. *Am J Pathol* **148**, 1435–43

Law, M.L., Kao, F.T.,Wei, Q. *et al.* (1987) The progesterone receptor gene maps to human chromosome band 11q13, the site of the mammary oncogene int-2. *Proc Natl Acad Sci USA* **84**, 2877–81

Macintosh, M.C.M., Brambati, B., Chard, T. and Grudzinskas, J.G. (1993) First trimester maternal serum Schwangerschafts protein 1 (SP1), in pregnancies associated with chromosomal abnormalities. *Prenat Diagn* **13**, 567–8

Mantzavinos, T., Phocas, I., Chrelias, H., Sarandakou, A. and Zourlas, P.A. (1991) Serum levels of steroids and placental proteins in ectopic pregnancy. *Eur J Obstet Gynecol Reprod Biol* **39**, 117–22

Morgan, F.J., Birkan, S. and Canfield, R.E. (1975) The amino acid sequence of human chorionic gonadotrophin. The alpha and beta subunit. *J Biol Chem* **250**, 5247–58

Naylor, S.L., Chin, W.W., Goodman, H.M., Lalley, P.A., Grzeschik, K.H. and Sakaguchi, A.Y. (1983) Chromosome assignment of genes encoding the α and β subunits of glycoprotein hormones in man and mouse. *Somat Cell Genet* **9**, 757–70

Niemann, S.C., Schonk, D., van Dijk, P., Wieinga, B., Grzeschik, K.H. and Bartels, I. (1989) Regional localization of the gene encoding pregnancy specific beta 1 glycoprotein (PSBG-1) to human chromosome 19q 13.1 *Cytogenet Cell Genet* **52**, 95–7

Nylund, L., Gustafson, O., Lindblom, B. *et al.* (1992) Placental protein 14 in human *in-vitro* fertilization early pregnancies. *Hum Reprod* **7**, 128–30

Owerbach, D., Rutter, W.J., Cooke, N.E., Martzal, J.A. and Shows, T.B. (1981) The prolactin gene is located on chromosome 6 in humans. *Science* **212**, 815-16

Price, K.M., Silman, R. and Grudzinskas, J.G. (1994) Isolation of fetal antigen 2 assay standard. *Clin Chim Acta* **226**, 83–8

Price, K.M., Silman, R., Armstrong, P., Teisner, B. and Grudzinskas, J.G. (1995a) The typing of fetal antigen 2 in human amniotic fluid. *Clin Chim Acta* **236**, 181–94

Price, K.M., Silman, R., Armstrong, P. and Grudzinskas, J.G. (1995b) Abnormal amniotic fetal antigen 2 levels in trisomy 18 and 21. *Hum Reprod* **10**, 2438–40

Rasmussen, H.B., Teisner, B., Andersen, J.A., Yde-Andersen, E. and Leigh, I. (1992a) Fetal antigen 2 (FA2) in relation to wound healing and fibroblast proliferation. *Br J Dermatol* **126**, 148–53

Rasmussen, H.B., Teisner, B., Bangsgaard-Petersen, F., Yde-Andersen, E. and Kassem, M. (1992b) Quantification of fetal antigen 2 (FA2) in supernatants of cultured osteoblasts, normal human serum, and serum from patients with chronic renal failure. *Nephrol Dial Transplant* **7**, 902–7

Roberts, C.J. and Lowe, C.R. (1975) Where have all the conceptions gone? *Lancet* **i**, 498–9

Ruge, S., Sorensen, S., Vejtorp, M. and Vejerslev, L.O. (1992) The secretory endometrial protein, placental protein 14, in women with ectopic pregnancy. *Fertil Steril* **57**, 102–6

Rutanen, E.-M., Bohn, H. and Seppala, M. (1982) Radioimmunoassay of placental protein 12: levels in amniotic fluid, cord blood and serum of healthy adults, pregnant women and patients with trophoblastic disease. *Am J Obstet Gynecol* **144**, 460–3

Rutanen, E.-M., Koistinen, R., Wahlstrom, T., Sjoberg, J., Stenman, U.H. and Seppala, M. (1984) Placental protein 12 (PP12) in the human endometrium: tissue concentration in relation to histology and serum levels of PP12, progesterone and oestradiol. *Br J Obstet Gynaecol* **91**, 377–81

Seppala, M., Venesmma, P. and Rutanen, E.-M. (1980) Pregnancy-specific beta-1 glycoprotein in ectopic pregnancy. *Am J Obstet Gynecol* **136**, 189–93

Seppala, M., Julkunen, M., Riittinen, L. *et al.* (1992) Endometrial proteins: a reappraisal. *Hum Reprod* **7**, 31–40

Shearman, R.P. (1979) 'Endocrinology of the feto-maternal unit' in R.P. Shearman (Ed.) *Human Reproductive Physiology*, pp.97–126. Oxford: Blackwell Scientific

Siiteri, P.K. and MacDonald, P.C. (1966) Placental oestrogen biosynthesis during human pregnancy. *J Clin Endocrinol Metabol* **26**, 751–62

Silahtoraglu, A.N., Tumer, Z., Kristensen, T., Sottrup-Jensen, L. and Tommerup, N. (1993) Assignment of the human gene for pregnancy-associated plasma protein A (PAPP-A) to 9q33.1 by fluorescence *in situ* hybridization to mitotic and meiotic chromosomes. *Cytogenet Cell Genet* **61**, 214–16

Spencer, K. (1994) 'Is the measurement of unconjugated oestriol of value in screening for Down's syndrome?' in J.G. Grudzinskas *et al.* (Eds) *Screening for Down's Syndrome*, pp. 141–61. Cambridge: Cambridge University Press

Spencer, K., Macri, J.N., Aitken, D. and Connor, J.M. (1992) Free beta hCG as a first trimester marker for fetal trisomy. *Lancet* **339**, 1480

Stabile, I. and Grudzinskas, J.G. (1994) 'Ectopic pregnancy: What's new?' in J.W.W. Studd (Ed.) *Progress in Obstetrics and Gynaecology*, vol. 11, pp.291–309. Edinburgh: Churchill Livingstone

Stabile, I., Grudzinskas, J.G. and Chard, T. (1988) Clinical applications of pregnancy protein estimations with particular reference to PAPP-A. *Obstet Gynecol Surv* **49**, 73–89

Stabile, I. Grudzinskas, J.G. and Chard, T. (1992) *Spontaneous Abortion: Diagnosis and Treatment*. London: Springer Verlag

Teisner, B., Rasmussen, H.B., Hojrup, P., Yde-Andersen, E. and Skjodt, K. (1992) Fetal antigen 2: an amniotic protein identified as the aminopropeptide of the $\alpha 1$ chain of human procollagen type I. *APMIS* **100**, 1106–14

Than, G.N., Tatra, G., Bohn, H. *et al.* (1987) Placental protein 14 serum levels following conception. *Med Sci Res* **15**, 1243

Tornehave, D., Fay, R.N., Teisner, B., Chemnitz, J., Westergaard, J.G. and Grudzinskas, J.G. (1989) Two fetal antigens (FA-1 and FA-2) and endometrial proteins (PP12 and PP14) isolated from amniotic fluid: localisation in the fetus and adult female genital tract. *Eur J Obstet Gynecol Reprod Biol* **30**, 221–32

Tornehave, D., Jensen, P., Teisner, B., Rasmussen, H.B., Chemnitz, J. and Moscoso, G. (1993) Fetal antigen 1 (FA-1) in the human pancreas. Cell type expression, topological and quantitative variations during development. *Anat Embryol* **187**, 335–46

Van Cong, N., Vaisse, C., Gross, M.S., Slim, R., Milgrom, E. and Bernheim, A. (1991) The human placental protein 14 gene is localised to chromosome 9q34. *Hum Genet* **86**, 515–18

Wahlstrom, T., Koskimies, A.I., Tenhunen, A. *et al.* (1985) Pregnancy proteins in the endometrium after follicle aspiration for *in vitro* fertilisation. *Ann NY Acad Sci* **442**, 402

Waites, G.T., Bell, S.C., Walker, R.A. *et al.* (1990) Immunohistological distribution of the secretory endometrial protein, 'pregnancy-associated endometrial α2-globulin', a glycosylated β-lactoglobulin, homologue, in the human fetus and adult employing monoclonal antibodies. *Hum Reprod* **5**, 105

Wald, N.J., Stone, R., Cuckle, H.S. *et al.* (1992) First trimester concentrations of pregnancy associated plasma protein A and placental protein 14 in Down's syndrome. *BMJ* **305**, 28

Wald, N.J., George, L., Smith, D., Densem, J.W. and Petterson, K. (1996) Serum screening for Down's syndrome between 8 and 14 weeks of pregnancy. International Prenatal Screening Research Group. *Br J Obstet Gynaecol* **103**, 407–12

Watkins, P.C., Eddy, R., Beck, A.K. *et al.* (1987) DNA sequence and regional assignment of the human follicle-stimulating hormone beta-subunit gene to the short arm of human chromosome 11. *DNA* **6**, 205–12

Chapter 3

The social and ethical issues of risk assessment

Robert Silman

Introduction

The social and ethical issues which are most commonly discussed with regard to screening for Down syndrome are those which relate to the consequence of screening; i.e. the termination of a Down fetus.

1. The anti-abortionist argument is that the termination of a fetus is a close approximation to murder because the fetus is an unborn human being. There is no moral distinction between terminating a fetus, at whatever stage in development, and killing a child. Consequently, there is no moral or social distinction between terminating a fetus with a disability, such as a Down fetus, and killing a Down child. For the anti-abortionist, the detection of disability through a screening programme is simply the first step on the road to eugenic murder.

2. The counter-argument relies on two factors. The first is that the fetus is not an 'unborn' child. There is a true moral distinction between the reality of humanness which is the newborn child, and the potentiality of humanness which is the fetus. The pro-abortionist will argue that the potentiality argument is essentially absurd. If a fetus is a potential human being, why not sperm and eggs? And if sperm and eggs are potential human beings, we should be encouraging widespread promiscuity to convert them into live children. The argument *ad absurdio* is complemented by the further factor which is that we have a duty to respect the autonomy of the mother. The woman's real human right to determine whether she wishes to carry a fetus takes precedence over the potential human rights of the fetus.

One can usually discover which argument is being espoused by the vocabulary which is used. Both sides express themselves in positivist language. Thus the anti-abortionists describe themselves as pro-life, and their adversaries describe themselves as pro-choice. For the pro-life movement, the unborn child is adjectivally removed from the newborn child. They are therefore of one and the same substance. For the pro-choice movement fetus is nominally distinct from baby. There is therefore a substantive difference between the two.

The argument waged at the level of individual rights and responsibilities is also reflected in social and political ideology. However, here there is greater confusion. The current political rhetoric is often self-contradictory. For example, the exhortation that you should accept responsibility for your pregnancy and therefore bear your child to term, is contradicted by the lament that you should not have children irresponsibly, especially if you are a single mother and the State has to support you and your child.

There is nothing new or interesting which can be added to these arguments. They are debated endlessly, and it is unlikely that anything in this chapter will influence anyone's opinion on any of these fundamental issues.

However, there is a topic which is rarely commented on, and which is at the heart of the debate concerning the screening for Down syndrome. This is the social and ethical issue concerning the very notion of risk estimation itself. Whether it is the risk estimation associated with winning the lottery, or taking the contraceptive pill, or eating infected beef, or having a Down child, there is an alarming divergence between the calculations of the statisticians/scientists and the response of individual members of the public to those calculations. If risk estimation were the only issue in deciding whether to take a risk, no one would play the lottery. But, virtually everyone plays the lottery. The purpose of this chapter is to address the moral and social dimension of this seeming paradox.

A personal example

When I was a first MB medical student, I was given a genetic problem to solve. The genetics were rudimentary as befitted a novice. Essentially the problem was as illustrated in Fig. 3.1, and was expressed as follows: '(a) Your patient has one parent who carries a dominant genetic disease. (b) Your patient wishes to have children by a partner who has no genetic disease. (c) What is the risk that your patient will have a child with that genetic disease?'

The answer is obvious. There is a one in two risk that the patient carries the genetic disease, consequently there is a one in four risk that the patient's offspring will carry the genetic disease.

Nonetheless I entered into a furious argument with my teacher about the nature of the advice which should be given to this theoretical patient. For my teacher, the advice followed the facts and therefore should be, 'You have a one in four risk that you will have an affected child.' My argument was that the facts were only true of a population. If, as a doctor, I had a population of such patients (Fig. 3.2a) then I would advise my population that one in four of their children would be affected by the genetic disease. However, if, as a doctor, I was dealing with an individual (Fig. 3.2b), the risk was either one in two that my individual patient was going to have an affected child or there was no risk whatsoever. In other words what was true for the population was untrue for the individual.

The argument between me and my teacher was waged around the issue of population versus individual. For my teacher, the patient was simply a member of the population and must necessarily identify with the population. My argument

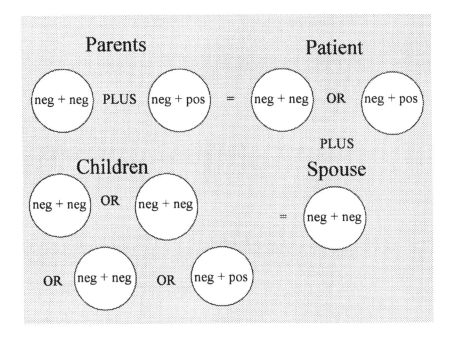

Fig. 3.1. The patient has one parent with genetic disease (neg+pos) and one parent without genetic disease (neg+neg). The patient wishes to have a child by a partner who has no genetic disease (neg+neg).

was that individuals do not behave like populations, nor should they. For an individual there is only one concept of risk which is either it will happen or it won't, i.e. all or none. Consequently if I tell my patient there is a one in four risk, my patient will think it is likely to happen, and just about as likely as a one in two risk. However, if I tell my patient there is a one in two chance of there being no risk whatsoever, it opens the possibility of escaping all risk. Whereas the advice to the population has to be doomsday advice, i.e. the population is condemned to having one in four of their children affected by the genetic disease, the individual patient is not part of this doomsday scenario, i.e. the individual patient has a very high chance of having no children affected by the genetic disease.

This debate between me and my teacher about what advice was appropriate in these circumstances happened many years ago. It, nonetheless, contained the seeds of the unresolved issues of risk estimation as they apply today.

The lottery

The analysis of the different interests of a population versus those of an individual can be best dissected using an example which stares us in the face each week, namely the lottery. The lottery is an ideal tool for this analysis, because: (a) it is not about risk but about chance (and we should not forget that when we talk

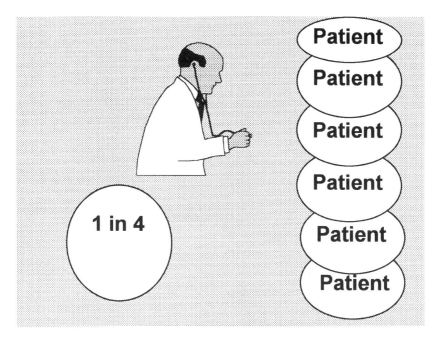

Fig. 3.2(a).   The doctor's advice to a population of such patients.

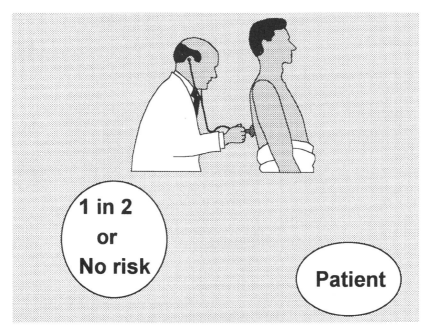

Fig. 3.2(b).   The doctor's advice to an individual patient within the population.

about risk we are simply adding an emotive element to the concept of chance), and (b) the statistics are not in doubt.

Example one: For a one pound stake there is a twenty million to one chance of winning ten million pounds.

It is clear that the odds are against me. If I was representing a population, e.g. if I was a fund manager, I would be certain to lose. Consequently, if I invested my client's funds in the lottery under such terms, I would be criminally incompetent.

The individual who stakes an individual one pound in such circumstances can be similarly criticised, if the individual is considered exclusively as a member of the population. The individual's excuse 'I don't mind losing one pound if I have a chance of winning ten million pounds' is simply childlike naiveté. For the statistician/scientist the individual has failed to understand the reality behind the numbers, and the individual is behaving irrationally.

Example two: For a one pound stake there is a five million to one chance of winning ten million pounds.

Now, as a fund manager, everything has changed. Under these terms the odds are with me. If I invest my client's funds I am bound to win and win handsomely. I could not ask for a better return on my investment. The consequence of these odds is that the fund will rapidly show an immense profit and Camelot, the lottery organisers, will soon become bankrupt.

But has anything changed for the individual? The prize is still the same, it is still ten million pounds. The odds have changed. But is it any more rational to bet one pound on five million to one odds versus one pound on twenty million to one odds? If the goal is to win ten million pounds, and it is rational to bet at five million to one odds, then the individual can become rational by simply staking four pounds instead of one. If, on the contrary, the statistician/scientist considers it irrational to bet one pound at five million to one odds, at what point does it become rational? Somewhere between five million to one and evens, it must be a rational act to stake one pound to win ten million pounds!

The purpose of these examples is to illustrate the inevitable and necessary distinction between the cost benefit analysis of chance (risk) which is made by statisticians/scientists on populations, versus the cost benefit analysis of an individual. In my example, the cut-off point for the population is startling clear. It is ten million to one. The Government has legislated that the cut-off point will always remain in Camelot's favour, just like a roulette wheel in a Casino, otherwise the lottery, as an institution, cannot survive. Hence fund managers do not invest in the lottery (or on roulette). But that is of no concern to an individual, nor should it be. For an individual, the cut-off point is not defined by the population odds. An individual who says, at twenty million to one, 'I don't mind losing one pound if I have a chance of winning ten million pounds,' is just as rational as an individual who says it at five million to one, or at five to one. The statistician/ scientist cannot dictate, and is incapable of dictating, the cut-off point for an individual, and the statistician/scientist who attempts to do so is behaving irrationally.

Of course this does not mean that individuals are always rational. An individual who says, 'I am spending more than I can afford because I desperately want to win ten million pounds and I don't believe the odds are as bad as they seem,' is irrational. But the irrationality has nothing to do with the cut-off point of population statistics. It has to do with the unrealistic nature of the individual's personal expectations.

Cost benefit and cut off

We are therefore led back to the issue of risk assessment in screening for Down syndrome, and the divergent meaning of the word 'risk' for a population of mothers versus an individual mother within that population.

Let us suppose, for the sake of argument, that the individual mother belongs to a population of 25 000 mothers where the risk of having a Down child is one in 250. Let us further suppose that this risk estimation is accurate.

Fractions and unity

For the population of 25 000 such mothers, if no action is taken to thwart the event, approximately 100 children will be born with Down syndrome. This is an inevitable consequence of an accurate risk estimation. The 100 children with Down syndrome will be a fact. The 100 children will exist, i.e. there will be a real fraction.

For the individual mother within this population, if no action is taken to thwart the event, one child will be born. This single child will have Down syndrome or will not have Down syndrome. This is a fact. It does not matter about the population statistics, the mother will not give birth to a child which is one two hundred and fiftieth part Down syndrome, i.e. there is no fraction. It is all or none.

Public policy and personal choice

The cost benefit analysis of risk estimation on populations is a political act. How much does it cost to screen the pregnant population? How much does it cost to provide further tests for the one in 250 sub-group? What is the benefit of such a screening programme in reducing the number of Down children in the population at large? What is the benefit to society (e.g. to the social services or the NHS) in reducing the number of Down children? The cost benefit analysis is made on the reality of fractions. Whether the risk is worth taking is calculated on the cost of increasing the denominator versus the benefit in having a smaller fraction.

The individual mother is provided with the same risk estimate as the population, but it serves a different purpose. The cost benefit analysis of the risk is quite different. It has nothing to do with fractions. It is about unity. How much does it matter to me if I have a Down child? What is the cost (emotional/financial/familial) to me if my baby is a Down child? What is the benefit (emotional/financial/familial) if I can prevent this event? How much will it cost me in emotional and personal terms if I sacrifice a healthy fetus in finding out if I have a Down fetus? What is the cost to me if my healthy baby is destroyed by an unnecessary amniocentesis? Whether I can afford to take a risk of one in 250 can only be decided by me in the context of my individual circumstances, and even then with great difficulty.

The hidden dogmatism of *test positive/test negative*

There is nothing undemocratic about a political analysis of risk estimation. Social engineering is not totalitarian dogmatism so long as it is not imposed. There is nothing to suggest that we (i.e. politicians/doctors/scientists) intend to impose a screening programme on individuals. It is provided as a service. A pregnant mother is free to accept or reject it. If she accepts a screening test, she is free to interpret the statistics in her own way.

None the less, the divergence between the interests of the statistician/scientist compared with the interest of the individual has sometimes led to an improper presentation of the service. For example, a one in 250 risk may be an appropriate cut-off point for the population as determined by scientists/statisticians. What is dogmatic about such a cut-off is that individual patients are expected to comply. It is like the old Stalinist concept of the Party. The Party knew what was good for society, and rejection of the Party line by an individual was condemned as petit bourgeois subjectivism. Similarly, the statistician/scientist determines an appropriate level of 'test positive' or 'test negative' for a given population, and the patient is expected to concur. Like any form of dogmatism, it is stupid. It is stupid because it fails to recognise that the cost benefit analysis of an individual is necessarily different from that of the population. And it is stupid because, anyway, most forms of cost benefit analysis on populations are flawed. Just as the Communist Party did not know what was good for the population, so statistician/scientists do not necessarily have it right for their populations. That is not to say that we should not attempt a cost benefit analysis, it is simply that we should not be dogmatic about our recommendations.

Conclusion

If we leave aside the notion that the word 'risk' carries a judgement, we can all agree that risk estimations are neutral. They are based on probability statistics. How we use the numbers does not change them. The triumph of the new tests in screening for Down syndrome is that they provide us with better and better risk estimations.

Risk estimates are the same whether provided for populations or for the individuals within those populations. For example, if a population of 25,000 mothers has a risk estimate of one in 250 of carrying a Down child, every individual mother within that population of 25 000 mothers carries the same risk.

The risk estimate carries a different prediction for the population than for the individual. For the population of 25 000 mothers, we can accurately predict the outcome, i.e. there will be approximately 100 children born with Down syndrome. For any individual mother within that population we can also accurately predict the outcome. It will be independent of the risk estimate, i.e. the mother will, or will not, give birth to a Down child.

How we use a risk estimate is a matter of judgement. The judgement for a population is necessarily different from the judgement for the individual because the prediction is different. In the case of a population, the judgement has to do with the cost of reducing the 100 Down births versus the benefit. In the case of an individual mother, the judgement has to do with 'Can I afford to take a risk of one in 250 of having a Down child?'

Cost benefit analyses on populations may be flawed. However, they are a legitimate exercise. It is appropriate that statisticians/scientists should attempt to provide the social services and the NHS with judgements on when risks should be acted upon and when risks should be ignored.

Cost benefit analyses by individuals may be flawed. However, they are a legitimate exercise. It is appropriate that an individual mother should attempt to provide herself with a judgement on when a risk should be acted upon and when a risk should be ignored.

The judgement on when a risk should be acted on and when a risk should be ignored is necessarily different for the population taken as a whole than for any individual within that population. Though they are different, they are both legitimate.

What is illegitimate is that statisticians/scientists should try to impose their judgements on individuals.

The practical consequences of these axioms are:

1. A screening test should not be presented to all patients as 'risk'. It is insulting to those who do not choose to undergo the test, especially those who do not consider the outcome to be 'tragedy' or 'disease'.
2. Patients should be counselled as to what is going to happen when they are offered a screening test. They should be encouraged to begin the process of exploring what level of risk they consider appropriate for their circumstances prior to being given any actual risk data.
3. Patients should provide their personal cut-off point before they receive a test result. It should not be dependent on the test result.
4. The result of the screening test should be presented in the form of a risk estimate without any judgement as to whether the risk is worth taking or not. Whether the risk is worth taking is decided by whether the risk estimate has fallen above or below the patient's personal cut-off point.
5. Doctors should not impose a universal cut-off point. They should tailor the cut off to suit the judgement of the patient rather than to comply with notional resource implications for the NHS.

Chapter 4

General aspects

Discussion

Chard: Professor Grudzinskas did not mention what to my mind is the sole known gene locus which might be related to the endocrinology of Down syndrome. That gene locus is the locus for the interferon alpha receptor which resides on chromosome 21. There is also well-published evidence that interferon alpha can in a somewhat artificial tissue culture system promote the secretion of hCG. If one wanted to be simplistic one could put that together in a mechanism. I do not want to advocate that for a moment, but I thought I might briefly expose that matter. The reference for the record is Iles and Chard (1989).

Adinolfi: I have two questions to Professor Cuckle. The first one is about the paternal age effect. As you know, many studies have been done on the incidence of trisomy or diploidy in spermatozoa using the FISH (fluorescent *in situ* hybridisation) technique. Is there any evidence that there is an increased incidence of trisomy 21 in older men? Incidentally, if there is a paternal age effect it should be very evident in cases of 47 XYY since they are all of paternal origin.

Cuckle: I am not very expert in this area. The empiric studies that have been done in the past have sometimes seen them, and sometimes they have not. That is because it is a small effect, and also because they have had to look at paternal age independently of maternal age and the correlation is very high. You would have to get lots of older fathers and younger mothers really to show it.

Adinolfi: That is why I suggested the 47 XYY because there is not a general effect there. I have another question about epidemiology and screening. Do you think we should recognise a group of women who are not at risk for age or IQ level? They are women who have normal chromosomes in peripheral blood, they are not at risk for age and yet they have fetuses or neonates with trisomy 21. In these cases we should suspect that they have a gonadal mosaicism and if tested by FISH their oocytes will show a high incidence of chromosomal disorders such as an extra chromatid or chromosome 21. The origin of the chromosomal defects in

34

the offspring of these patients is different from other cases and the only useful screening is that performed at the oocyte level after stimulation. No other test can document why they have such a high incidence of trisomy 21.

Cuckle: I am sorry, I did not quite understand who these women were. In women who are having *in vitro* fertilisation (IVF), there may be other ways of quantifying the risk. In particular, in women who are having IVF with a donor egg, there is a whole question about Down syndrome screening risk of those women: whether we are using the age of the mother of the egg donor at the time of donation – that sort of issue. We all do, but there are no real data on that. It may be that the seed versus soil argument is not fully answered. So, yes, I am aware of that measurement.

Ward: Might I ask about the issue of refinements and a repeat test. I know this was a difficult area with second trimester screening.

Cuckle: That is more of a biochemical point than an epidemiology point. The correct way of interpreting a repeat test statistically is to take account of the prior test as well as the repeat test and use all the information. It certainly does come up more and more because of first trimester testing, and will in the future because we shall be screening in the first trimester, as is being done now by Professor Nicolaides. Then they come to us.

This is now private screening: we have plenty of women who want a 'belt-and-braces' approach. Professor Nicolaides gives them a negative result and then they come to us for a serum screening without telling us that they have been to have ultrasound. Obviously you have to take account of the fact that you have assessed nuchal translucency, so you need some correlations between first trimester ultrasound and second trimester biochemistry that we do not have. We make assumptions of independence which may not be valid, but that is the best one can do.

I was not raising the question of these refinements from the biochemistry aspect or the likelihood ratio calculation aspect but I am concerned that there might be epidemiological issues to do with bias. Repeat testing is not a very good example; let's look at the smoking one because it is the most powerful one and I did not have time to go into it. Smoking affects all of the markers to some degree and some of the markers to a great degree, and you might want to take account of it. Probably it is not worth it: it is not a big effect, so if you were trying to increase detection by doing so you would not have a big impact on detection and the current opinion is that you should not adjust for smoking.

This relates to what Dr Silman was saying. If you take the view that I am not so interested in population here as in the individual, and I am interested in giving every individual the best estimate of risk that I can get for her rather than maximising detection necessarily, then you may want to take account of smoking in interpreting the biochemistry. The point I make is that if you do that, beware – you must be particularly careful that you do not bias the risk. In fact, you can bias it in such a way that you would lose detection if you were not careful. You have to take account of the prior risk, and in smokers it would seem that the prior risk is reduced. So if you are doing it you have to use the best estimate of the extent of reduction from the literature.

Another caveat to that is that all of those data and of predominantly second trimester data, given that smoking is an abortifacient, it may be that the prior risk calculation is wrong if you try to use it in any pregnancy.

Wald: Has Professor Cuckle any evidence on why there is an age effect on the birth prevalence of Down syndrome.

Cuckle: I don't think there is any evidence. There are all sorts of hypotheses and there are bits of epidemiological information that go one way or the other way. I was intrigued by some work looking at the number of eggs according to maternal age. This is by sampling ovaries and looking at oocytes. It seems extraordinary, but the curve is almost the inverse of the Down syndrome risk curve.

That supports the production line hypothesis, because it would suggest that there are a fixed number of eggs that if fertilised will lead to Down syndrome and they do not get used up as quickly as normal eggs, so there are more of those to drop proportionally as the pool of eggs reduces. So it is probabilistic but it is based on differential usage of good and bad eggs. The production line hypothesis, for those who do not know, is that the eggs that are made first *in utero* when the mother herself was *in utero* are the better eggs, and they are used first.

Adinolfi: I think that Polani and Crolla (1991) have shown in mice that there is a reduction of chiasmata in the older eggs' oocytes. That is why non-disjunction occurs more frequently in older oocytes. This has not been established in humans but there is some evidence in favour of this non-disjunction.

Simpson: I have some comments. First, additional support of the production line hypothesis is the fact that from DNA decreased recombinance in the non-disjunctional chromosomes has been reported. That is consistent with the previous cytological studies that show decreased chiasmata.

My second comment is that there is really not a good alternative hypothesis. One that geneticists have posed for years has been of delayed fertilisation, involving a sperm or egg that has been present *in vivo* for several days prior to conception which would have an increased likelihood of leading to aneuploidy. As we know, that is well established in a host of mammals but it has been difficult to prove in humans.

My colleagues and I have been involved in a South American study of natural family planning populations for about a decade and now have about a thousand cases in which the timing of conception can be accurately determined. It looks as though there will be no increased prevalence of Down syndrome. We have also found the same in a case controlled population that has been published recently (Phillips *et al.* 1995).

I have one other comment relevant to Dr Silman's presentation. It seems to me that there is something that, if not new on pregnancy termination, needs to be put into the record. The complication rate differs between first versus second trimester pregnancy termination – in the United States, the public does not recognise that the CDC (Center for Disease Control) figures in the United States show the death rate from first trimester pregnancy terminations is about 1 per 100 000, whereas the death rate from second trimester terminations, either by D&E or by instillation, is of the order of 6–8 per 100 000. This is a six-fold difference at the minimum between the complication rates in the second versus the first trimester.

Cuckle: One point that Dr Silman did not make about termination is that we are a society in which we accept terminations in the UK. So what is wrong with terminating a Down fetus if you are willing to terminate so many other pregnancies for not as good a reason? One argument against, that is not often made, is that this is selective termination: you are selectively identifying a fetus of a particular type.

Silman: I hoped I had covered that point because what I think the anti-abortionists would argue is that abortion is murder and if you are using termination for Down, then it is eugenic murder. So it is just a different quality of murder. In the first case it is murder for social convenience, in the second case it is murder for eugenics and there is a qualitative difference in those two forms of murder for the anti-abortionists.

Cuckle: My point is that you do not have to believe that abortion is murder to still feel uncomfortable with selectively terminating particular types of individuals. I must say, I feel slightly ambivalent.

Torgerson: A question to Professor Cuckle about the age incidence of Down syndrome. Could it be that, rather than chronological age, it is reproductive, fertility age? For example, if a woman was aged 40 and was getting to her menopause at 45, she would have the same risk as a woman at age 45 who would have a menopause at age 50?

Cuckle: If we were right about the number of oocytes reducing with age, when the number gets below a certain level you get the menopause. So the menopause – or the perimenopause – is actually related to the pool of eggs left. You would expect an effect of some sort, but you would need to do big studies really to see it.
   Another thing that has not been mentioned is the possibility of gonadal mosaicism, on which I have also corresponded with Paul Polani and we have not got very far. It would be nice to have a look at the numbers of eggs in the ovaries of mothers of Down children and see if there is some specific mosaicism in the ovary.

Simpson: On the reproductive age as opposed to the chronological age, this is another example of where the experimental evidence in mammals has not proved to be extrapolatable to humans. There are data in the mouse that would suggest that that would be valid. We have looked at this in humans (Phillips *et al.* 1995) in two ways. We took the younger mothers who had had children with Down syndrome, say, in their twenties or so to look to see whether there was an increased frequency of premature variant failure in the subsequent 15 years compared to controls; we did not find any. Then in older women who had had Down syndrome children in the 35–45 age cohort we looked to see the actual age of menopause and compared it to various control US populations, and they showed a virtually identical age of menopause. So in neither of those two ways did we find any evidence.

Whittle: I wonder if I could draw Professor Cuckle back to the data on the loss calculations for Down syndrome at various gestation ages. He showed us a number of models to figure out those losses. I think I know the data on which some of those were based, but they were very neat curves. I guess they have confidence limits as well, and I wonder whether you can indicate those to us?

Cuckle: For Down syndrome the best information on the overall fetal loss rate comes from Hook (Hook *et al.* 1989). In this series of 110 women who refused termination following a second trimester prenatal diagnosis of Down syndrome the fetal loss rate is 29% (95% confidence interval 22–37%). The loss rate varies with gestation and this can be estimated from a recent analysis of a similar series of 168 women from Professor Alberman's register (Hook *et al.* 1995). The number of pregnancies at risk of fetal loss is relatively small at some gestations and so the authors have fitted a model to allow more precise estimation of gestation-specific loss rates. For the earlier gestations the confidence interval will be quite wide.

I prefer to use both this direct information on the fetal loss rate and the indirect information derived by comparing the observed Down syndrome prevalence at amniocentesis with the expected birth prevalence from the maternal age-specific rates. Taking both together, we can be confident that about one-third of fetuses with Down syndrome known to be alive at mid-trimester will not survive to term.

Information about the loss rate in affected fetuses known to be alive in the first trimester is much sparser. There are hardly any published data from women who refuse termination at this time so one has to rely on the comparison of the observed prevalence at CVS with the expected birth prevalence. Two studies have done this calculation (Macintosh *et al.* 1995; Snijders *et al.* 1994), using overlapping data sets, and get the same fetal loss rate 54%.

Macintosh: In our data set, which was a meta-analysis and also involved the Danish cytogenetic register, there was no evidence for an increasing miscarriage rate in older women. But one is very constrained by the age range you are looking at, between 35 and 46. It is a statistical problem that, looking at models, you cannot really tell whether there is a differential miscarriage rate in older women for Down syndrome pregnancies. There is one paper that did find one in the 1990s. It was in the *American Journal of Human Genetics* (Kratzer *et al.* 1992). I believe it is to do with statistical handling that they found a difference in miscarriage rates, and it is difficult to know absolutely whether the miscarriage rate for Down syndrome pregnancies in young women is exactly the same as in older women. But we have to make that assumption if we are to give first trimester risks to younger women.

Cuckle: I agree. That study is in Snijders' meta-analysis (Snijders *et al.* 1994), showing that in the narrow age window of 35–45 years old there was no apparent age effect. But it is consistent with there being one at younger ages. Does it really matter?

This brings me to another point to do with what Dr Silman has been saying. What is risk? A risk is simply just saying that you don't know. In terms of Down syndrome, if you knew, a fraction of the population would have 100% risk and the rest of the population would have 0% risk. That is the same as your argument. It is obvious that some people will have 100% risk and some will have 0%. So the risk that we give to the woman is the best estimate that we have on the basis of all the information that we have, that her baby has Down syndrome or that she will deliver a baby with Down syndrome. I favour making statements like, 'You will deliver a baby with Down syndrome,' rather than, 'You've got one now,' but I know that in America they take the reverse position.

As I also said before, there are two purposes of all this. One is to maximise detection by using risk in an optimum way; the other is to inform individuals. And it may be that the latter use requires you to tell them what the risk is now.

Chard: I wonder if I could return to Dr Silman's lottery model again and ask for his comment on what I think could reasonably be, a *reductio ad absurdum* of that particular model. He correctly points out that when people are addressing something like a lottery they do not use risk in the manner in which we discuss it in this room today, in that quantitative, probabilistic sense at all. Therefore, would we not be better in our counselling – and it would certainly greatly simplify it – to follow that line to eliminate any question of a quantification of risk and simply ask the individual women: which do you prefer – a miscarriage or a Down syndrome baby? That is the sole question that needs to be asked. Logically it does not differ from the situation of someone saying I will spend a pound, because I don't really mind a pound on the lottery, versus winning £10 million, because I regard that as a positive outcome.

Silman: That is exactly what I was trying to argue, and this is where I take issue with Professor Cuckle. As far as the individual patient is concerned, either she is going to have a Down fetus or she is not. She is not going to have one in a hundred. She is either going to have a Down child or she is not going to have a Down child. So I suppose what I was trying to argue is that the risk benefit analysis from the patient's point of view has virtually nothing to do with your risk benefit analysis. As far as the patient is concerned, the question is: how much does it matter if I am going to have a Down child? What am I prepared to sacrifice in order not to have a Down child?

I guess if I was a mother I would say I would want to be certain I was not going to have a Down child. I don't care if the risk is 1 in 10, 1 in 30, 1 in 200 or 1 in 1000.

Wald: I was going to support Professor Cuckle's view on the use of risk. Risk is really a quantitative measure for expressing uncertainty. If there is one group that definitely is going to have it and another group that has a one in two chance, and they are put together, then it is one in four.

On the ethical issue, Professor Cuckle is absolutely right. There is a distinction between non-selective and selective abortion. Dr Silman indicated that if one's view of termination was murder of the fetus, that meant eugenics. I do not believe that is the case. Even if you took that extreme view, the definition of eugenics is the purpose for taking away the life of the fetus. If that purpose is determined by the mother or the couple as an individual choice, it is not a feature of state policy or collective social policy. If it is a feature of state or collective social policy with pressure, then it does become eugenics. In the whole ethical discussion it is extremely important to distinguish the purpose for termination and whether it is a society-driven thing and an aspect of state policy, which is reprehensible, or whether it is a matter of personal choice by individual couples, which in our society is acceptable.

Hicks: I want to draw attention to what I think Professor Cuckle said – that there were two main reasons for this whole enterprise. One was to maximise detection rates and the other was to do as well as possible by individual women.

That is a very crucial issue. I will declare a personal view. I think this enterprise is about doing as well as possible by individual women, not about maximising the detection rate for the population.

Silman: What I was trying to argue in terms of the socio-ethical issues was that your position I would see as a sort of Stalinist-populationist position. I do not believe that I, as an individual, want to hear from you that I have a one in four chance when in fact the breakdown of that would be that either I am unaffected or I have a one in two. I would much rather, as an individual, have that piece of individual information rather than information on population.

As far as social eugenics is concerned, there is clearly a whole movement at the moment towards screening for all sorts of features about the possible offspring – features of sexuality, of perfection and so on. I agree entirely with Professor Cuckle: this is a quite distinct area which raises its own moral dilemmas and moral issues. If we think that it is not state-driven that we have termination for Down syndrome, I would contest that completely. This very focus, this very forum is the sort of forum which has been supported by the state because the state has an interest in not having Down syndrome children. One of the things that was argued very strongly by Dominic Lawson, when he had a Down child, was that there was extraordinary pressure that it is better not to have Down children. There is a pressure for that answer. I am not saying that that is wrong but I am saying it exists, and I do not think that just by saying that the state is not involved in this actually removes state pressure.

Marteau: I would like to endorse the comments that Dr Silman has just made, which draw our attention to the political, economic and social context within which screening takes place. I think we will return to that as the meeting continues. I would like to come back to the more specific point about the term 'risk'. Probably all of us in the room are using it in different ways. My own view about risk is that it comprises a likelihood of some adverse event. So when Dr Silman was talking I was thinking that he was drawing our attention to the fact that statisticians tend to trade in likelihoods or frequencies and perhaps patients are more interested in the nature of the outcome.

Although that is a position to take, if we look at what the empirical evidence looks like, certainly women place a greater emphasis on the nature of the outcome but they are also sensitive to frequencies. So people do not think in a completely binary way; people behave differently according to the frequencies that they are given. But if we just tease out those two parts of risk that helps us.

Ward: On that note, can I thank the three speakers and all the discussants.

References

Hook, E.B., Topol, B.B. and Cross, P.K. (1989) The natural history of cytogenetically abnormal fetuses detected at midtrimester amniocentesis which are not terminated electively: New data and estimates of the excess and relative risk of late fetal death associated with 47,+21 and some other abnormal karyotypes. *Am J Hum Genet* **45**, 855–61

Hook, E.B., Mutton, D.E., Ide, R., Alberman, E. and Bobrow, M. (1995) The natural history of Down Syndrome conceptuses diagnosed prenatally that are not electively terminated. *Am J Hum Genet* **57**, 875–81

Iles, R.K. and Chard, T. (1989) Enhancement of ectopic β-human chorionic gonadotrophin expression by interferon-α. *J Endocrinol* **123**, 501–7

Kratzer, P. G., Golbus, M. S., Schonberg, S. A., Heilbron, D. C. and Taylor, R. N. (1992) Cytogenetic evidence for enhanced selective miscarriage of trisomy 21 pregnancies with advancing maternal age. *Am J Hum Genet* **44,** 657–63

Macintosh, M.C.M., Wald, N.J., Chard, T. *et al.* (1995) Selective miscarriage of Down's syndrome fetuses in women aged 35 years and older. *Br J Obstet Gynaecol* **102**, 798–801

Phillips, O. P., Cromwell, S., Rivas, M., Simpson, J. L. and Elias, S. (1995) Trisomy 21 and maternal age of menopause: does reproductive age rather than chronological age influence risk of nodisjunction? *Hum Genet* **95,** 117–18

Polani, P. E. and Crolla, J. (1991) A test of the production line hypothesis of a mammalian oogenesis. *Hum Genet* **88,** 64–70

Snijders, R.J.M., Holzgreve, W., Cuckle, H. and Nicolaides, K.H. (1994) Maternal age-specific risks for Trisomies at 9–14 weeks' gestation. *Prenat Diagn* **14**, 543–52

SECTION 2

STATISTICAL ASPECTS OF SCREENING FOR DOWN SYNDROME

Chapter 5

Screening using risk estimation: uses and abuses of the method

Nicholas J. Wald and Allan Hackshaw

Introduction

The systematic application of 'risk' as a screening variable is a relatively new concept in public health practice. It uses information that predicts the presence or absence of a disorder to estimate the probability (or odds) of having that disorder and then uses a risk cut-off level to separate the screened population into a 'positive' and a 'negative' group. Risk screening has a number of uses but it is subject to a number of abuses which, once identified, can be avoided. This chapter covers some of the uses and abuses associated with antenatal screening for Down syndrome, using risk calculated on the basis of maternal age with serum markers.

Uses

The combination of different tests on a common scale

This is, perhaps, the most important use of risk. It enables several factors or 'markers', each of which is associated with a particular disorder, to be used in combination to distinguish individuals who are likely to have that disorder from others who are not. When combining markers, the concentrations of one marker (such as the concentration of α-fetoprotein (AFP) in defining the overlapping frequency distributions of Down syndrome and unaffected pregnancies) is replaced by the corresponding distributions of risk estimates based on several markers. The method, when appropriately used, allows for the fact that one marker may be correlated with other markers, so that the information from each on the probability of being affected is not completely independent of that for the others.

Fig. 5.1 is an example of the distributions of risk in Down syndrome screening using the four marker test based on AFP, unconjugated oestriol (uE₃), total human chorionic gonadotrophin (total hCG) and inhibin-A (all adjusted for maternal weight), together with maternal age and gestational age based on 'dates' (time since the first day of the last menstrual period). Adopting a risk cut-off level of 1 in 240, 70% of pregnancies with Down syndrome would be detected for a 5% false-positive rate (that is, as well as classifying 5% of unaffected pregnancies as positive). The distributions cover a risk range of about 1:1 to 1:1 million. This range provides an indication of the discriminatory potential of the screening method – the wider the range of risk, the greater the efficacy of the screening method. Fig. 5.2 shows in a similar way the distributions of risk based on free

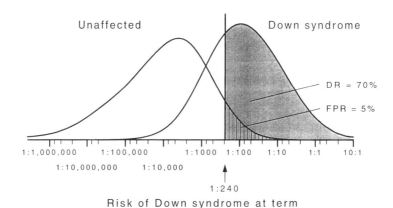

Fig. 5.1. Second trimester distribution of risk of Down syndrome in affected and unaffected pregnancies using alphafetoprotein (AFP), unconjugated oestriol (uE₃), total human chorionic gonadotrophin (hCG), and inhibin-A with maternal age.

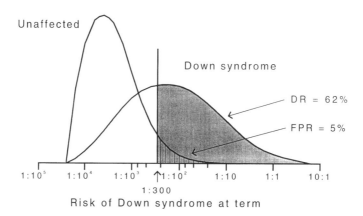

Fig. 5.2. First trimester risk screening: distribution of risk of Down syndrome in affected and unaffected pregnancies using free β-hCG and PAPP-A with maternal age.

β-hCG, and pregnancy associated plasma protein A (PAPP-A) with maternal age at 8–14 weeks of pregnancy. At a risk cut-off level of 1 to 300, 62% of Down syndrome pregnancies will be detected for a false-positive rate of 5%.

Risk is efficient

The use of risk calculated using the appropriate statistical methodology is the most efficient way of combining different tests, in that it maximises the detection rate for a given false-positive rate. This is a major objective in screening because it maximises the efficacy and safety of screening. It is best achieved by using each marker as a separate variable with due allowance for any association between markers, otherwise there may be a loss of detection for a given false-positive rate. For example, this can happen if the ratio of two markers is used and, say, 5% of subjects with the highest values are classified as 'positive' without calculating risk. Data from the Bart's screening service (based on 100 pregnancies with Down syndrome and setting the false-positive rate at 5%; St Bartholomew's Hospital, London) illustrate the loss of efficiency: the detection rate would have been 47% when using the ratio of AFP and hCG and 51% when combining the two markers by means of a single risk estimate. Using the ratio is not appropriate because it gives equal weight to each marker, and so does not allow for the fact that each marker has a different discriminatory potential.

Risk is relevant

Reporting risks is directly relevant to patients. For example, saying that a woman has a 1 in 100 chance of having an affected pregnancy is direct and clear. It is easy to understand; it provides the information needed to help a woman reach a decision on whether to have an invasive diagnostic test. Reporting risks encourages informed choice.

Risk indicates the error rate of the test

Reporting a risk intrinsically indicates the error rate of the test. For example, a risk of 1 in 100 means that if this is judged positive, 1 will be a true positive and 99 will be false positives. Conversely if it is judged to be negative, 99 will be true negatives and 1 will be a false negative.

Risk can be empirically validated

It is important that the method of calculating risk can be validated in a way that is readily understood, so that there is confidence in its use. This can be done simply using data from a screening programme, by ranking the women according to their predicted risk at term and dividing them into groups, each with approximately equal numbers of Down syndrome pregnancies. The mean predicted risk of all women in each group can then be compared with the prevalence of Down syndrome at birth in that group. The prevalence is calculated as the observed number of Down syndrome pregnancies divided by the total number of pregnancies and adjusted for the spontaneous fetal loss rate (23%) of affected pregnancies with screen-positive results which, in the absence of screening, would not have gone to term (Wald *et al.* 1996). Table 5.1 shows the validation of risk using the quadruple test at Bart's. Fig. 5.3 compares the predicted risk at term

Table 5.1. Quadruple test: predicted risk at term and prevalence of Down syndrome at birth

Predicted risk at term		Observed no. of Down syndrome pregnancies (a)	Observed no. no. of unaffected pregnancies (b)	Prevalence of Down syndrome at birth[d] (1 in (a+b)/a)
Category	Mean			
1 in 1–6	1 in 3.3	11 (8.5)[c]	14	1 in 2.6
1 in 7–40	1 in 19	9 (6.9)[c]	210	1 in 31
1 in 41–150	1 in 88	11 (8.5)[c]	645	1 in 77
1 in 151–700	1 in 348	9 (8.1)[c]	2481	1 in 307
<1 in 700	1 in 2979	7	16200	1 in 2315
All	1 in 504	47 (39)[c]	19550	1 in 502

[c] The number in parentheses is the observed number of women with Down syndrome pregnancies with screen-positive results (that is, those with risks ≥1 in 250) discounted by 0.23 to allow for the excess spontaneous fetal loss of affected pregnancies had screening not been carried out.
[d] Using the discounted number of Down syndrome pregnancies in column (a).

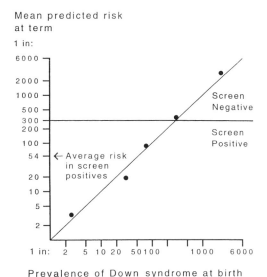

Fig. 5.3. Quadruple test: validation of risk estimates. Dots represent quintiles of predicted risk in Down syndrome pregnancies.

with the prevalence at birth. The diagonal line is the line of identity between the predicted risk and the prevalence. There is a strikingly high level of agreement between the two, showing that the method of risk estimation is accurate.

Abuses

Changing risk

There is no single (or 'true') estimate of risk for a woman. The risk value will change in light of additional information. Changing risk with new information can create the impression of improvement or deterioration in prognosis. This is a false impression because prognosis is unaltered. A woman either has an affected pregnancy or she does not; risk is a measure of uncertainty regarding her prognosis. The risk estimate that uses all the available information is the most accurate estimate, and should replace a previous one based on less information. If a woman aged 30 (with a risk of a term pregnancy with Down syndrome of about 1:1000) has a triple test and her individual risk estimate is 1:500 her risk has 'increased'. Another woman aged 40 with an approximate age specific risk of a term pregnancy with Down syndrome of about 1:100 might have a triple test result which also gives her an individual risk estimate of 1:500. Her risk has 'decreased'. Once the triple test result is known, the advice given to the two women should be the same. The fact that more detailed information has led to an increased risk estimation in one patient and a decreased risk in another is immaterial. It is only the final estimate of risk that is useful, not the history of risk estimation. In this respect, it can be misleading to report an age-specific risk as well as the triple test risk, and this practice is best avoided.

Use of average risk in women with screen-positive results

Some centres report results to women with positive screening results by giving them the 'average risk' in this group of women, although precise estimates of risk are available. This is unsatisfactory and misleading. The estimates of individual risk across the entire range of risk estimation are accurate (as shown by Fig. 5.2), so the woman is losing information of value. Many women will be given an incorrect risk estimate. The average risk for women with positive results using the triple test is about 1 in 50. Using this estimate instead of an individual risk estimate would mean that women with a risk estimate of 1 in 10 would be given the same information as women with a risk estimate of 1 in 200. This is of practical importance because among women with positive results, those with a lower risk (say 1 in 200) are more likely to decline the offer of an amniocentesis than are women with a higher risk (of, say 1 in 10) (Wald *et al.* 1992; Haddow *et al.* 1992).

Stepwise screening

Stepwise screening involves administering more than one screening test for the same disorder to the same person in sequence. This approach is inefficient when compared with screening using the tests simultaneously (one-step screening) because it increases the false-positive rate for a given detection rate. This means that the screening programme is less safe, as there are more fetal losses associated with the invasive diagnostic procedure (Wald and Cuckle 1991; Wald and Kennard 1997).

Stepwise screening for Down syndrome, where it exists, commonly uses two tests (two-step screening). There are two types of two-step screening. One involves the further screening of screen-positives and the other involves the further screening of screen-negatives.

Two-step screening: further screening of screen-positives

An example is age screening followed by the further screening of positives using serum tests. In this example, determining maternal age is, in effect, the first screening test. Only women above a specified age, say 30, that is, screen-positive, are offered serum screening. Those who have positive results after the serum test are then offered a diagnostic test. This approach is carried out in a few districts in Britain. Fig. 5.4(a) illustrates the screening performance using the triple test as the serum test; the detection rate is 42% for a 3% false-positive rate. Fig. 5.4(b) shows

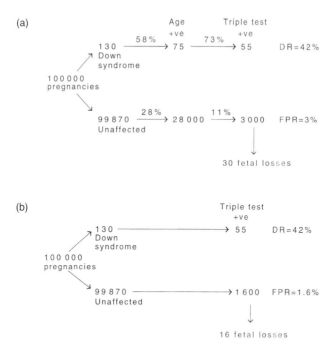

Fig. 5.4. (a) Example of the two-step screening of 're-screen positives' type: age screening followed by re-screening of positives (age ≥30 years) using the triple test (+ve if risk ≥1 in 250). (b) One-step equivalent to screening in (a). Set detection rate at 42% (triple test +ve if risk ≥1 in 100). (DR=detection rate, FPR=false-positive rate.)

the one-step equivalent in which all women, regardless of age, are offered a serum test. If the detection rate is also set at 42% (as in Fig. 5.4(a)) to allow a comparison of like with like, the false-positive rate is 1.6%. There would be half the number of false-positives (1.6 vs 3.0%), half the number of amniocenteses, and half the number of losses of healthy fetuses due to amniocentesis. The two-step approach has been adopted in some centres because it is less expensive, although it is less safe (more healthy fetuses lost for a given detection rate).

Two-step screening: further screening of screen-negatives

An example is age screening followed by a diagnostic test in positives and the further screening of negatives using serum tests. Maternal age is again the first screening test. All women above a specified age, say 35, that is, screen-positive, are offered a diagnostic test. Serum testing is not done. Women below 35 years, that is, screen-negative, are offered serum testing and those with positive serum results are offered a diagnostic test. This approach (Fig. 5.5(a)), is widely used in the United States. The overall detection rate is 65% and the false-positive rate is 11%. The one-step equivalent (Fig. 5.5(b)), in which the detection rate also is set at 65%, would yield a false-positive rate of 7.3%. There would be one-third less false-

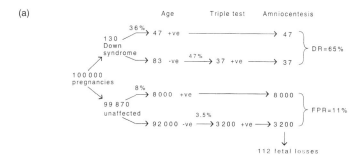

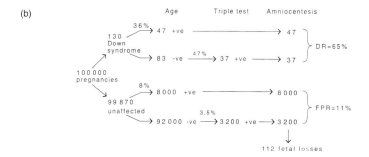

Fig. 5.5. (a) Example of two-step screening of the 're-screen negatives' type. Age screening followed by a diagnostic test in positives (age ≥35 years) and the re-screening of negatives using the triple test (+ve if risk ≥1 in 250). (b) One-step equivalent to screening in (a). Set detection rate at 65% (triple test +ve if risk ≥1 in 350). (DR=detection rate, FPR=false-positive rate.)

positives (7.3 vs 11%), one-third less amniocenteses, and one-third less fetal losses. The two-step approach has been adopted because of an uncritical adherence to historical screening practice (age only screening), even though it is more expensive and less safe.

Though not often perceived as such, a variation of two-step screening of the 'further screening of positives' type is the practice of using an ultrasound scan at 18–20 weeks in women with a positive serum test to revise risk. Screen-positive women who have undergone serum screening are offered a detailed 18–20 week ultrasound anomaly scan (which is, in effect, a second screening test). In the absence of ultrasound markers indicative of Down syndrome, a woman's risk based on the serum test is lowered, and there will be a tendency for her to be reassured and not undergo an invasive diagnostic test (that is, amniocentesis or chorionic villus sampling). The effect of this could be that about half the originally screen-positive pregnancies with Down syndrome would be missed, assuming that the anomaly scan has a detection rate of 50% for a 5% false-positive rate. This is illustrated in Fig. 5.6, in which women with a risk of one in 200 based on the serum test would have their risk halved to one in 400 if the anomaly scan was negative. This practice is unsatisfactory because it will tend to give false reassurance to a woman who was screen-positive on the first test, and became screen-negative after the second test, but proceeded to have an affected birth. As well as being inefficient, this adds to the emotional stress of the woman. A diagnostic test should be offered to all women with a positive result after the serum test, regardless of a subsequent ultrasound scan result.

Two-step screening is always less effective than its one-step equivalent. One-step screening maintains the advantage of risk screening in that it maximises the detection rate for a given false-positive rate. It also avoids the distress of missing affected cases in persons who have been identified through screening as being at increased risk.

Conclusion

The use of 'risk' as a screening variable is particularly useful if the results of two or more tests need to be combined simultaneously. Experience with the use of 'risk' as a screening variable is evolving. Patients and health professionals are becoming familiar with the concept. It allows patients to make informed choices.

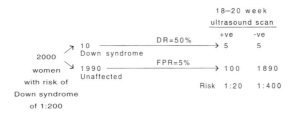

Fig. 5.6. Variation of two-step screening of the 're-screen positives' type: use of an anomaly scan in women with positive serum screening results. (DR=detection rate, FPR=false-positive rate.)

Abuses such as stepwise screening need to be avoided. One of the main strengths of risk screening is that it makes uncertainty explicit, and therefore will encourage a better understanding of medical practice and its limitations. At the same time, the overall performance of a test needs to be quantitatively specified before being introduced into routine practice. The overall consequences of screening should be predictable in spite of the uncertainty associated with the result for any individual person.

Acknowledgement. We thank Hilary Watt for statistical help.

References

Haddow, J.E., Palomaki, G.E., Knight, G.J. *et al.* (1992) Prenatal screening for Down syndrome with use of maternal serum markers. *N Engl J Med* **327**, 588–93

Wald, N. and Cuckle, H. (1991) 'Biochemical screening for Down's syndrome' in M. Chapman, G. Grudzinskas and T. Chard (Eds) *The Embryo,* pp.251–9. London: Springer-Verlag

Wald, N.J. and Kennard, A. (1997) 'Antenatal screening for neural tube defects and Down syndrome' in D.L. Rimoin, J.M. Connor and R.E. Pyeritz (Eds) *Emery and Rimoin's Principles and Practice of Medical Genetics* (3rd ed.). Edinburgh: Churchill Livingstone

Wald, N.J., Hackshaw, A.K., Huttly, W. and Kennard, A. (1996) Empirical validation of risk screening for Down syndrome. *J Med Screen* **3**, 185–7

Wald, N.J., Kennard, A., Densem, J.W., Cuckle, H.S., Chard, T. and Butler, L. (1992) Antenatal maternal serum screening for Down syndrome: Results of a demonstration project. *BMJ* **305**, 391–4

Chapter 6

The Mahalanobis distance: should atypicality be a feature of all Down syndrome screening programmes or would a specific screening test for trisomy 18 be better?

Timothy M. Reynolds

Introduction

This book deals primarily with screening in the first trimester of pregnancy. However, routine screening in the first trimester is not yet established so data on the less common chromosomal anomalies are not yet available. This chapter is based entirely on data collected from second trimester pregnancies but the basic mathematical principles will be the same whether screening is carried out in the first or second trimester.

The mathematics: how to calculate the Mahalanobis distance

The Mahalanobis distance is already calculated in every multivariate Gaussian Down syndrome screening test carried out (Wright *et al.* 1993). It is essentially a standard normal deviate which defines the distance from the mean in the Gaussian distribution formula in terms of standard deviations. For simplicity this will first be explained using the general Gaussian formula and then with the specific example of the bivariate case.

$$f(x_1, x_2, \ldots x_n) = (2\pi)^{-n/2} \cdot |V\text{-}1|^{\frac{1}{2}} \cdot e^{-\frac{1}{2}\{(x-\mu)' \cdot V^{-1} \cdot (x-\mu)\}}$$

In the equation the bold typed section in curly brackets { } to the right is the section which calculates the Mahalanobis distance. This is expressed in matrix algebra because otherwise it would be too cumbersome. To explain: $(x-\mu)$ is a matrix containing the values of the patient result minus the appropriate mean for all analytes and V^{-1} is a matrix containing all of the covariance data, i.e. the combination of the standard deviations and correlation coefficients. The $'$ indicates the shape of the matrix; $(x-\mu)'$ having three columns and one row whilst $(x-\mu)$ has three rows and one column; V^{-1} has three rows and three columns so that the result of multiplying all three matrices together is a single numeric value. In the bivariate case the equation is simpler and can therefore be written out in full:

$$f(x,y) = \frac{1}{2\pi \cdot \sigma_x \sigma_y \cdot \sqrt{(1-\rho^2)}} \cdot e^{-1/2 \left\{ \left(\frac{x-\mu_x}{\sigma_x}\right)^2 + \left(\frac{y-\mu_y}{\sigma_y}\right)^2 - \left(2\rho \cdot \left(\frac{x-\mu_x}{\sigma_x}\right)^2 \cdot \left(\frac{y-\mu_y}{\sigma_y}\right)\right)\right\}}$$

Once again the Mahalanobis distance is in bold and is enclosed within the curly brackets. Fig. 6.1 demonstrates the situation. The contour map shows the way that

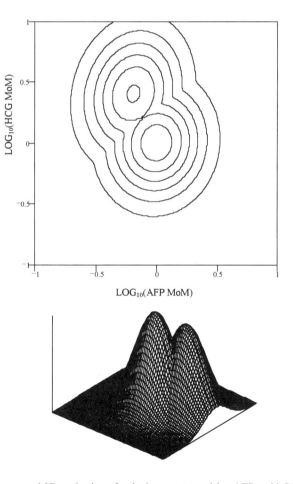

Fig. 6.1.   Contour map and 3D projection of a dual screen comprising AFP and hCG.

Down and unaffected distributions overlap but at the centre there are two pairs of concentric circles which, just as a weather map shows points having equal pressures (isobars), shows points having the same Mahalanobis distance. The 3-dimensional projection shows the effect of the other parts of the equation which define the shape of the distribution and the height of each peak.

Interpretation: how is the Mahalanobis distance interpreted?

Essentially, the Mahalanobis distance tells us how far a particular set of results is from the mean defined by the population distribution. The bigger the distance, the less likely the sample is to come from the defined population. Interpretation of just how likely is easy because the Mahalanobis distance has a defined distribution of its own: the χ^2 distribution. To determine any cut off you simply need to look in a statistical table for the probability you require at the same number of degrees of freedom as there are analytes. Thus for two analytes and a 99% probability of normality (alternatively a 1% probability of atypicality) the cut off is 9.210. For the rest of this chapter this cut off will be used wherever estimates of the effect of using the Mahalanobis distance in screening are quoted.

In Down syndrome screening, the only Mahalanobis distance which needs to be considered is the one relating to the unaffected population because the aim is to detect patients whose results cannot be considered to be 'normal'. Therefore, any Mahalanobis distance which exceeds the cut off is considered to be so atypical of normal that further investigation of that patient is necessary. Depending on the screening procedures used, this may simply indicate that the gestation dates have been estimated wrongly and that recalculation of the Down risk is all that is necessary but if the dates are correct it indicates that there may be something different about that pregnancy and that special care is needed to exclude other conditions.

Fig. 6.2 shows how this method can be integrated with other biochemical screening modalities to detect abnormalities. The trisomy 18 risk calculation stage has been defined as optional because later in this chapter estimates will be given of the detection rates for non-Down chromosomal abnormalities that can be achieved by a specific Down syndrome screen and of how performance changes when an additional specific screen for trisomy 18 or test for atypicality is added to the screening process.

Integration of trisomy 21, trisomy 18 and atypicality protocols. How does it work in practice? What are the effects on false positive rates?

Down screening works by trying to decide which of two very similar distributions a result is more likely to have come from. Fig. 6.3(a) shows just how similar the two distributions are and Fig. 6.3(b) shows the same diagram but on a log scale to

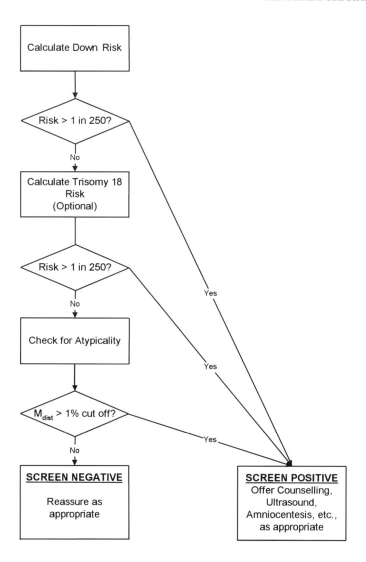

Fig. 6.2. Flow chart showing how trisomy 18 and atypicality screen are applied.

demonstrate why data are always log-transformed in Down screening – transformation converts the data into a 'regular' area which can be described mathematically with more precision. The diagrams show the 50% and 99%-centiles of the unaffected distribution and the 50%-centiles of the Down syndrome and trisomy 18 distributions. It can be seen that all of the most typical 50% of Down cases lie within the 99%-centile of normality as does a significant part of the most typical 50% of trisomy 18. Also shown on the diagram are four lines, each labelled with an age. These lines are the age-related threshold values such that if a patient of that age has α-fetoprotein (AFP) and human chorionic gonadotrophin (hCG) levels which place them above and to the left of that line, then they have a screen-

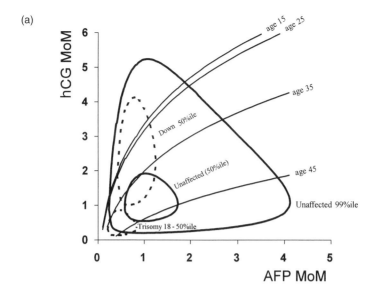

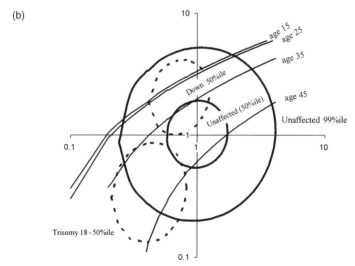

Fig. 6.3.   (a) Diagram showing the relative positions of normality, trisomy 18 and Down syndrome distributions with age-related threshold lines for positivity of Down risk screening at a 1 in 250 cut off. (b) Diagram of the same distributions as (a) but expressed on a Log scale.

positive Down risk (cut off=1:250). This illustrates a very important point: for a young woman, a large part of the most typical 50% of Down cases lies below and to the right of the threshold line which means that a significant proportion of Down syndrome cases cannot be detected. Conversely, for an older woman, in addition to the majority of the Down distribution, a large part of the unaffected distribution lies above and to the left of the threshold meaning that although there will be a high detection rate there must be a high false positive rate. A number of other research groups have proposed specific screens for trisomy 18 (Staples *et al.* 1991; Spencer *et al.* 1993; Crossley *et al.* 1995), so a similar set of lines could be drawn to isolate the trisomy 18 area but these are not shown for clarity.

Fig. 6.4 shows the areas selected by Down screening (lighter shading) and by atypicality screening (darker shading) for a 15-year-old woman, leaving the 'screen negative' area unshaded. For a 45-year-old, the area of light shading would expand to the 45 year threshold line and the darker shaded, and unshaded areas would shrink. This implies that as well as the age effects described above, there is also an age effect for atypicality screening; whereas in Down screening the false positive rate increases with age, in atypicality screening it decreases.

False positive rates in trisomy 18 and atypicality screening

False positive rates (FPR) using the different modalities of screening were evaluated by calculating likelihood ratios for Down syndrome and trisomy 18 and associated Mahalanobis distances for a set of 5080 patient results for a double screen of AFP plus total β-hCG (Reynolds, submitted). The likelihood ratios were multiplied by the age-specific risk for Down syndrome and for trisomy 18 (derived as 10% of the risk for Down syndrome (Spencer *et al.* 1993)) for each age in turn and the number of results 'detected' by a 1 in 250 risk or 1% atypicality cut off were counted to determine FPR. Table 6.1 shows age-related FPRs for two

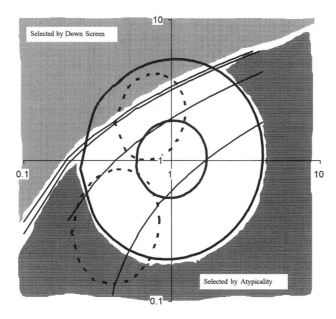

Fig. 6.4. Diagram to show area selected by a Down screen and by atypicality screening in a 15-year-old woman.

Table 6.1. Age-related false positive rates for Down screening with atypicality screening or with trisomy 18 and atypicality screening.

Age	Down screen FPR (%)	Atypicality FPR (%)	Trisomy 18 FPR (%)	Atypicality FPR after trisomy 18 screen (%)
16	1.22	0.94	0.30	0.65
18	1.26	0.94	0.30	0.65
20	1.32	0.92	0.30	0.63
22	1.40	0.92	0.30	0.63
24	1.52	0.92	0.31	0.61
26	1.79	0.92	0.31	0.61
28	2.16	0.92	0.37	0.55
30	3.13	0.91	0.53	0.41
32	4.82	0.89	0.73	0.31
34	8.50	0.85	0.87	0.28
36	15.0	0.81	1.36	0.24
38	25.4	0.75	1.99	0.22
40	40.8	0.73	2.91	0.18
41	49.5	0.73	3.76	0.18
42	58.2	0.67	4.45	0.14
43	67.0	0.65	5.65	0.12
44	75.0	0.63	6.57	0.08
45	81.6	0.63	7.46	0.08
46	86.8	0.61	7.36	0.06
47	91.1	0.55	6.89	0.01

screening methods: Down screen + atypicality, and Down screen + trisomy 18 screen + atypicality.

The results in Table 6.1 are particularly noteworthy in the older aged, trisomy 18 women. It can be seen numerically that the FPR increases until age 44 and then begins to decrease. This is more clearly shown graphically in Fig. 6.5. This effect is because the rate of increase of inclusion of results in the Down positive group is

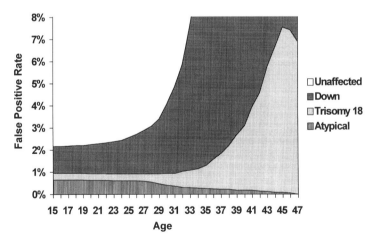

Fig. 6.5. Age-related false positive rates for a screen consisting of Down syndrome, trisomy 18 and atypicality.

Table 6.2.   Estimate of numbers of patients in a population of 1 million who would be assessed as being screen positive for Down screening with trisomy 18 and atypicality screens using cut off of 1 in 250 and 1% respectively

	Down screen + atypicality	Down screen + trisomy 18 screen + atypicality
Population	1 000 000	1 000 000
Screen −ve	950 224 (95.02%)	948 887 (94.89%)
Screen +ve: Down	40 743 (4.07%)	40 743 (4.07%)
Screen +ve: Trisomy 18	–	5246 (0.52%)
Screen +ve: Atypicality	9032 (0.90%)	5123 (0.51%)
Total screen +ve	49 775 (4.98%)	51 115 (5.11%)

so great that potential candidates for the trisomy 18 screen have already been defined as a positive Down risk before their trisomy 18 risk is assessed. Interesting as these figures may be, the crucial figure that concerns all screening programmes is the overall effect on FPR within a population. Table 6.2 shows an assessment of the total numbers of people who would be expected to be given positive results in a population of 1 million having the same age distribution as the pregnant population of Gwent in 1992. This shows that adding a trisomy 18 screen alone would increase the screen positive rate by 0.52% and that adding atypicality screening would increase it by 0.51% or 0.90% depending on whether a trisomy 18 screen is used or not.

Detection rates in trisomy 18 and atypicality screening

Now that I have shown the effect of adding trisomy 18 and atypicality screening on false positive rates, the next consideration has to be how good the two screening tests are at detecting a variety of chromosomal defects (Reynolds, 1997; Reynolds, submitted). I shall describe the effectiveness of trisomy 18 and atypicality screening on a set of 190 'non-Down' chromosomal anomalies (Bogart *et al.* 1987; Johnson *et al.* 1991; Staples *et al.* 1991; Burton *et al.* 1993; Aitken *et al.* 1994; Wenstrom *et al.* 1994; Benn *et al.* 1995; J. Crossley and D. Worthington personal communications) and on 144 cases of Down syndrome (Zimmermann *et al.* 1996). These cases are illustrated graphically in Fig. 6.6(a–g).

The data were assessed by calculating the likelihood ratios for Down syndrome and trisomy 18 screening and using these to calculate risk estimates by multiplication with a range of age-specific risk estimates (risk for trisomy 18 derived as 10% of the risk for Down syndrome (Spencer *et al.* 1993)). Thus a matrix of risks for all probable ages was produced which allows numerical integration against the pregnant population age distribution to give an overall detection rate for each condition. Table 6.3 shows the detection rates achieved for the different screening protocols.

For some anomalies it appears that adding atypicality or a trisomy 18 screen may be a good idea. However, the table does not take into account the incidences of the different conditions which occur less frequently than Down syndrome.

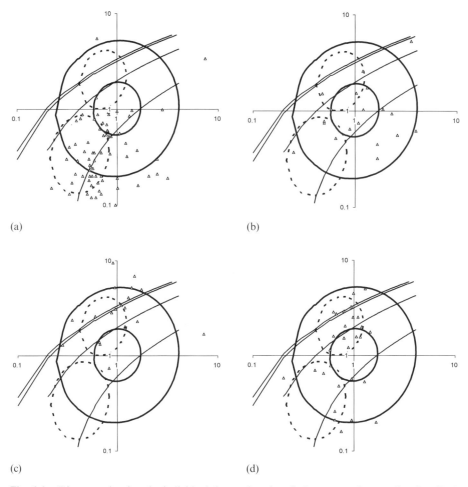

(a)   (b)

(c)   (d)

Fig. 6.6. Diagrams showing the individual data points for all chromosomal anomalies described. (a) trisomy 18, (b) trisomy 13, (c) Turner's syndrome, (d) other sex chromosome anomalies.

Consequently it cannot yet be stated whether the extra screen positives identified by the extra screen are in proportion to the extra benefit gained from better detection. Therefore, it is necessary to try to estimate the numbers of cases which would be detected by each screening protocol. Since the expected number of Down cases for a population can be easily estimated from the same formula used to calculate age-related Down risks, all that is needed is an estimate of the relative incidence of the other anomalies. These data are readily available (Ferguson-Smith and Yates 1984) with the exception of the incidence of triploidy. Taking the incidence of Down syndrome to be 1, the relative incidences for the other chromosomal anomalies were; trisomy 18=0.20; trisomy 13=0.06; Turner's syndrome=0.03; misc. sex=0.33; others=0.32. Since the number of cases of triploidy in the data set was only eight, the relative incidence of this condition was estimated at 0.01. Table 6.4 shows the estimated number of cases of each type of

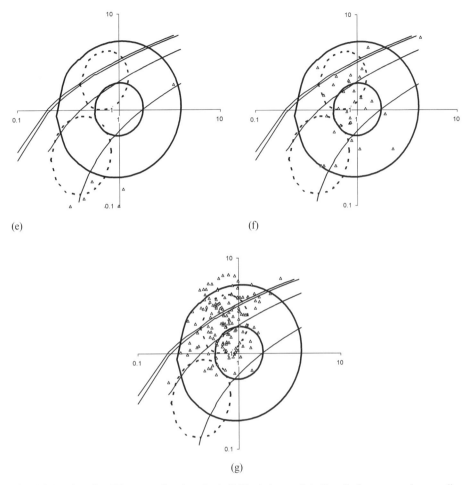

(e)   (f)

(g)

Fig. 6.6 (continued).   Diagrams showing the individual data points for all chromosomal anomalies described. (e) triploidy, (f) miscellaneous other chromosomal anomalies, (g) Down syndrome.

anomaly that would be expected in a population of 1 million and gives estimates of the number of cases that would be detected by a Down screen alone and the expected extra detection if trisomy 18 or atypicality screens were added.

The data in Table 6.4 are very interesting because they apparently show that the addition of a trisomy 18 screen can be achieved with a better detection hit rate than Down screening achieves. It also shows that although atypicality does add detection it does it at the expense of approximately 25% more false positives per detected case. However, this raises an ethical dilemma: is it right to screen for sex chromosome anomalies which in general do not cause significant handicap? Therefore the figures have been recalculated excluding sex chromosome anomalies. After this restatement, the detection rate for Down screening alone decreases to 1 in 45 compared to the detection rate for trisomy 18 screening of 1 in 40.8. Atypicality becomes even less effective with a detection rate of 1 in 71.1 if used

Table 6.3. Detection rates for different chromosomal anomalies for Down screening alone and in combination with a specific trisomy 18 screen and atypicality

	n	Down only (%)	Down + atypicality (%)	Down + trisomy 18 (%)	All three (%)
Down syndrome	144	58.9	59.3	58.9	59.3
Trisomy 13	20	19.9	30.2	22.0	31.0
Trisomy 18	79	6.3	45.8	45.4	51.1
Turner's	20	66.0	71.0	66.2	71.0
Misc. sex	29	34.8	45.5	44.9	48.7
Triploidy	8	14.3	88.1	88.1	88.1
Others	34	27.9	28.6	32.0	32.7
Overall (excl. Down)	190	22.6	45.5	44.5	49.0
Screen +ve rate		4.07	4.98	4.59	5.11

Table 6.4. Estimated numbers of cases detected by different screening protocols. Detection rate represents the expected number of true positives for that protocol; i.e. adding atypicality should provide extra detection of 174 cases but costs 9032 extra positives. The detection rate in that group of patients is 1 in 51.8 whilst the detection rate of the main screening test is 1 in 37.8.

	n	Down only	Extra detection from atypicality	Extra detection from trisomy 18 screen	Extra detection from trisomy 18 and atypicality
Down syndrome	1285.4	757.1	5.1	0	5.1
Trisomy 13	77.1	15.3	7.9	1.6	8.6
Trisomy 18	257.1	16.2	101.6	100.5	115.2
Turner's	38.6	25.5	1.9	0.1	1.9
Misc. sex	424.0	147.6	45.4	42.8	58.9
Triploidy	12.9	1.8	9.5	9.5	9.5
Others	411.0	114.7	2.9	16.9	19.7
Overall (incl. Down)	2506.1	1078.2	174.3	171.4	218.9
Screen positives		40743.0	9032.0	5246.0	10369.0
Detection rate		1 in 37.8	1 in 51.8	1 in 30.6	1 in 47.4
Excluding sex anomalies	2043.5	905.1	127.0	128.5	158.1
Detection rate		1 in 45.0	1 in 71.1	1 in 40.8	1 in 65.6
Marginal benefit of atypicality				incl. sex	47.5
				excl. sex	30.0
Detection rate				incl. sex	1 in 107.8
				excl. sex	1 in 173

alone or 1 in 65.6 if used with a trisomy 18 screen. However, this overestimates the benefit of using atypicality as we should be looking at the marginal improvement that it generates. In fact if a trisomy 18 screen is used, the additional benefit of adding atypicality is only 47.5 cases for 5123 extra screen positives or only 30 cases if sex chromosome anomalies are excluded – a hit rate of only 1 in 107.8 or 1 in 173, respectively.

Conclusion

When Down screening was introduced there was little information available about serum marker levels in other chromosomal abnormalities. This meant that any abnormality that gave serum results atypical of Down syndrome and especially those whose results were diametrically opposite (e.g. raised AFP and low hCG) appeared to be 'more normal than normal' so gave very low Down syndrome risks. In the first paper to describe atypicality screening (Wright *et al.* 1993), an instance where the estimated maternal Down risk for a trisomy 18 sample was less than 1 in 150,000 was quoted. This is obviously misleading and cannot be accepted because it could give the mother considerable reassurance only to result in her confidence being shattered later when the trisomy 18 is discovered. This is an inevitable effect of a screen looking for a specific condition and classifying everything else as 'not that condition'; in a world of apples and oranges, a grapefruit would be an orange.

Therefore in the early days of a screening programme, it is sensible to have a non-specific screen which detects when a result is not normal. There is to my knowledge only one report of a large scale trial of atypicality screening in the literature (Buchanan *et al.* 1994). This showed that using a 1% atypicality cut off in conjunction with a Down screen generated a 0.3% false positive rate in women aged less than 35 who had negative Down and NTD risks. Since an upper cut off was applied to the AFP level, this is consistent with the age-related false positive rates for atypicality presented here. Now, however, more data are available about other chromosomal anomalies in the second trimester so a specific screen can be designed for the next major group (trisomy 18). There have been at least four reports of screening for trisomy 18 in the literature with variable effect. Staples *et al.* (1991) demonstrated a 58.3% detection rate with a 0.3% false positive rate. Spencer *et al.* (1993) demonstrated a 50% detection rate for a 1% false positive rate; Crossley *et al.* (1995) demonstrated a 65% detection rate for a 0.55% false positive rate; Palomaki *et al.* (1995) demonstrated a 60% detection rate with a 0.2% false positive rate. These are in line with the data presented here that a 45.4% detection rate can be achieved with a specific trisomy 18 screen for a 0.51% false positive rate. Overall, therefore, there is corroborative evidence that the estimates of detection and false positive rates for a specific trisomy 18 screen and for an atypicality screen presented here are true.

Thus, a specific trisomy 18 screen detects almost as many as, or more cases than, an atypicality screen can but for half the false positive rate. Furthermore, in the second trimester there is already a third specific screen which looks at the far right side of the distribution, thus reducing the area over which atypicality operates: serum AFP screening for neural tube defects takes out those samples for which the AFP exceeds a certain cut off level (2.0–2.5 MoM depending on local choice). Consequently, it can be conclusively stated that there is no longer any place for atypicality screening in the second trimester.

In the first trimester, however, there are currently few available data on non-Down chromosomal abnormalities so it is difficult to design a specific screening test. It is, therefore, probable that if first trimester screening becomes widespread there will be a place for atypicality for the first few years until sufficient data to carry out extra specific screens are available.

References

Aitken, R., King, J. and George, P. (1994) Screening for Down syndrome. *Ann Clin Biochem* **31**, 300–1

Benn, P., Horne, D., Briganti, S. and Greenstein, R. (1995) Prenatal diagnosis of diverse chromosome abnormalities in a population of patients identified by triple marker testing as screen positive for Down syndrome. *Am J Obstet Gynecol* **173**, 496–501

Bogart, M., Pandian, M. and Jones, O. (1987) Abnormal maternal serum chorionic gonadotropin levels in pregnancies with fetal chromosome abnormalities. *Prenat Diagn* **7**, 623–30

Buchanan, P., Krantz, D., Kasturi, R., Cook, E. and Macri J. (1994) Identification of trisomy 18, triploidy and other abnormalities: the use of an atypicality index incorporating maternal serum FreeBeta and AFP. *Am J Hum Genet* A277

Burton, B., Prins, G. and Verp, M. (1993) A prospective trial of prenatal screening for Down's syndrome by means of maternal serum α-fetoprotein, human chorionic gonadotropin and unconjugated estriol. *Am J Obstet Gynecol* **169**, 526–30

Crossley, J., Aitken, D., Berry, E. and Connor, J. (1995) Screening for trisomy 18: a practical addition to biochemical screening for Down's syndrome. *Proceedings of the ACB National meeting, Focus 95*, A68

Ferguson-Smith, M. and Yates, J. (1984). Maternal age specific rates for chromosomal aberrations and factors influencing them: Report of a collaborative European study on 52,965 amniocenteses. *Prenat Diagn* **4**, 5–44

Johnson, A., Cowchock, F., Darby, M., Wapner, R. and Jackson, L. (1991) First trimester maternal serum alpha-fetoprotein and chorionic gonadotropin in aneuploid pregnancies. *Prenat Diagn* **11**, 443–50

Palomaki, G., Haddow, J., Knight, G. *et al.* (1995) Risk-based prenatal screening for trisomy 18 using alpha-fetoprotein, unconjugated oestriol and human chorionic gonadotropin. *Prenat Diagn*, **15**, 713–23

Reynolds, T. (1997) Atypicality revisited: further data on the effectiveness of the Mahalanobis distance in Down's syndrome screening. *Ann Clin Biochem* (in press)

Spencer, K., Mallard, A., Coombes, E. and Macri, J. (1993) Prenatal screening for trisomy 18 with free β human chorionic gonadotrophin as a marker. *BMJ* **307**, 1455–8

Staples, A., Robertson, E., Ranieri, E., Ryall, R. and Haan, E. (1991) A maternal screen for trisomy 18: an extension of maternal serum screening for Down's syndrome. *Am J Hum Genet* **49**, 1025–33

Wenstrom, K., Williamson, R. and Grant, S. (1994) Detection of fetal Turner's syndrome with multiple marker screening. *Am J Obstet Gynecol* **170**, 570–3

Wright, D., Reynolds, T. and Donovan, C. (1993) Assessment of atypicality: an adjunct to screening for Down syndrome that facilitates detection of other chromosomal defects. *Ann Clin Biochem* **30**, 578–83

Zimmermann, R., Reynolds, T., John, R. *et al.* (1996) Age-independent indices in second-trimester serum screening for Down's syndrome are useless. *Prenat Diagn* **16**, 79–82

Chapter 7

The Glasgow ratio method

David A. Aitken and Jennifer A. Crossley

Introduction

The advent of biochemical screening for Down syndrome in the second trimester of pregnancy has revolutionised the process of identifying pregnancies at increased risk. Lower than normal levels of alphafetoprotein (AFP) and unconjugated oestriol (uE$_3$), and higher than normal levels of intact human chorionic gonadotrophin (ihCG) and free beta subunit of hCG (FβhCG) are associated with Down syndrome pregnancies. However, as there is no complete separation of the distribution of levels of these markers in Down syndrome and unaffected pregnancies, none can be considered an absolute predictor of affected pregnancies. Instead, the results from serum marker screening can be used to estimate the likelihood that a specific marker level is associated with a Down syndrome pregnancy in individual women.

The prior probability that a woman will have a pregnancy with Down syndrome is dependent on her age. Before 25 years this risk is low but increases rapidly beyond 35 years. A screening policy based solely on maternal age as a method of selecting pregnancies for diagnostic fetal chromosome analysis is inequitable and inefficient as in practice all women younger than 35–37 years of age are excluded and a maximum of only 30% of Down syndrome pregnancies can be diagnosed. Serum marker analysis extends screening to women of all ages by providing a posterior probability of an affected pregnancy which can be used to modify the maternal age risk. This results in at least double the overall detection efficiency for affected pregnancies at a reduced follow-up rate compared with 'age-only' screening. However, detection rate varies with maternal age being higher in older mothers and this has prompted the investigation of different methods of using marker data to optimise screening performance.

Modifying maternal age risks

The predictive value of a marker depends on the magnitude of the shift from normal of the median value in Down syndrome pregnancies, the width of the distribution of values in normal and affected pregnancies and the degree of association of the marker with any others used together. A mathematical method of deriving a risk from marker variables and combining that with maternal age to give an overall risk (usually expressed as an odds ratio 1: n) of Down syndrome in individual pregnancies was proposed by Cuckle *et al.* (1987) using maternal age and maternal serum AFP and extended by Wald *et al.* (1988) for multiple markers with maternal age. The method is underpinned by the conversion of all analyte values to multiples of the median (MoM) and the log transformation of these MoM values to give Gaussian distributions. Provided the data are normally distributed, a ratio can be determined from the relative heights of the overlapping distributions of analyte levels in Down syndrome and unaffected pregnancies at a specific analyte value which effectively converts that analyte value into a risk (termed the likelihood ratio). A combined risk with maternal age is then calculated by dividing the right hand side of the maternal age odds ratio by the likelihood ratio. The same approach can be used for two or more markers taking into account any significant correlation between the markers (Wald *et al.* 1988; Reynolds and Penney 1989; Crossley *et al.* 1991). By selecting an appropriate threshold risk as the decision point for amniocentesis a proportion of affected pregnancies can be identified within a fixed proportion of the screened population with the highest risks, termed the false positive rate. Such multivariate analysis with two or three markers and maternal age has produced estimated detection rates of around 60% of Down syndrome pregnancies at a 5% false positive rate in several retrospective studies (Wald *et al.* 1988; Crossley *et al.* 1991; Spencer *et al.* 1992). This 'standard likelihood ratio method' (SLRM) has been widely adopted in routine screening where detection rates for various combinations of markers reflect those found in retrospective studies (Haddow *et al.* 1992; Wald *et al.* 1992a; Spencer and Carpenter 1993; Goodburn *et al.* 1994).

Further refinement to screening and the calculation of risk can be added. For example, various maternal factors (weight, race, insulin dependent diabetes mellitus, smoking, previously affected pregnancy, parity) and pregnancy factors (accuracy of the gestational estimate, threatened abortion, multiple pregnancy, fetal abnormality, metabolic disorder) can affect maternal serum marker levels and appropriate

Table 7.1. Detection rates (DR) for Down syndrome and corresponding false positive rates (FPR) from two studies using non-parametric ratio methods

Study	Ratio value cut-off	Down syndrome		
		DR	(%)	FPR %
Arab *et al.* (1988)	>100	15/29	(62)	10
	>135	11/29	(38)	2
White *et al.* (1989)	≥ 40	15/15	(100)	11
	≥ 50	11/15	(73)	4

correction of the MoM values is possible for some of these complications which leads to small but useful improvements in performance. In general, taking account of such variables tends to reduce the variance associated with the distribution of marker levels in Down syndrome and unaffected pregnancies.

Ratios of analyte levels

As there is substantial overlap in the distribution of analyte levels in Down syndrome and unaffected pregnancies, no method of deriving risk from one or more serum marker measurements can produce a 100% detection rate without classifying the majority of women as screen positive. In an effort to maximise the detection rate and minimise the false positive rate alternative screening algorithms have been investigated. One of the first proposals was a ratio of AFP and hCG results to distinguish between Down syndrome and unaffected pregnancies. Arab *et al.* (1988) and White *et al.* (1989) each suggested a screening algorithm using the function: hCG (in concentration units, IU/ml) divided by AFP (in MoM). The higher ratio values were associated with Down syndrome pregnancies and an empirically chosen cut-off value was used to select pregnancies for diagnostic testing (Table 7.1). However, as this ratio value cannot be used as an odds modifier, neither study incorporated information from the risk associated with maternal age. Also, the use of hCG in concentration units and AFP in MoMs means that no allowance is being made for the change in median level of hCG with gestation and therefore higher ratio values will be generated at 15 weeks than at say, 20 weeks' gestation. Nevertheless, these two small studies suggested that such an approach using analyte levels alone might provide reasonable sensitivity and specificity. This was further investigated by Cuckle *et al.* (1989) using the hCG and AFP results from a previously reported study of 77 Down syndrome and 385 unaffected pregnancies (Wald *et al.* 1988). Detection rates, obtained by direct observation at a series of fixed false positive rates determined by threshold ratio values from the function hCG(MoM)/AFP(MoM), were lower than the comparable detection rates obtained using the SLRM for the same combination of markers without the incorporation of maternal age. When age risks were included, SLRM detection was further increased.

Benz *et al.* (1993) have proposed the use of an age risk-independent ratio (the 'Ulm index') derived from a three-marker function hCG(MoM)^2/AFP(MoM)× uE$_3$(MoM) to improve detection of Down syndrome pregnancies in women under 35 years of age. This approach has been criticised by Zimmermann *et al.* (1996) who pointed out that any gain in detection using this method would be dependent on a better separation of the distribution of analyte values (in median MoM and/or by reduced variance) in Down syndrome and unaffected pregnancies in younger women. However, in a study of analyte levels in 161 Down syndrome pregnancies and a series of unaffected pregnancies, they could find no relationship between maternal age and MoM distributions for AFP, uE$_3$, ihCG (intact or total hCG), or FβhCG (free β-hCG). Other studies have confirmed the independence of marker levels and maternal age (Wald and Watt 1996). Zimmermann *et al.* (1996) conclude that detection cannot be improved by omitting maternal age risk information.

The Glasgow ratio method

Crossley *et al.* (1991) first proposed an alternative method of using ratios of analyte levels to produce an odds modifier which allowed maternal age risks to be included in the combined risk estimate. In a retrospective study of AFP and ihCG levels in second trimester maternal serum samples from 49 Down syndrome and 410 unaffected pregnancies, the ratio hCG(MoM)/AFP(MoM) was used as a new variable. Frequency distributions of these ratio values were found to have a log Gaussian distribution by probability plot and Kolmogorov–Smirnov test in both Down syndrome and unaffected pregnancies. The parameters of the ratio distributions (Fig. 7.1) are presented in Table 7.2 along with the parameters of the

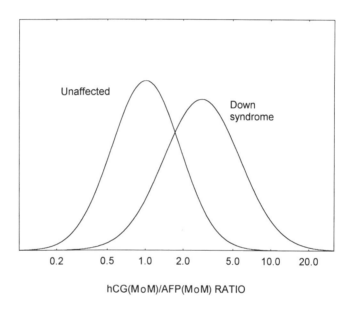

Fig. 7.1. Log Gaussian distributions of the hCG(MoM)/AFP(MoM) ratio values derived from the analysis of ihCG and AFP in 49 Down syndrome cases and 410 controls at 15–20 weeks' gestation. (Data from Crossley *et al.* 1991.)

Table 7.2. Medians of AFP and ihCG results (in MoM) and hCG(MoM)/AFP(MoM) ratios in 49 Down syndrome cases and 410 controls at 15–20 weeks of gestation. Means and standard deviations (SD) are of the log Gaussian distributions (data from Crossley *et al.* 1991)

Variable	Down syndrome			Controls		
	Median	Mean	SD	Median	Mean	SD
AFP	0.80	−0.0969	0.1864	1.00	−0.0177	0.1438
ihCG	2.18	0.3385	0.3127	1.00	0.0043	0.2499
hCG/AFP	2.85	0.4502	0.3046	1.01	0.0043	0.2714

individual AFP and ihCG distributions from which the ratios were derived. The median ratio in unaffected cases was 1.01 and in the Down syndrome cases 2.85. For any combination of AFP and hCG results, an odds modifier (likelihood ratio) can be obtained from the overlapping hCG(MoM)/AFP(MoM) distributions and, as in the SLRM, a combined risk with maternal age can be calculated by dividing the right hand side of the maternal age odds ratio by the likelihood ratio. A comparison of the corresponding detection and false positive rates obtained by the SLRM and 'Glasgow ratio method' (GRM) using the results from this study and a population model of the age distribution of pregnancies in the west of Scotland is given in Table 7.3. Marginally improved detection was obtained using the GRM and a higher threshold risk was required to determine a 5% follow-up rate.

Others have examined the performance of the GRM using marker data from case-control studies. Spencer *et al.* (1992) used AFP, ihCG and FβhCG results from a multicentre study of 90 Down syndrome cases and 2800 unaffected pregnancies to investigate ihCG(MoM)/AFP(MoM) and FβhCG(MoM)/AFP(MoM) ratios. Both ratio distributions were found to be log Gaussian in trisomic and unaffected pregnancies with median MoMs for the Down syndrome distributions of 2.85 for the ratio with ihCG and 3.63 for the ratio with FβhCG. When detection and false positive rates were modelled using the SLRM and GRM for each pair of markers and maternal age, virtually identical detection (50%) at a 5% false positive rate was obtained for the combination of ihCG and AFP by each method whereas the figures for FβhCG/AFP were 59% detection by the SLRM and 54% detection by GRM.

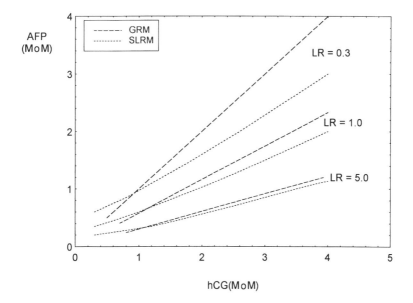

Fig. 7.2. Combinations of AFP(MoM) and hCG(MoM) required to generate the same likelihood ratio values (iso-risks) using the Glasgow ratio method (GRM) and standard likelihood ratio method (SLRM).

Table 7.3. Detection rates (DR) and corresponding false positive rates (FPR) obtained for AFP, ihCG and maternal age using the Glasgow ratio method (GRM) and standard likelihood ratio method (SLRM) (data from Crossley *et al.* 1991)

Method	5% false positive rate		60% detection rate	
	Cut-off risk[a]	DR	Cut-off risk[a]	DR
GRM	1:235	57%	1:280	5.9%
SLRM	1:265	56%	1:320	6.2%

[a] Mid-trimester risk

Table 7.4. Maternal and marker parameters of Down syndrome and unaffected pregnancies screened prospectively in west of Scotland over a four year period. Means and standard deviations (SD) are of the log Gaussian distributions

	Down syndrome ($n=144$)	Unaffected pregnancies ($n=109,903$)
Proportion of samples at each gestation		
15 weeks	30.6%	27.6%
16 weeks	40.3%	45.5%
17 weeks	19.4%	17.8%
18 weeks	7.6%	5.7%
19 weeks	0%	2.1%
20 weeks	2.1%	1.0%
21 weeks	0%	0.3%
Maternal age		
Median	33 years	27 years
Range	17–44 years	13–49 years
≥35 years	38.2%	8.0%
Median maternal weight	64.0 kg	63.0 kg
AFP MoM		
Median	0.70	0.97
Mean	−0.1549	−0.0132
SD	0.1569	0.1625
hCG MoM		
Median	2.15	1.00
Mean	0.3324	0.00
SD	0.2730	0.2285
hCG MoM/AFP MoM ratio		
Median	3.23	1.03
Mean	0.5095	0.0120
SD	0.2856	0.2635

Evans *et al.* (1995) compared the performance of the GRM, the SLRM and a new method of discriminant analysis termed 'DADs' (discriminant aneuploidy detection) using AFP and ihCG results from the routine prospective analysis of 17,042 unaffected and 28 Down syndrome pregnancies. Although the DADs model was found to outperform either of the Gaussian models on this particular data set, it was observed that at fixed risk cut-off points the GRM gave higher detection rates than the SLRM but with correspondingly higher follow-up rates. When the false positive rates were held constant, the GRM and SLRM gave identical detection rates (68% at a 5% false positive rate).

The difference in performance between the GRM and SLRM noted above and in the original study by Crossley *et al.* (1991), has its origin in the slightly different likelihood ratios generated by each method for the same combination of AFP and hCG MoMs. This is illustrated in Fig. 7.2 which shows three pairs of constant likelihood ratios (0.3, 1.0, 5.0) obtained by the SLRM and GRM plotted against the AFP MoM and hCG MoM required to generate them. The pairs of 'iso-risk' lines derived by each method intersect at an hCG level of about 1.0–1.2 MoM and at varying AFP levels below 1.0 MoM. At hCG MoMs above the intersection point and at fixed AFP MoMs, progressively higher likelihood ratios are generated by the GRM than by the SLRM for the same hCG MoM. At hCG MoMs below the intersection point the opposite is found, with lower likelihood ratios being generated by the GRM.

Routine second trimester screening with the Glasgow ratio algorithm

From September 1991 to September 1996, over 135,000 pregnancies were screened in the west of Scotland using AFP and ihCG. We have analysed the results obtained in the first 110,000 singleton pregnancies screened over a four-year period (which includes data from the first 30,084 pregnancies previously reported (Crossley *et al.* 1994)) using the GRM and SLRM. Within this screened popu-

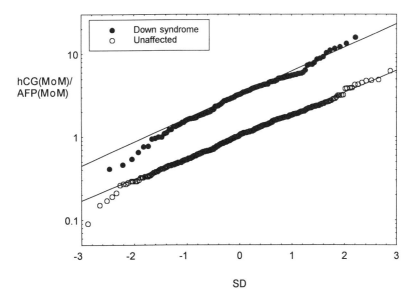

Fig. 7.3. Probability plots of the frequency distributions of the hCG(MoM)/AFP(MoM) ratio values in 144 Down syndrome pregnancies and a subset of 500 unaffected pregnancies selected at random from 110 000 pregnancies analysed prospectively for ihCG and AFP. The continuous lines are those defined by log Gaussian distributions with means and standard deviations (SD) given in Table 7.4.

lation there were 144 cases of Down syndrome. A summary of the population, pregnancy and marker parameters in the Down syndrome and unaffected cases is given in Table 7.4. Probability plots of the frequency distributions of the hCG(MoM)/AFP(MoM) ratio values in the Down syndrome cases and a randomly selected subset of 500 unaffected pregnancies are shown in Fig. 7.3. Both fit log Gaussian distributions (Kolmogorov Smirnov test: $D=0.0734$, $p=0.42$ for Down syndrome; $D=0.0395$, $p=0.42$ for unaffected pregnancies). The median of the distribution of likelihood ratios generated by the GRM was 4.94 in the Down syndrome pregnancies compared with 3.94 by the SLRM. The corresponding figures for unaffected pregnancies were identical for each method (0.317).

In routine screening using the GRM to estimate risk in individual pregnancies, 98 of the 144 Down syndrome pregnancies (68%) were identified within an initial screen positive group of 6.4% defined by a mid trimester cut-off risk of 1:220. After re-assessment of gestation, the final false positive rate was 5.2%. Re-analysis of the marker data using the SLRM to produce an identical initial false positive rate yielded the same level of Down syndrome detection (98/144) although a lower threshold risk was required to define the high risk group (Table 7.5). Of the 98 detected cases, 96 were identified by both methods whereas two Down syndrome

Table 7.5. Detection rates (DR) and corresponding false positive rates obtained with AFP, ihCG and maternal age using the Glasgow ratio method (GRM) and standard likelihood ratio method (SLRM) in 110,047 pregnancies, including 144 cases of Down syndrome, screened prospectively

Method	Cut-off risk[a]	DR	FPR Initial	FPR Final
GRM	1:220	68%	6.4%	5.2%
SLRM	1:260	68%	6.4%	–

[a] Mid-trimester risk

Table 7.6. Parameters of Down syndrome cases and controls (a) classified in the high risk group by GRM and the low risk group by SLRM and (b) classified in the low risk group by GRM and the high risk group by SLRM. The threshold risk for the GRM was 1:220 and for the SLRM 1:260. The values for the unaffected pregnancies in each category are the medians for the 409 pregnancies in each series. LR = likelihood ratio, risk = n

	AFP MoM	hCG MoM	Maternal age (years)	GRM LR	GRM risk (1:n)	SLRM LR	SLRM risk (1:n)
(a)							
Down case 1	0.85	2.00	33	2.15	200	1.71	270
Down case 2	0.80	2.56	24	4.18	210	3.75	300
Unaffected ($n=409$)	0.86	2.20	30	3.38	215	2.71	274
(b)							
Down case 3	0.58	0.70	39	0.45	270	0.65	180
Down case 4	0.48	0.67	37	0.62	310	0.97	200
Unaffected ($n=409$)	0.53	0.91	36	0.96	259	1.19	238

cases which were classified in the high risk group by GRM were low risk by SLRM, and two cases which were low risk by GRM were classified as high risk by SLRM. Examination of these four Down syndrome pregnancies (Table 7.6) shows that the two additional cases detected by the GRM are pregnancies in younger women with relatively high hCG MoMs and neutral AFP MoMs whereas the two cases classified as low risk by the GRM are pregnancies in older women with low hCG MoMs and low AFP MoMs. Unaffected pregnancies with similar classification differences show the same age and analyte patterns as the Down syndrome cases. This is in agreement with the prediction from the iso-risk data presented in Fig. 7.2. When the likelihood ratios generated by the GRM for the 144 Down syndrome cases are superimposed on the iso-risk plot (Fig. 7.4), the two additional cases detected by GRM plot to the right of the intersection points of the iso-risk lines and have a higher odds modifier by that calculation method. The two missed cases plot to the left and have a lower odds modifier by the GRM. From the unaffected pregnancies in Table 7.6 it can be seen that a slightly different population of women with respect to maternal age is recruited by each method into the high risk group. A higher proportion of younger women and a lower proportion of older women are classified as screen positive by the GRM than by the SLRM and this results in additional detection of Down syndrome cases among younger women using the GRM. However, detection in older women is correspondingly reduced.

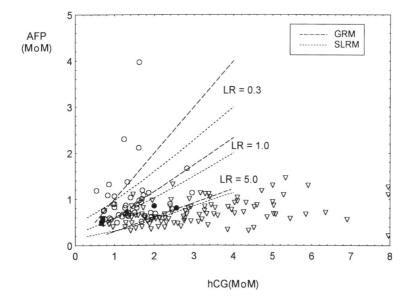

Fig. 7.4. Likelihood ratios in 144 Down syndrome pregnancies derived from ihCG and AFP results using the Glasgow ratio method (GRM). The cases are identified according to their final classification into high risk or low risk groups by the GRM and SLRM after the incorporation of maternal age risks. ($\bigtriangledown$=high risk group by GRM and SLRM; $\bigcirc$=low risk group by GRM and SLRM; ●=high risk group by GRM, low risk group by SLRM; ■=low risk group by GRM, high risk group by SLRM).

Although these results suggest that there is little to choose between the GRM and SLRM in overall screening performance, this may be affected by the age distribution of the population and there may be some advantage in using the GRM in double marker hCG/AFP screening in women under 35 years of age. In principle, the GRM can be used for any pair of markers where one has increased levels and the other reduced levels in relation to Down syndrome pregnancies and there is no significant correlation between them. For example, the method may perform satisfactorily with hCG and uE_3 where the latter is used as an alternative to AFP (e.g. Herrou *et al.* 1992). However, deriving a likelihood ratio or odds modifier from the overlapping ratio distributions is based on the assumption that the distributions are normal. If the individual markers have a normal distribution this would be expected but since the fit for some markers (e.g. uE_3, Crossley *et al.* 1993) is poor, it is important to assess the ratio distribution by probability plot to confirm that it is suitable for the derivation of an odds modifier.

First trimester screening using the Glasgow ratio method

Several studies suggest that FβhCG and pregnancy associated plasma protein (PAPP-A) are the best biochemical predictors of Down syndrome in the first trimester. FβhCG levels are increased (Aitken *et al.* 1993a) and PAPP-A levels are reduced (Wald *et al.* 1992b; Brambati *et al.* 1994; Spencer *et al.* 1994) in Down syndrome pregnancies between 7 and 14 weeks of gestation. As in the second trimester, these marker changes can be used to generate an odds modifier to

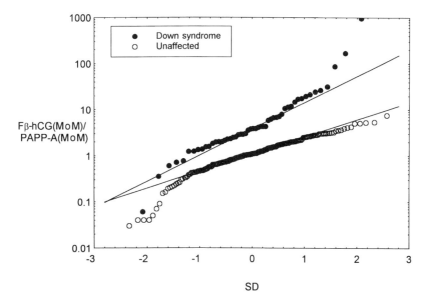

Fig. 7.5. Probability plots of the frequency distributions of the FβhCG(MoM)/PAPP-A(MoM) ratio values in 52 Down syndrome cases and a subset of 227 controls selected at random from 10 600 unaffected pregnancies. The continuous lines are those defined by log Gaussian distributions with means and standard deviations (SD) given in Table 7.7.

produce a combined risk with maternal age using appropriate algorithms (Spencer *et al.* 1994; Krantz *et al.* 1996; Wald *et al.* 1996). However, calculation of risk is complicated by the magnitude of the change in levels of PAPP-A in Down syndrome pregnancies which becomes less as gestation advances (Aitken *et al.* 1993b).

We have investigated the use of the GRM in first trimester screening in a study of FβhCG and PAPP-A levels in a series of 54 cases of Down syndrome and 10,600 unaffected pregnancies at 7–14 weeks' gestation (Berry *et al.* 1997). The number of Down syndrome cases at each week of gestation was 2 at 7 weeks, 7 at 8 weeks, 4 at 9 weeks, 10 at 10 weeks, 10 at 11 weeks, 12 at 12 weeks, 6 at 13 weeks, 3 at 14 weeks. PAPP-A results were not available in two Down syndrome cases due to insufficient sample. The study shows that although PAPP-A levels are reduced in the 52 Down syndrome cases for which results were available (0.50 MoM), the levels change with gestation from 0.48 MoM at 7–9 weeks, to 0.63 MoM at 13–14 weeks' gestation. Paired second trimester Down syndrome pregnancies had a PAPP-A median MoM of 0.94 at 15–17 weeks. The elevation in FβhCG levels was found to be virtually constant across the 7–14 week gestational range with an overall median MoM of 1.99. Detection and false positive rates were compared using the SLRM and the GRM based on the ratio FβhCG(MoM)/PAPP-A(MoM). The parameters of the individual FβhCG and PAPP-A distributions and the ratio distribution are given in Table 7.7. Probability plots (Fig. 7.5)

Table 7.7. Medians of FβhCG and PAPP-A results (in MoM) and FβhCG(MoM)/PAPP-A(MoM) ratios in a series of Down syndrome and unaffected pregnancies at 7–14 weeks' gestation. Means and standard deviations (SD) are of the log Gaussian distributions (data from Berry *et al.* 1997)

Variable	Down syndrome			Controls		
	Median	Mean	SD	Median	Mean	SD
FβhCG	1.99	0.299	0.306	0.99	−0.003	0.289
PAPP-A	0.50	−0.305	0.481	0.98	−0.011	0.236
FβhCG/PAPP-A	3.82	0.538	0.571	1.10	0.039	0.373

Table 7.8. Modelled Down syndrome detection rates at a 5% false positive rate estimated by the standard likelihood ratio method (SLRM) and Glasgow ratio method (GRM) using FβhCG and PAPP-A results in combination with maternal age at 7–14 and 10–12 weeks' gestation. Data from a retrospective analysis of 54 Down syndrome and 10,600 unaffected pregnancies (Berry *et al.* 1997)

Calculation method	Detection rate at	
	7–14 weeks	10–12 weeks
GRM	55%	62%
SLRM	49%	60%

confirm that the ratio values in the Down syndrome and unaffected pregnancies have a reasonable fit to log Gaussian distributions. Using a population model, detection rates at a 5% false positive rate based on the 52 cases with complete analyte data were 49% for the SLRM and 54% for the GRM. Detection rates improved when these were modelled using the marker parameters derived from the analysis of samples at 10–12 weeks' gestation when a maximum detection rate of 62% was obtained using the GRM (Table 7.8).

Summary and conclusion

The above studies suggest that combining data from two screening markers using a MoM ratio can provide detection rates for Down syndrome at least equivalent to those obtained using the SLRM. However, any screening algorithm which makes use of a ratio of analyte values must provide an index which can be combined with the maternal age risk if screening performance is to be maximised. Initial proposals for the use of analyte ratios (Arab *et al.* 1988; White *et al.* 1989) did not allow age risks to be incorporated which can only lead to loss of sensitivity and specificity in routine screening. The GRM approach derives a likelihood ratio from overlapping normal ratio distributions and thereafter the calculation of a combined risk with maternal age is the same as the SLRM.

Although the GRM and SLRM have much in common and in routine second trimester screening give virtually identical detection rates, a slightly different subset of Down syndrome pregnancies is selected into the high risk group by each method. There is a tendency for the GRM to detect more affected pregnancies in younger women and the SLRM to detect more affected pregnancies in older women. Thus the GRM may be more appropriate in centres where the policy is to restrict screening to women under 35 years of age or where the age distribution of the population is biased towards younger women.

References

Aitken, D.A., McCaw, G., Crossley, J.A. *et al.* (1993a) First-trimester biochemical screening for fetal chromosome abnormalities and neural tube defects. *Prenat Diagn* **13,** 681–9

Aitken, D.A., McKinnon, D., Crossley, J.A. *et al.* (1993b) Changes in the maternal serum concentrations of PAPP-A and SP-1 in Down's syndrome pregnancies between first and second trimesters. *Proceedings of the ACB National Meeting, Birmingham 1993.* Abstract B7, p.72

Arab, H., Siegel-Bartelt, J., Wong, P.Y. and Doran, T. (1988) Maternal serum beta human chorionic gonadotropin (MSHCG) combined with maternal serum alpha-fetoprotein (MSAFP) appears superior for prenatal screening for Down syndrome (DS) than either test alone. *Am J Hum Genet* **43**, (Suppl) A225

Benz, R., Muller, U., Krahner, P.M., Wagner, G.S. and Terinde, R. (1993) Serum-screening auf Down-syndrom bei Frauen unter 35 jahren mit einem altersunabhangigen index. *Z Geburtshilfe Perinatol* **197**, 205–8

Berry, E., Aitken, D.A., Crossley, J.A., Macri, J.N. and Connor, J.M. (1997) Screening for Down's syndrome: changes in marker levels and detection rates between first and second trimesters. *Br J Obstet Gynaecol* (in press)

Brambati, B., Tului, L., Bonacchi, I., Shrimanker, K., Suzuki, Y. and Grudzinskas, J.G. (1994) Serum PAPP-A and free βhCG are first trimester screening markers for Down syndrome. *Prenat Diagn* **14**, 1043–7

Crossley, J.A., Aitken, D.A. and Connor, J.M. (1991). Prenatal screening for chromosome abnormalities using maternal serum chorionic gonadotrophin, alphafetoprotein, and age. *Prenat Diagn* **11**, 83–101

Crossley, J.A., Aitken, D.A. and Connor, J.M. (1993) Second-trimester unconjugated oestriol levels in maternal serum from chromosomally abnormal pregnancies using an optimised assay. *Prenat Diagn* **13**, 271–80

Crossley, J.A., Aitken, D.A., Berry, E. and Connor, J.M. (1994) Impact of a regional screening programme using maternal serum α fetoprotein (AFP) and human chorionic gonadotrophin (hCG) on the birth incidence of Down's syndrome in the west of Scotland. *J Med Screen* **1**, 180–3

Cuckle, H.S., Wald, N.J. and Thomson. S.G. (1987) Estimating a woman's risk of having a pregnancy associated with Down's syndrome using her age and serum alphafetoprotein level. *Br J Obstet Gynaecol* **94**, 387–402

Cuckle, H.S., Densem, J.W. and Wald, N.J. (1989) Simplification of biochemical screening for Down syndrome. *Am J Hum Genet* **45**, 979–80

Evans, M.I., Chik, L., O'Brien, J.E. *et al.* (1995) MoMs (multiples of the median) and DADs (discriminant aneuploidy detection): improved specificity and cost-effectiveness of biochemical screening for aneuploidy with DADs. *Am J Obstet Gynecol* **172**, 1138–47

Goodburn, S.F., Yates, J.R.W., Raggatt, P.R. *et al.* (1994) Second trimester maternal serum screening using alpha-fetoprotein, human chorionic gonadotrophin, and unconjugated oestriol: experience of a regional programme. *Prenat Diagn* **14**, 391–402

Haddow, J.E., Palomaki, G.E. and Knight, G.J. (1992) Prenatal screening for Down's syndrome with the use of maternal serum markers. *N Engl J Med* **327**, 588–93

Herrou, M., Leporrier, N. and Leymarie, P. (1992) Screening for fetal Down syndrome with maternal serum hCG and oestriol: a prospective study. *Prenat Diagn* **12**, 887–92

Krantz, D.A., Larsen, J.W., Buchanan, P.D. and Macri, J.N. (1996) First-trimester Down syndrome screening: free β-human chorionic gonadotrophin and pregnancy-associated plasma protein A. *Am J Obstet Gynecol* **174**, 612–16

Reynolds, T.M. and Penney, M.D. (1989) The mathematical basis of multivariate risk screening: with special reference to screening for Down's syndrome associated pregnancy. *Ann Clin Biochem* **27**, 452–8

Spencer, K. and Carpenter, P. (1993) Prospective study of prenatal screening for Down's syndrome with free β human chorionic gonadotrophin. *BMJ* **307**, 764–9

Spencer, K., Coombes, A.J., Mallard, A.S. and Ward, A.M. (1992) Free beta human chorionic gonadotropin in Down's syndrome screening: a multicentre study of its role compared with other biochemical markers. *Ann Clin Biochem* **29**, 506–18

Spencer, K., Aitken, D.A., Crossley J.A. *et al.* (1994) First trimester biochemical screening for trisomy 21: the role of free beta hCG, alphafetoprotein and pregnancy associated plasma protein A. *Ann Clin Biochem* **31**, 447–54

Wald, N.J. and Watt, H.C. (1996) Serum markers for Down's syndrome in relation to number of previous births and maternal age. *Prenat Diagn* **16**, 699–703

Wald, N.J., Cuckle, H.S., Densem, J.M. *et al.* (1988) Maternal serum screening for Down's syndrome in early pregnancy. *BMJ* **297**, 883–7

Wald, N.J., Kennard, A., Densem, J.W., Cuckle, H.S., Chard, T. and Butler, L. (1992a) Antenatal maternal serum screening for Down's syndrome: results of a demonstration project. *BMJ* **305**, 391–4

Wald, N.J., Stone, R., Cuckle, H.S. *et al.* (1992b) First trimester concentrations of pregnancy associated plasma protein A and placental protein 14 in Down's syndrome. *BMJ* **305**, 28

Wald, N.J., George, L., Smith, D., Densem, J.W. and Petterson, K. (1996) Serum screening for Down's syndrome between 8 and 14 weeks of pregnancy. *Br J Obstet Gynaecol* **103**, 407–12

White, I., Papiha, S.S. and Magnay, D. (1989) Improving methods of screening for Down's syndrome. *N Engl J Med* **320**, 401–2

Zimmermann, R., Reynolds, T.M., John, R. *et al.* (1996) Age-independent indices in second-trimester serum screening for Down's syndrome are useless. *Prenat Diagn* **16**, 79–82

Chapter 8

Statistical aspects of screening for Down syndrome

Discussion

Nicolaides: Dr Reynolds, how do you diagnose the various abnormalities that you discussed?

Reynolds: I did not diagnose them myself. I was given various sets of data from about 10 different groups, collected them together into a set and that is what I was told they were.

Nicolaides: There are two problems with chromosomal defects other than Down's. The sex chromosome abnormalities – nobody knows who they are because they do not have any features at birth to recognise them. And a lot of the others like triploidy will be highly lethal and they will die before you see them at birth. So I am not quite sure what the denominator was in your calculations unless they were incidental diagnoses in those who happened to have had invasive tests because they were screened positive for something else.

Reynolds: I have said these were data I received from elsewhere, so it was all I had to look at. How effective atypicality in any of the trisomy 18 screenings were – I acknowledge that many of them will have spontaneously aborted and also with the sex chromosome patients, I separate those out and extrapolate them because I don't know whether it is even ethical for them to be considered for termination. The data are biased, I will agree with that; but you can only work with what you have.

Nicolaides: But what you have may be completely useless.

Reynolds: What I have shows that I do not believe atypicality is useful and therefore that is actually of benefit, because these were diagnosed from other people's screening programmes, so they are cases that we know about which have been picked up for various conditions.

Nicolaides: Sorry. The mechanism of the screening is completely inadequate in detecting the abnormalities that you were examining. A simple example: if we take Klinefelter's syndrome, nobody would recognise that at birth. The only ones that you would have identified and therefore used in your calculations would be the subgroup that by default happened to have been screened positive for Down syndrome and had amniocentesis. Similarly, the triploidies, because they are almost never born alive and are quite common early on in pregnancy, may give you a false elevated prevalence at the time of the invasive test in the subgroup that you have examined, and therefore a very high screen positive rate.

Chard: If I may defend Dr Reynolds, he probably does not necessarily have – nor does anybody – the information that could completely answer your question. He is in the somewhat unfortunate position in that he is the only person today who has actually addressed the non-21 situation, so it is a bit hard on him. I am sure what Professor Nicolaides is coming round to saying is that of course if you are doing nuchal translucencies, which I firmly agree we should, you will be picking up all these without any doubt or difficulty at all, so why are we necessarily wasting our time with biochemistry and atypicality?

That is a matter to which we will undoubtedly return but with respect to the current discussions could we perhaps move on to some other topics?

Cuckle: The first thing about atypicality is that we do not use it in Leeds but I am glad you came to the conclusion that it is useful. But in any kind of clinical chemistry I do not see how you can really avoid it because you look at the results and if you see a result that looks very peculiar it is hard just to sit on it. It goes against the principles of screening to do anything about it because screening should be for a well-defined end point and we are screening for Down syndrome and trisomy 18. These other conditions are accidental so that we have to pick them up coincidentally but we sometimes don't want to pick them up. It causes more trouble than it is worth – that is the conclusion you have come to and I suppose I have come to the same one. I don't think it is entirely avoidable. If you have a MoM of 50 for hCG what are you going to do about it? You do tend to do something about it. When Professor Nicolaides sees a nuchal translucency of 15 mm he cannot ignore it. It is a similar sort of situation.

Regarding subtle signs, first of all, we should not be making very strong statements about detection rates and false positive rates on the basis of a single series. People do that in papers: they fit a model to their own data and they quickly draw a conclusion about relative detection rates. That is dangerous.

Having said that, I agree with it in principle and I think it is best to add together different series to produce meta-analysis wherever possible. If you look at all the prospective studies, the models that we are using seem to fit. There are 17 prospective studies published with either two or three-marker screening, all of them using hCG ± AFP. The observed false positive detection rate in those studies combined is pretty much on the model predictions, so however bad the models are – and there may be bad tails or some other bits of them – they are not bad.

Wald: A short point. Although the issues are complicated, we all know that, the trick in this field is to try to make complicated issues simple so that they can be used in screening as long as they are reasonably robust. The concern right down through the model is mainly in the tails of the distribution and they are a problem. There are a number of suggested methods for dealing with the problem but none are entirely satisfactory. It is quite extraordinary, given the initial uncertainty and the sample sizes, how well the predictions have been brought out in practice, so it basically works.

Macintosh: I would like to get away from tables and go back to trisomy 18. There are some data from the Chromosome Abnormal Database at the Oxford Medical Laboratory that indicate the majority of cases of trisomy 18 are picked up prenatally and the indication for why they are picked up prenatally was because of the obvious markers with ultrasound. For a condition that is likely to be lethal within six months if the fetus does survive at term we should not be screening using a technique such as biochemistry, which is clearly less helpful than ultrasound – if indeed we should be screening for this at all. So I do not agree that all laboratories should be giving risks for trisomy 18.

I shall be talking about this later but along with the NEQAS questionnaire of laboratories in the UK that are providing risks for trisomy 18. Out of 75 there are only four laboratories that routinely provide a risk for Edwards' syndrome and 30 of the 75 would alert the clinician if they thought there was some abnormality when looking at the biochemistry.

Chard: There is a good contentious statement: don't do trisomy 18 screening.

Wald: I don't think you are right, Dr Macintosh. I don't like calling it screening for trisomy 18 because we do not intend to screen for that; it is a spin-off from Down syndrome. As you point out, most of our screening of pregnancy is for an extremely lethal condition. Having said that, you can get about 60% detection for about a 0.2% false positive rate. It is an incredibly powerful test. Unfortunately, it is not something you would want to go out and screen for. But I doubt if ultrasound would do better than that. It is an extremely high ratio, 60% for 0.2%.

Macintosh: I like the theory but I don't think much of the practice. I am saying that a review of the risks that are coming out from laboratories regarding trisomy 18, which are not screening for this condition but alerting clinicians, shows that there is absolutely no consensus to the cut off value used. I would be surprised if there was audit on the false positive rates and screen positive rates that were being brought about by alerting clinicians to the abnormal biochemistry. If the theory is carried out it may be a different question, but it is not.

Cuckle: I am a big advocate and we do do it. People are not very consistent in their ultrasound policy of screening for trisomy 18 either. So to say there is inconsistency is not criticism; it just means they have not come to consensus yet, which they could do through the National External Quality Assurance Scheme (NEQAS). I believe it is here to stay, it is an obvious spin-off and you will do it. People are doing it increasingly. I would disagree with extending it to Turner's syndrome, for example, because that is a condition that you do not necessarily want to pick up but you do it accidentally. There is concern about whether some of the mid-trimester Turner's really are Turner's syndrome.

Reynolds: I am from a lab that does not screen for trisomy 18. In fact, we do not use atypicality either, we work from the gut feeling principle. What I wanted to comment on was Dr Macintosh's point about lack of consistency in cut-offs. There is also a problem with lack of consistency in cut-offs for trisomy 21. In my area we have one boundary using 1 in 100; we use 1 in 150; the next boundary uses 1 in 250 and the next one uses 1 in 300.

Hicks: That is a nice point about the variation in cut-offs. In a way it brings us back to what are the aims of testing for Down syndrome: was it about minimising the birth rate of Down syndrome for the population or was it about optimising the position of individual women? When I said I thought it was about optimising the position of individual women, I saw some nods round the table. But it is easy for us sometimes to lose the implications of that as we talk. For example, Professor Wald had a valid definition of the efficiency of the programme over maximising a given detection rate for a given false positive rate. But that is a population definition which is valid for the population and it may be valid for individuals, but it may not if values among the individuals differ widely.

I am into fund manager definitions. If our population consisted only of widows and orphans on one extreme and wealthy entrepreneurs at the opposite extreme, picking a fund in the middle that pays a moderate rate of return with a moderate risk may be inappropriate for everybody. I suggest that we can only be confident of Professor Wald's definition being accurate if we are also confident that the values in the population were not very disparately distributed.

Similarly, as we talk about false positive and detection rate pairs, it is also important that we remember what are the implications for the way in which the results are presented to individual women because often the consequence is that we have to vary the cut-off on which we report a risk as positive to an individual woman.

You raise the point about there being variations in cut-offs in your geographical area. I don't know why those rates were set but it may be that they reflect the values of the obstetricians' thinking of what they perceive as high risk. It may be for cost reasons, it may be for other reasons. But ultimately those values are set at what somebody thinks is the right balance of risk or benefit that an individual woman should accept.

My point is that as we talk we should not forget the implications of what we are saying for individual women.

Reynolds: Can I come back on that? In a wider survey of why people have different risks we found there was one category of high risk cut-off because they were trying to save money. Another chose 1 in 150 because they decided that that was the risk of fetal loss from amniocentesis and therefore they would match the two together. Another chose the risk because the obstetrician did not like doing amniocentesis and they were using it as a way to reduce their amniocentesis rate. There was a whole wide range of what seemed very dubious risks but some seemed genuine.

Nicolaides: I have some comments on Professor Wald's concept of abuses. The first is exactly the same point of view that has been raised: there is the abuse of the system to offer somebody an individualised statistical risk and respond to the inevitable question that any clinician experiences every day with every patient who asks the question, 'What was my risk before?' I consider it to be a strongly indicated use of giving both the previous and the new risk. You cannot refuse to give it rather than label it as an abuse.

Secondly, there is the issue of sequential screening. Sequential screening is clinical medicine where you see somebody and you ask them a series of questions; then you undertake a clinical examination; then you do a series of investigations; then, depending on your findings, you do a series of new investigations and eventually you arrive at a diagnosis or perhaps a probability diagnosis. It is a reality that women have scans; it is a reality that women have biochemical tests; and it is a reality that those who believe in ultrasound can provide evidence that you can diagnose certain abnormalities and those who believe in biochemistry similarly can do the same.

The reality is that you definitely need to be able to combine the findings from the two methods rather than arbitrarily classify people into positive and negative and, once you have classified them and put them in a corner, not allow them the luxury of knowing what that positivity and negativity means, and have the option of further tests that would clarify that statistical risk. So the two are actually together.

The reality is whether you decide that you will offer the medical screening and, by certain completely arbitrary and almost certainly false economic assumptions made about 30 years ago, classify the population into positive and negative, or try to estimate risks and accept that those risks can be changed by other aspects of their examination and then let them decide whether they consider that risk to be high or low.

Wald: Of course if a woman says 'what was my risk before the triple test, just on age?' she is entitled to know. If you have information and someone asks for it you can give it. My concern with that is that it is so easily misunderstood. If a woman happened to ask you 'What was the risk on the hCG alone before it was combined with the AFP and the uE$_3$?' do you give that? That is just as rational. What is the point of knowing what the age-only risk is, the AFP-only risk is, the oestriol-only risk is? It is meaningless. So if you encourage it you are encouraging a rather meaningless exercise.

You said sequential screening is clinical medicine. To that extent it is an indictment against clinical medicine that a number of people in the western world are trying to put it right to try to make it more rational, more evidence-based as the time passes, while at the same time preserving ultimately choice. If I had one method of performing an appendectomy that killed one in 10,000 people and another one that killed one in 1000 people, and I could afford both, which should I offer? All I am saying is that it is a method of screening that will save half the number of babies, so why not use that? It is as simple as that. It is a safety element, if you like.

Cuckle: I would like to address some of the points that Professor Nicolaides and Dr Hicks have raised – to put them in the right perspective we need to make a clear distinction between screening and clinical practice. We are talking about screening. Screening is a public health measure; it is not like ordinary clinical medicine. To devise a screening policy is a public health issue: it is about rationing of a scarce or dangerous resource. Once a woman is positive she becomes a patient, and so there is this funny relationship between the screening programme and its policy that has been worked out nicely to get the 5% false positive rate in a certain detection rate and then what happens after that point is that clinical medicine gets its hands on the results of the policy. That is where you are both raising those kinds of concerns.

But that is the real world. The policy as a policy has to be designed to optimise detection, because that is the public health aim, at the same time as providing information and clinicians with information, which the clinicians then feed back to the woman. So it is messy but you have to make that distinction.

What is the full consequence of what you are saying, Dr Hicks? Are you saying that we should not even use cut-offs, that we should just give risks? If you do that, which may seem more humane or more clinical than screening, it becomes a bit unpredictable and you cannot really have an unpredictable screening policy. If you roll it on a few years it may become more predictable and you would find that false positive rates would stay at 5% or the amniocentesis rate would stay at 5% and that would be OK.

Nørgaard-Pedersen: The perception of risk is important, and it is important for the health personnel to understand what it is all about. Therefore we need to explain this to the doctors who use the test system. Furthermore, we need also to take into account that neural tube defects should be linked to Down syndrome. The advice we have given doctors is to say that the risk for Down syndrome and malformation at under 35 years of age is 3 in 1000, and above that age it is 7 in 1000.

Then we have some guidelines concerning the interpretation of the particular risk. We give a risk report for Down syndrome but we also give whether the results are normal or whether the AFP is slightly elevated or significantly elevated or the risk of Down syndrome is greater than 1 in 400 at birth. Then you can put these things together and say that when the risk of Down syndrome is increasing you have a decreased risk for neural tube defect and vice versa. Our health personnel are able to understand the issues better presented in this way. With respect to ultrasound, not all centres are able to screen for malformation and not at 15–16 weeks. So it is important keep in mind not only the Down syndrome screening but also see it together with neural tube defect screening because it may also have some benefit for the woman who is waiting for the results and she may eventually decide that although the risk may be greater than 1 in 400 she finally declines to have further invasive tests because this particular child will be precious to a 36- or 37-year-old woman. The whole process should take all of this into account. Many doctors do not understand the whole process.

Reynolds: It seems to me that this discussion is a reflection of what went on earlier, the debate about whether it is the population or the individual that you are treating. Statisticians are on the side of the population; doctors look at the patient, we want to give the patients the information they need. To my mind it makes sense to give people the age risk and their individual risk because, particularly in older women, they actually want the babies and will only opt to have a primary amniocentesis if they are at much higher risk than the one they have prepared themselves for. So the pure population view of it does not come into patient psychology.

The other interesting thing, which I don't know if anybody has looked at and it is perhaps a study that should be done, is to find out what risk people feel is acceptable rather than what we feel is acceptable to impose on them

Macri: A stark example of the negative impact of sequential types of testing is unfortunately still going on in some areas of the United States, namely the terrible practice of obtaining a serum AFP-only evaluation, which provides perhaps some rudimentary form of risk for Down syndrome, and then the clinician goes on and asks at that point for multiple marker assessment. One need not be a mathematician to understand the absurdity of that kind of approach, but it is still proceeding in the United States where in some areas there is still AFP-only testing going on.

Silman: Professor Cuckle was talking about a screening programme being a social policy, and it seems to me that that is entirely appropriate. But there is a 'meta-language' being used at the same time, and Professor Wald was using that language, talking about irrational decisions as though a decision that did not coincide with the social policy by an individual was in some way irrational. I come back to his example because if we can pinpoint it with a lottery we can certainly do it with Down syndrome. It is presumably irrational for me to take one pound with the chance of winning £10 million if there is 22 million:1 against me. But does it become rational for me to take one pound and to put it on to win £10 million if there is 9 million:1 against me? Does that become a rational decision by me as an individual with my one pound?

   If it really does suddenly become rational, then surely it would be rational for me to put two pounds on and to bring down the odds to that 9 million:1 and I am now becoming rational. What I am trying to say is that the cost and benefit analysis of the individual is subject to the choice of that individual – how important something is to them and how important is the cost to them. And the information that we need in terms of risk estimate is for them to use within their own judgement criteria, and it should not be condemned.

Nicolaides: That is completely obvious and you are right. I have done the survey that was requested; I do it every month when I run a course. The participants are doctors and nurses, and never has anybody chosen the cut-off risk of 1 in 300 for having an invasive test. People vary from 1 in 10 because they believe that having a baby with Down syndrome is not such a bad thing, but having a iatrogenic death of a normal baby is a dreadful sin, and others choose a cut-off risk of 1 in 2000 because under no circumstances would they tolerate having a baby with Down syndrome whereas they could cope with a miscarriage.

   The second thing is that it is also a reality that we have ultrasound scanning in 1996. It is also a reality that a lot of defect features will be interpreted at ultrasound scan and, through very bad research unfortunately over the last 20 years, a lot of those markers are given statistical risks to the patients for having invasive tests. The only thing we can support is a mechanism of combining the various risks and accepting the absolute reality that there will be sequential screening. If you do not correct for the biochemical results at 16 weeks, and you ignore those in interpreting the ultrasound findings at 20 weeks, the only thing that you will achieve is to double or quadruple the invasive testing rate. If you accept the reality that there should be sequential screening, a lot of the patients with mild hydronephrosis, choroid plexus cysts, short femur or echogenic bowel for which today we are offering invasive tests, if you took into account the biochemical result that would have modified the current risks dramatically downwards, you would avoid an invasive test.

SECTION 3

CONSEQUENCES FROM SECOND TRIMESTER SCREENING

Chapter 9

Lessons from the second trimester

Timothy Chard

There are a number of important features of Down syndrome screening for which experience already gained from second trimester programmes may assist in implementation of first trimester programmes. These features are discussed here. For detailed references the reader is recommended to other chapters in this book, and to recent reviews (e.g. Chard and Macintosh 1995).

Screening for Down syndrome by maternal serum biochemistry in the second trimester was introduced in the late 1980s and by the mid-1990s it had become routine in many Obstetric Units throughout the developed World. Over the same period there were numerous studies of tests, both biochemical and biophysical, which might prove equally effective in the first trimester. Sufficient evidence has now accumulated to suggest that first trimester screening (10–13 weeks) is both feasible and probably equally or more effective than second trimester screening. It is also generally agreed that, all other things being equal, first trimester screening would be preferable to second trimester screening from the point of view of the woman and her family. Thus, it is likely that within the next few years there will be a progressive switch from the second to the first trimester, later testing being reserved only for those who do not present at the appropriate time. That being the case, it is reasonable to ask whether experience gained from the implementation of second trimester programmes can be applied to their first trimester counterparts.

Clinical trials of Down syndrome screening

In an ideal world, all diagnostic and therapeutic modalities, including screening tests, would be subjected to randomised controlled trials before routine implementation. This ideal is difficult to achieve in a screening programme, especially one in which the adverse outcome is a relatively rare event. A partial substitute is that a prospective study of the test be carried out, without intervention on the basis of test results, before routine implementation. However, none of the very influential studies which led to the introduction of second trimester screening met even these limited criteria for 'controlled' studies. Most investigations were the subject of practical implementation from the outset, with intervention based on theoretical extrapolation from a very limited database.

It appears that this story will be repeated with the introduction of first trimester screening. In particular, the information already gained from 'interventional' studies is now so substantial and cogent that it would probably be unethical not to act immediately on any results in new progress. Appeals for prospective, non-interventional studies are likely to be ignored.

Regional and national policies

As in the past, there will continue to be calls for the establishment of regional or even national policies for Down syndrome screening in the first trimester. Superficially, such demands are entirely logical and desirable. In the US, in particular, there is a remarkable homogeneity of practice, arising from the existence of the excellent guidelines regularly published by the American College of Obstetricians and Gynecologists (ACOG), and by the fact that most clinicians would be averse to deviating from these guidelines for fear of medico-legal consequences. However, experience from the second trimester suggests that such overall coherence of approach is unlikely to occur in the UK. Despite a decade of experience, there are still no broad agreements or recommendations which serve to guide detailed second trimester screening policy within an individual health district. Each district purchaser or provider is largely left to determine local policy. This may include the decision as to whether to screen or not (often driven by financial considerations), the type of screening (whole population or selected subgroups), and the screening method (combinations of biochemical analytes, ultrasound etc.). Indeed, it is by no means uncommon to find substantial differences in policy within a single Unit, individual clinicians having their own, often very disparate ideas.

Which methods will be used?

Both biophysical (e.g. femur length) and biochemical methods were originally proposed for Down syndrome screening in the second trimester. However, it rapidly became apparent that the biochemical parameters were much superior. There is now no doubt that maternal serum biochemistry has become the gold-standard against which all other approaches must be judged.

The same argument (biophysical versus biochemical) has arisen in respect of the first trimester. Here, however, there is extremely cogent evidence that a biophysical test (measurement of nuchal translucency) is equal, possibly even superior, to biochemical tests both in the first and second trimesters. The criticism is that performance is poor unless there is appropriate equipment, protocols, training of personnel and audit. These criticisms can be answered by meticulous attention to guidelines in the setting up of such programmes, an approach which has already proved successful in at least 20 district general hospitals in the UK (see Chapter 19). The further criticism that results can vary greatly between observers and Units can also be answered by the same rigorous implementation of quality control to ultrasound services. Indeed, the performance of biochemistry in this respect is often, on careful inspection, disappointingly poor (see Chapter 28).

The choice of biochemical tests in the second trimester still remains contentious. The pre-eminent test is measurement of hCG, in particular, the free β-subunit of this molecule. The addition of other parameters appears to yield diminishing returns. Most Units include AFP and some also add oestriol. Other parameters (e.g. α-subunit of hCG, inhibin) may yield marginal improvements, but the numbers required to confirm these improvements are impractically large. Indeed, some have suggested that the incorporation of additional analytes may actually *decrease* the efficiency of screening, as well as adding to costs.

In the first trimester the situation appears rather more clear-cut. Two analytes – free β-subunit of hCG and PAPP-A – are particularly effective. However, other analytes, notably AFP and oestriol, also exhibit significant deviation in cases of fetal Down syndrome and might, therefore, be candidates for part of a multi-marker screen (see Chapters 15 and 16).

One basic rule of the biochemical tests is that the only analytes which will be routinely applied are those for which reagents are provided by a commercial manufacturer. In the past, primary development and even routine screening has been performed with materials prepared 'in-house' in the laboratory itself, notable examples including the 'Barts/London' assays for hCG, AFP and PAPP-A. However, the demands of regulatory bodies, such as the FDA and its equivalents in Europe, dictate stringent conditions for the manufacture of such materials (e.g. Good Manufacturing Practice (GMP)). These regulations are entirely desirable and appropriate, but require resources which are not justified by the usage of a single Unit. Furthermore, and with occasional exceptions, manufacturers may only elect to proceed if they have a proprietary position (e.g. patent rights) in respect of the analyte in question. Such rights have played a significant role in the introduction and development of assays for hCG, the free β-subunit of hCG and oestriol, and urine β-core of hCG. Similar proprietary arrangements also affect the role and distribution of software for analysis of the results (e.g. the 'Alpha' programme for analysis of biochemical tests; the Fetal Medicine Foundation programme for analysis of nuchal translucency).[1]

Cost-effectiveness

Intuitively, it would seem that the economic gains to be achieved by pre-empting a costly life-time disability such as Down syndrome would be readily provable. Most published attempts at this exercise seem to support this view. Perhaps more important, given the general agreement as to the overall desirability of this area of

---

[1]These observations in no sense imply disapproval of such arrangements by the author who, indeed, is a co-holder of one potentially relevant patent.

practice, is the question of choosing the most cost-effective approach to screening. This includes factors such as whether testing is offered to the whole population or only selected groups (e.g. women under the age of 35). Other matters with cost implications include the number and choice of biochemical analytes, and the question as to whether measurement of nuchal translucency is a relatively simple addition to an existing dating scan, or represents an entirely new procedure. There is no doubt that the findings of such costing exercises for first trimester screening will prove as contentious as has been the case for second trimester screening programmes. In the UK, where there are no national policies, the decision to offer screening or not and the type of screening, is almost entirely at the whim of individuals within either the provider or purchaser groups.

Ethical aspects of screening

It is generally agreed that screening programmes such as those for Down syndrome will generate ethical questions. Furthermore, it is commonly believed that extensive discussion by all parties involved might reach some sort of resolution of these questions. Experience in the second trimester suggests that such discussions can occupy as much or more time than that of all other activities involved in the implementation of a screening programme. Experience also suggests that no resolution will ever be reached, or even approached (see Chapter 3). Views basically polarise between those who, on personal or religious grounds, are opposed to termination of pregnancy (approximately 20% of the population) and those who, although never commending the process, nevertheless believe it to be acceptable under specific circumstances (the remainder of the population). It can be confidently predicted that, in ten years time, arguments identical to those heard today will still be rehearsed, and will apply equally to testing at all stages of pregnancy.

Counselling

It is unarguable that any women offered Down syndrome screening should be provided with adequate information for her and her partner to make decisions both about the initial test and the possible subsequent follow-up. However, the amount and content and method of delivery of that information is the subject of ongoing discussion (see Chapter 29). Probably the most contentious area is how to describe 'risk' (see Chapter 28). Should this be as an absolute value, or a binary statement ('negative' or 'positive') or should it be something else?

Failure of counselling is one of the commonest criticisms made by consumers of the screening process. There are numerous, sometimes amusing, anecdotes illustrating total lack of understanding by women who have been counselled or even, on occasion, on the part of their counsellors. As with most activities, the solution is better training. The latter would be greatly helped if there were a single agreed counselling protocol.

In the UK, but not apparently elsewhere, the need for counselling has often been the grounds on which a screening programme has been rejected. Faced with extreme demands for extra staff, purchasers may easily become discouraged and determine to allocate scarce resources to other purposes.

Risks of invasive tests

When second trimester screening was introduced the diagnostic (invasive) test, amniocentesis, was very well established and its risks were believed to be well known. By contrast, the invasive tests of the first trimester, chorion villus sampling (CVS) and early amniocentesis are less well characterised. There is a strongly held view that CVS carries a much more substantial risk of causing miscarriage than does later amniocentesis. But the best current evidence does not support this view, rather pointing towards similar procedure-related risks for both techniques at any stage of pregnancy (see Chapter 26). It will undoubtedly take some time for these views to be confirmed and publicised in such a way as to be reassuring to both women and their advisers.

Because there are constant changes in techniques, equipment and operator experience, it is almost impossible to extrapolate from the past to either present or future practice in this topic. If there is any overall practical conclusion, it is that the relative risks of the invasive procedures are *not* considered to be a significant factor in deciding between first and second trimester screening programmes. However, an essential part of setting up a new first trimester programme is to ensure that there are staff appropriately trained to perform the early invasive procedures, if necessary by referring patients to a testing centre whilst local skills are acquired.

Practical implementation

At the time when second trimester screening was being introduced, reservations were expressed as to whether women would present at the appropriate stage of pregnancy (15–18 weeks). In fact, this problem had already been largely solved by the widespread application, since the 1970s, of AFP measurement for the detection of neural tube defects within the same time-window. But there is no comparable routine and well-established event in the late first trimester. There is no doubt that substantial efforts will have to be made to educate women and their advisers about such a change in policy. Equally, this should not be an excuse for inaction.

Fetal cells in the maternal circulation

The ideal screening test, or even diagnostic test, for Down syndrome would be examination of fetal cells in the maternal circulation. At many times over the past decade it has seemed that this entirely laudable aim would be achieved within a relatively short space of time, thereby rendering all other techniques superfluous. The state-of-the-art in such procedures is reviewed in Chapters 10 and 24. There is no doubt that this area includes some of the most important basic science which is presently taking place in Down syndrome research. That being said, progress towards a practical procedure has been shown but it is unlikely that any such test will become practicable until well into the next century.

Problems unique to first trimester screening

Introduction of first trimester testing differs from that in the second trimester in that it follows-on from an already successful system, albeit that its superiority is generally agreed. Almost certainly the switch from the second to the first trimester will necessitate a period of parallel operation, with great potential for confusion on the part of both providers and consumers. Several authors in this volume describe the problems which may occur with serial testing: an increase in the total number of screen positives, and a major decrease in the detection rates of tests performed later in the sequence. There is no obvious answer to this problem, until and unless a firm decision can be made to opt for one or the other form of screening. Furthermore, second trimester testing must continue to be available to those who do not present in the first trimester window.

Conclusions

A progressive move towards first trimester screening for Down syndrome is inevitable. It is also obvious that much can be learnt from the implementation of Down syndrome screening in the second trimester which can be applied to screening in the first trimester. Equally, it must be recognised that there are important questions which have still not been resolved after ten years of routine application. Many of these questions will not be resolved as part of a switch to first trimester testing.

Reference

Chard, T. and Macintosh, M.C.M. (1995) Screening for Down's syndrome *J Perinat Med* **23**, 421–36

Chapter 10

Maternal serum screening in the United States: current perspective (1996)

Joe Leigh Simpson

In the United States maternal serum analyte screening for the detection of Down syndrome is recommended by the American College of Obstetricians and Gynecologists, the American College of Medical Genetics, and other authoritative organisations. However, the manner in which screening is performed differs from those in the United Kingdom and other countries. This reflects only in part the differences between health-care delivery system in the United States and elsewhere.

The purpose of this chapter is to consider current standards and practices in the United States with respect to maternal serum screening for Down syndrome. In order to appreciate how these US policies evolved, it may be useful to review the historical development of prenatal diagnosis in the United States.

Introducing prenatal genetic diagnosis in the United States (1968–76)

Amniocentesis was first used widely in obstetrics to monitor pregnancies with Rh-isoimmunisation (Bevis 1952). For this purpose amniotic fluid liquor was analysed. Prenatal genetic diagnosis and amniocentesis were first coupled in 1955–56, when separate groups in Israel, United States and Denmark used the procedure in pregnancies at risk for X-linked recessive disorders (Serr *et al.* 1955; Makowski *et al.* 1956; Fuchs and Riis 1956). X-chromatin analysis was performed on amniotic fluid cells, techniques for complete chromosomal analysis not then being available. Application was limited to X-linked recessive conditions; however, the principle of prenatal genetic diagnosis was established.

There were relatively few applications over the next decade, probably reflecting the lack of awareness of medical genetics in general and by obstetrician/

gynaecologists in particular. Recall also that during this era pregnancy termination in the United States was illegal, even for genetic malformations. Doubtless the inability to act upon results contributed also to a relative lack of enthusiasm.

Soon after Tjio and Levan (1956) showed that the human chromosome number was 46, techniques were developed that enabled the chromosomal complement to be determined from blood (lymphocytes). The chromosomal basis of Turner's syndrome, Klinefelter's syndrome, Down syndrome and other autosomal trisomies was soon recognised. Not surprisingly, interest in prenatal genetic diagnosis was kindled. Childhood-onset X-linked recessive conditions might have been considered mere curiosities, but all obstetricians recall delivering infants with Down syndrome. Avoiding this unfortunate circumstance was attractive.

Initially amniotic fluid cells proved difficult to culture, but Steele and Breg (1966) showed that these cells could indeed be successfully cultured. Metaphase preparations thus became possible. Using cells obtained by amniocentesis, the first prenatal diagnosis of Down syndrome was reported in 1967 by Jacobson and Barter (1967) and by Nadler (1967). Nadler and Messina (1969), were the first to detect a metabolic disorder *in utero*. Later, that group from Northwestern University (Chicago) were the first to publish a series of cases demonstrating the practicality of performing prenatal genetic diagnosis (Nadler and Gerbie 1970). The Northwestern group was widely considered to have provided evidence of the relative safety and accuracy of amniocentesis for prenatal genetic diagnosis.

In the early 1970s the question was whether amniocentesis was sufficiently safe to be offered routinely, and if so, to women of what age? In considering how this question was answered, recall that the only aneuploidy risk figures then available were based on five-year intervals. From age 30–34 years the risk was 1 in 880, from 35–39 1 in 290, and from 40–44 1 per 100 (Collmann and Stoller 1962). Thus, the only choices for that maternal age above which amniocentesis would be offered routinely were 30, 35 or 40 years. The 1970 publication of Nadler and Gerbie had presented a favourable benefit: risks analysis for women aged 35 and above, although limited capacity of US labs to culture and analyse cells precluded widespread availability.

To determine the safety of amniocentesis in the United States and thus define the age at which the procedure should be offered routinely, NICHD sponsored a multi-centre collaborative study of women undergoing amniocentesis. During 1972–75, the loss rate proved to be 3.5% in 1045 women who underwent amniocentesis and 3.2% in 992 controls; this small difference was not statistically significant, and disappeared completely when corrected for maternal age. A Canadian study concurrently showed loss rates almost exactly identical to that in the United States; however, no control group was recruited (Simpson *et al.* 1976).

Although not statistically significant, the absolute difference of 0.3% in the US study somehow proved pivotal. Logically assuming the existence of some procedure-related losses, geneticists began to communicate to patients that the procedure-related loss rate with amniocentesis was approximately 0.5% (1 in 200). Aware also that the total risk of chromosome abnormalities was not restricted to Down syndrome, and further aware that the only aneuploidy risk figures available were in five-year intervals, the conclusion was reached that amniocentesis should be offered routinely only to women aged 35 years or older at delivery. Had the one year risk figures available later in the decade Hook (1981), existed earlier, it is quite possible that a different maternal age (e.g. 34, 36 or 37 years) would have been adopted in the US Irrespective, the NICHD Amniocentesis Study (1976) led to general acceptance in the US of amniocentesis for prenatal genetic diagnosis. The establishment of age 35 as that at which the procedure should be offered was also accepted. At least one well publicised lawsuit in the New York City region (*Becker* v. *Schwartz*) further served to spur adoption of this policy.

Incidentally, there is, in retrospect, reason to believe that the loss rate in the NICHD control group was spuriously high. The observed loss rates after 16 weeks of 3.2% is actually closer to that expected after only 8–9 weeks (Simpson *et al.* 1987). Ordinarily loss rates after 16 gestational weeks of perhaps only 1–2% would be expected Simpson (1990), even allotting for a maternal age effect. Perhaps some control subjects in the US NICHD study could have already experienced fetal demise at the time of registration, given that ultrasound was not then routine. Control subjects might also have volunteered for the study because of fear of adverse outcome (selection bias). It is for these and other reasons that many continue to counsel procedure-related loss rates of 0.5%, despite acceptance that concurrent ultrasound now practised should considerably decrease risk. However, a 1986 Danish randomised study showed that even with ultrasound the amniocentesis-related risk was still 1% (Tabor *et al.* 1986). This study is, incidentally, widely questioned in the US, being at odds with clinical impressions (Sicherman *et al.* 1995).

Maternal serum alpha fetoprotein (MSAFP) screening for neural tube defects (1977–85)

Amniocentesis was already being performed for advanced maternal age when Brock and Sutcliffe (1972) showed that amniotic fluid alpha fetoprotein (AFAFP) was elevated in pregnancies with an open neural tube defect (NTD). Almost immediately, amniocentesis was also offered to women at increased risk for NTDs (i.e. those having a previously affected offspring). United States laboratories usually assayed AFAFP in all specimens submitted for genetic tests as well. False positive AFAFP values were a problem until the invaluable specificity of amniotic fluid acetylcholinesterase in NTD was recognised later in the decade. Reliable ultrasound later became available as well.

In 1977 the UK collaborative study on maternal serum AFP screening was reported. The overall NTD detection rate proved to be approximately 80%. Similar data soon became available from the United States (Macri 1978). The propriety of routinely offering maternal serum alpha fetoprotein (MSAFP) screening in all US pregnancies was thus raised, at least for the perhaps 50% of the population who were presenting for prenatal care before 20 gestational weeks.

ACOG concerns

Perhaps surprisingly to some, the American College of Obstetricians and Gynecologists (ACOG) and American geneticists in general did not greet the advance of MSAFP screening with universal enthusiasm. By 1977 several manufacturers had already developed radioimmunoassay kits for MSAFP and had requested US Food and Drug Administration (FDA) approval. Although we and other American geneticists and obstetricians never doubted assay reliability, we were concerned about the ability of the US health-care system to handle problems. We were expressly concerned that the prerequisites for genetic screening, as espoused in 1975 with considerable publicity by the US National Academy of Sciences, could not be fulfilled (Macri 1978). Specifically, could the problems engendered by screening be met? Large numbers of women with an elevated MSAFP would exist compared to the relatively few who had an NTD. Relatively few obstetricians were knowledgeable about genetics at that time; thus, the burden of counselling would inevitably have fallen on geneticists. In July Nadler and Simpson (1979a,b) stated the consensus position in an editorial published concurrently in the two major US obstetrics and gynecology journals: the promise of MSAFP was 'not yet fulfilled'.

In 1979, the American College of Obstetricians and Gynecologists did not have its present Committee on Genetics. Rather, this author served as the 'Designated Person in Genetics', responsible for alerting ACOG to issues of genetic import-ance. I also served as a liaison between ACOG and the American Academy of Pediatrics (AAP) Committee on Genetics, a committee that did consider the issue formally. Not until 1981 did ACOG designate a Subcommittee on Genetics initiated, then reporting to the Committee on Obstetrics: Maternal–Fetal Medicine (now called Committee on Obstetrical Practice). Genetics Subcom-mittee Chairs were, in sequence, myself, Drs Mitchell S. Golbus, Sherman Elias and Michael Mennutti. The subcommittee mechanism was superseded by a Committee on Genetics, of which Dr Paul G. McDonough is the first Chairman. Depending upon the specific year, then, different lines of communication existed from the reproductive genetic community to ACOG. Irrespective, in the late 1970s ACOG agreed with its reproductive geneticists and petitioned the FDA against the unrestricted release of reagents for MSAFP testing; the American Academy of Pediatrics and its Committee on Genetics concurred.

FDA response

The FDA soon agreed that MSAFP reagents should not be released in un-restricted fashion. The FDA proposed that reagents be made available only to 'institutes' or 'commercial units' that could guarantee availability of the ancillary tests necessary for successful screening, e.g. ultrasound and genetic counselling. The medical community anticipated that screening could then begin in orderly fashion, incrementally or regionally if necessary. However, Health and Human Services (HHS) Secretary Patricia Harris chose not to sign the FDA regulations, nor did her successors. The practical effect was to hold MSAFP screening in limbo in the US, for no reagents were released.

In 1983 the FDA issued new guidelines, now with very few stipulations. Manufacturers were required only to mount an educational effort and to monitor the outcome of 1000 cases in each of five centres using their reagents. Commercial units and other laboratories were otherwise free to purchase reagents. We and others did so, reasoning that governmental approval of MSAFP reagents altered the equilibrium that prior to that time had not favoured MSAFP screening. Moreover, the intervening delay (1979–83) was salutary in several ways. Post-graduate obstetric forums had frequently discussed MSAFP screening, ultrasound quality had vastly improved and obstetricians had became more cognisant of genetic issues.

In May 1985 the Department of Professional Liability of the American College of Obstetricians and Gynecologists rather unexpectedly heightened dialogue by publishing an 'Alert' (ACOG 1985a). ACOG Fellows were advised that they should 'be offering MSAFP'. It was specifically suggested that patients be 'informed of the availability of this test', with the patient's decision documented in the chart. Although the wisdom of publishing this Alert has been questioned (Annas and Elias 1985), without question the 'standard' had been set or re-inforced. This was subsequently affirmed in an ACOG Technical Bulletin (1986), which superseded a Technical Bulletin (1982) that had stated that routine MSAFP screening in all pregnancies was of 'uncertain value' and 'should not be imple-mented' if counselling and follow-up services are not available. The next edition of the *ACOG Standards in Obstetrics and Gynecology* (1985b) and the *AAP/ACOG Guidelines in Perinatal Care* (1983) further codified practice. Simpson and Nadler (1987) wrote a sequel to their 1979 editorial (Nadler and Simpson 1979a,b), reminding readers that maternal serum screening was now clearly recommended.

Introducing maternal serum analyte screening (1984–94)

In 1984 Merkatz *et al.* (1984) reported the association between low MSAFP and fetal trisomy. This finding was soon confirmed in the United Kingdom and elsewhere. After the report by Merkatz *et al.* (1984), we and others began to pursue low MSAFP values (< 0.4 MoM) by offering amniocentesis to detect Down syndrome. In a 1986 report by our group, then at Northwestern University in Chicago, we detected one case Down syndrome and two trisomy 18 cases among 1421 screened women (Simpson *et al.* 1986). The women screened had primarily sought screening to detect NTDs. Simply applying a threshold below which amniocentesis was offered was clearly not optimal, however, because such an algorithm failed to take into account that the significance of a given value would vary proportional to the age of the mother. Associations between fetal trisomy and both elevated hCG and low unconjugated oestriol were later recognised, leading to construction of software that could take into account values of all three analytes as well as key potential confounding factors.

The first prospective US studies using triple marker screening were published in 1992. In a University of Tennessee study conducted between 1989 and 1992, our group (Phillips *et al.* 1992) prospectively explored the feasibility of detecting Down syndrome using the algorithm developed by Wald and colleagues. We continued to offer amniocentesis or chorionic villus sampling as the sole method of detecting Down syndrome in women over age 35 at delivery, but now offered triple analyte screening to detect Down syndrome in women less than age 35. Among 9530 women screened, four cases of Down syndrome were detected and three were missed. In the same year Haddow *et al.* (1992) reported results of their large prospective study in the New England region. In this study MSAFP was offered to the entire population; however, most women screened were less than 35 years of age. Detection rate approximated 90% in women over age 35 and 60% in women under 35 years.

By 1993, many US centres were offering multiple serum analyte screening for the detection of Down syndrome. By 1994 a policy change was communicated by an ACOG Committee Opinion Statement (ACOG Committee Opinion 1994), originating from the Committee on Obstetric Practice. In the latter document it was recommended that maternal serum screening for Down syndrome be offered to all women under 35. In the 1994 document no preference was stated concerning triple relative merits of double screening, and MSAFP alone even remained as an option. However, by late 1994 very few US labs were still offering single analyte (MSAFP) screening for the detection of Down syndrome.

Significantly, the ACOG Committee Opinion statement (1994) did not recommend universal maternal serum screening as an obligatory initial step. An invasive diagnostic procedure (i.e. amniocentesis or chorionic villus sampling) was still recommended for women age 35 years and older. This policy was more recently reinforced by an ACOG Education Bulletin (1996).

Current controversies (1996)

In the US, several controversies exist, although not all are of paramount concern to the practitioner. Some are looked upon by practitioners as trivial, primarily the province of laboratory workers. For example, there is little discussion among clinicians concerning the relative merits of a specific assay, e.g. free β-hCG v. total β-hCG. There is only limited interest in adding or replacing extant serum analytes, for example substituting or adding dimeric inhibin A. In general, the relative lack of interest in issues reflects most clinicians and patients seeing little difference between 80% v. 70% v. 60% sensitivity. If a new analyte could allow near 100% sensitivity, it would be accepted enthusiastically. Otherwise, interest in incremental improvement is limited. If adding another analyte were to increase costs, this reticence would be accentuated.

First trimester serum analyte screening

The propriety of serum screening in the first versus second trimester is not yet a major issue in the United States. After all, test kits for first trimester assays have not been made available to US laboratories. This will almost certainly soon change. Among other reasons NICHD has recently funded a multi-centre collaborative study to determine the relative safety and accuracy of early amniocentesis versus late CVS (10–14 weeks). As part of this study, NICHD study centres will doubtless begin to offer first trimester maternal serum screening to identify women at increased risk for Down syndrome. Assuming salutary performance, the assays utilised in this governmental-funded study should receive rapid FDA approval.

Ultrasound for anomaly or marker detection

Using ultrasound in lieu of maternal serum screening or routine invasive procedures is not usually considered an option in the US at this time. A few physicians advocate ultrasound to confirm or exclude NTD after detecting elevated MSAFP. However, the 1996 ACOG Educational Bulletin (1996) alluded to above urges caution with this approach, reminding practitioners that 'the prospective identification of NTDs may be limited by the location and extent of the lesion, fetal position, quality of the images, and experience of the ultrasonographer'. In that Bulletin it was noted that whereas 90% sensitivity by ultrasound is achievable, 'these studies have been conducted in specialised centres and include patients referred for elevation of elevated MSAFP levels'. 'In such specialised centres,' risk of NTDs can be 'decreased by 95%' with 'adequate visualisation of fetal anatomy'; however, proper visualisation may not be possible and scanning in a private office cannot approach expertise in a tertiary centre. Thus, the patient 'may or may not choose to undergo invasive diagnostic procedure'.

Other approaches

Several other potential approaches can be envisioned, but none are now considered practical. For example, there seems to be little enthusiasm for using ultrasound as the sole method to detect anomalies or markers indicative of Down syndrome, in lieu of invasive diagnostic procedure on maternal serum screening. However, one recent report suggests benefit in performing ultrasound for Down syndrome markers after results of serum analyte screening are known (Bahado-Singh *et al.* 1996). To my knowledge, no large-scale prospective studies in the US are assessing first trimester nuchal translucency as a sole alternative to maternal serum analyte programmes.

Recovery of fetal cells in maternal blood is still investigational (Chapter 23), although under active evaluation by NICHD (de la Cruz *et al.* 1995).

Screening for Down syndrome in the US: options in 1996

Current discussion concerns whether all women over 35 should be offered an invasive procedure, whether universal maternal serum analyte screening as an obligatory initial test is preferable for women of all ages, or whether still other options are best. The major options and the current US policy are reviewed here in an attempt to distinguish my own preferences.

Offering an invasive procedure to women ≥ age 35 years with no other screening

By this traditional policy one would set a maternal age cut off (e.g. 35 years), offering women at or above this age an invasive procedure. No one else would be screened for Down syndrome routinely, either by an invasive procedure or by maternal serum screening. Once standard, this approach has been now rejected in the United States. The 1994 ACOG Committee Opinion Statement (1994) removed this option formally. The policy was codified again by the September 1996 ACOG Educational Bulletin (1996).

Performing maternal serum screening as an obligatory first step in women of all ages

The age-specific threshold for offering an invasive procedure (35 years in the US) would be replaced with universal maternal serum screening. An invasive procedure would then be offered only if the calculated risk equals that of a 35-year-old woman at mid-trimester (1/270). The cost effectiveness of this approach is considered established in the UK and generally acknowledged in the US. Nonetheless, universal maternal serum screening as an obligatory first step seems unlikely to be adopted as policy in the United States.

For nearly 20 years US women over age 35 have become accustomed to exercising the option of having or not having an invasive prenatal diagnostic procedure for detection of Down syndrome. US women have a proven history of independence, for example declining to participate in randomised studies of types conducted without controversy in Canada and the UK (e.g. first trimester CVS versus second trimester amniocentesis). The likelihood of US women over age 35 accepting 85–90% detection for Down syndrome seems dim, when they have become accustomed to 100%. Most older pregnant women are well aware of the issues underlying invasive prenatal testing, having had friends who were tested or having undergone CVS or amniocentesis themselves for genetic or other reasons. It should also be recalled that in the US most women are still able to choose their physician and concomitantly switch physicians if displeased. The fee-for-service model of selecting a compatible health-care provider still exists for many women. Even in managed care plans one can still usually choose a provider from among a list of choices. Relatively few women are enrolled in fully capitated or closed staff health maintenance organisations that preclude meaningful options.

Could insurers dictate obligatory maternal serum screening as an initial step, in order to save money? In my opinion, managed care organisations would be foolish to force their members into an unpopular option merely to save relatively small amounts of money. Their clients would abandon the insurer for other plans at the next enrolment period, with any immediate financial gains. Those physicians who insist on dictating obligatory serum screening in order to generate a more favourable economic profile may find themselves with fewer obstetric patients, especially fewer healthy patients. Even women on Medicaid usually retain choices. The California Medicaid (MediCal) philosophy of attempting to dictate particular courses of action has thus not been followed in other states.

Obstetricians are also likely to be reticent in implementing universal maternal serum screening to women of all ages. Concerning potential financial savings, few obstetricians think globally concerning the best use of the US health-care dollar. Many fervently believe that obstetric patients and women in general should receive relatively more health-care funding, not be satisfied with a set amount. Much of the public would probably agree, as witnessed by the remarkably quick passage of federal legislation that now allows parturients 48 h hospitalisation after vaginal delivery and 96 h after caesarean section.

Malpractice allegations are another concern for US obstetricians, with the problem being more complicated than generally recognised outside the US. Blithe dismissals are offered that physicians should ignore the spectre of malpractice allegations and simply practice good medicine, but this advice often proves impractical. The US obstetrician's yearly liability premiums are usually one third to one quarter of his/her net income. Imagine, moreover, the probable scenario if obligatory maternal serum screening were to replace offering an invasive procedure in older women. Imagine a trial alleging failure to detect Down syndrome in a 36-year-old woman. Perhaps maternal serum screening had indeed been performed, but the patient's calculated risk was less than 1/270 at mid-trimester; amniocentesis was not recommended. The claim might be that all 36-year-old women should still have been offered an invasive procedure, as was formerly the routine. The defendant obstetrician would probably be asked to explain the rationale for his/her performing obligatory maternal serum analyte screening in lieu of offering an invasive procedure. The defendant physician is likely to be asked to explain to the court the concept of likelihood ratios; the lack of independence among various analytes and, hence, the requirement for complicated software; the differing sensitivity by maternal age; and the role of potential confounding factors. The defendant or his/her counsel would doubtless attempt to defer to experts, but this arabesque is likely to be interpreted by the jury as the defendant physician merely being poorly informed. If the jury reaches this conclusion, they are likely to reason, 'How can this physician recommend (i.e. 'dictate' to the vulnerable patient) a course of action if he/she cannot explain it to us?'

Importantly, many cases settled out of court are *de facto* considered 'lost' by US physicians. Even if no individual settlement costs are incurred, considerable loss of time occurs away from practice and considerable mental anguish is generated. Moreover, all settlements in excess of $50,000 are recorded in the National Practitioner Data Bank. Whenever hospital re-appointments or appointments are sought, a physician's profile must be queried. In some states (Massachusetts) the public can phone to obtain a physician's profile. Further recall that an insurance carrier can 'settle' cases without approbation of the defendant physician, including those for sums greater than $50,000.

Offering an invasive procedure to women of all ages

A strong case can be made for offering CVS or amniocentesis to women of all ages. Indeed, our centre and many others in the US have for years performed such procedures on all younger women who request it and are counselled properly. If an invasive procedure were offered to women of any age, this author believes that relatively few under age 35 would accept, mostly women 30–34 years. I suspect few women under age 30 will wish to be tested directly, i.e. without prior maternal serum screening. If as predicted lower utilisation occurs in younger women, a policy of universally offering an invasive procedure would probably prove cost effective. Other US voices have also called for lowering the age-related threshold, or abandoning it completely (US President's Commission 1983; Druzin *et al.* 1993; Sicherman *et al.* 1995).

An attractive benefit of universal invasive testing would be detecting all autosomal trisomies and all sex chromosomal aneuploidies. The incidence of chromosomal abnormalities at birth is 1 per 160 (Hook and Hamerton 1977); the incidence is about 50% higher at mid trimester. The morbidity of sex chromosomal abnormalities is greater than some imagine, for example major behavioural problems being common in Klinefelter's syndrome. Selected Mendelian disorders (e.g. cystic fibrosis) could be screened. If the procedure-related risks of amniocentesis were not 1 per 200 but rather the 1 per 400 or 500 that many of us believe but cannot prove (Sicherman et al. 1995), a policy of offering invasive testing to women of all ages is likely to be especially attractive to the younger public. Certainly greater patient autonomy would be popular and consistent with women's preferences and expectations.

Offering an invasive procedure to women ≥ 35 years and offering maternal serum screening to women < 35 years

A fourth policy would be to retain the practice of offering an invasive procedure to women age ≥35 but additionally to offer maternal serum analyte screening to all women under age 35 years. This is the current ACOG standard, as already discussed.

Offering an invasive procedure to women ≥ 35 years, offering maternal serum screening to women < 35 years, but allowing women of any age to exercise their choice

A final option is to recommend an invasive procedure as the first option in women ≥ 35 years, to recommend maternal serum screening as the first option in women < 35 years, *but* to inform women in both age categories of the alternatives. This variant of the extant US policy is, in the opinion of this author, highly attractive. Let older women choose serum screening if desired, and let younger women have amniocentesis or CVS if desired. To be fair and acceptable, women in each age group should be informed with equanimity of the two alternatives at the initial encounter. Raising alternative options only at a later time, e.g. offering an invasive test only after results of serum screening results become available, would not seem appropriate.

For years many obstetrician/gynaecologists have been willing to perform amniocentesis or CVS on women under 35 years who desire the procedure, insisting only that patients are aware of procedure-related risks and diagnostic limitations. If this option were routinely offered, some women under 35 might opt for an invasive procedure, but the number overall is not likely to be large. This has been discussed above.

Similarly, some women over 35 years may find attractive the option of maternal serum screening as a first step. A few do approach their own pregnancy in search of the statistical certitude some serum screening devotees envision, deriving aneuploidy risks and balancing arithmetically whether their specific risk does or does not justify an invasive procedure. In my opinion, the number of women ≥ 35 who will use maternal serum screening in this fashion will be limited. Few women/couples wishing to exclude Down syndrome rigidly balance numerically the risk of Down syndrome against the risk of amniocentesis/CVS. Moreover, the relative burden of a pregnancy loss versus a Down syndrome child are not equal. For example, a risk of 1 in 500 or 1 in 600 for Down syndrome is traditionally considered low by geneticists, but it is not necessarily negligible to a professional woman with two normal children and perhaps already ambivalent about another pregnancy. Older women attracted to maternal serum screening as an initial test are more likely to be those having a high-risk pregnancy or having only achieved pregnancy with great difficulty (e.g. *in vitro* fertilisation). This group will find maternal serum screening attractive as a first step, for they wish to avoid, at all costs, jeopardising their pregnancy by an invasive test.

Conclusion

Maternal serum screening as an obligatory first step in detecting Down syndrome does not seem likely to replace extant practices in the United States. The current US (ACOG) recommendation is to continue offering an invasive procedure (amniocentesis or chorionic villus sampling) for women ≥ 35, while offering maternal serum screening to younger women. This author personally finds great merit in simultaneously offering women in each age category the alternative option as well, i.e. invasive procedure for younger women and serum screening for older women. Women ≥ 35 years who have achieved a pregnancy only with difficulty will find maternal serum screening prior to any invasive test attractive. Women under 35 years of age for whom achieving a pregnancy is not a difficulty may bypass maternal serum screening to have an invasive test, especially if aged 30–34 years.

First-trimester maternal serum screening is not yet an option in the US, and first-trimester cohort studies assessing nuchal translucency have not yet generated the same interest in the US as in the UK. The two approaches could be pursued together, or with recovery of fetal cells in maternal blood.

References

American College of Obstetricians and Gynecologists (1982) Prenatal detection of neural tube defects. *ACOG Technical Bulletin*, no. 67. Chicago: ACOG

American College of Obstetricians and Gynecologists (1983) *Guidelines for Perinatal Care.* Washington, DC: ACOG

American College of Obstetricians and Gynecologists, Department of Professional Liability (1985a) *Professional Liability Implications of AFP Tests.* American College Obstetricians and Gynecologists

American College of Obstetricians and Gynecologists (1985b) *Standards for Obstetric-Gynecologic Services*, 6th edn. Washington, DC: ACOG

American College of Obstetricians and Gynecologists (1986) Prenatal detection of neural tube defects. *ACOG Technical Bulletin*, no. 99. Washington, DC: ACOG

American College of Obstetricians and Gynecologists (1994*) Down Syndrome Screening Committee Opinion*, no. 141. Washington, DC: ACOG

American College of Obstetricians and Gynecologists (1996) Maternal serum screening. *ACOG Education Bulletin*, no. 228. Washington, DC: ACOG

Annas, G.J. and Elias, S. (1985) Maternal serum AFP: educating physicians and the public. *Am J Pub Health* **75**, 1374–5

Bahado-Singh, R.O., Tan, A., Deren, O. *et al.* (1996) Risk of Down syndrome and any clinically significant chromosome defect in pregnancies with abnormal triple-screen and normal targeted ultrasonographic results. *Am J Obstet Gynecol* **175**, 824–9

Bevis, D.C.A. (1952) The antenatal prediction of haemolytic disease of the newborn. *Lancet* **i**, 395–8

Brock, D.J. and Sutcliffe, R.G. (1972) Alpha-fetoprotein in the antenatal diagnosis of anencephaly and spina bifida. *Lancet* **ii**, 197–9

Collmann, R.D. and Stoller, A. (1962) A survey of mongoloid births in Victoria, Australia, 1942–1957. *Am J Public Health* **52**, 813–29

de la Cruz, F., Shifrin, H., Elias, S. *et al.* (1995) Prenatal diagnosis by use of fetal cells isolated from maternal blood. *Am J Obstet Gynecol* **173**, 1354–5

Druzin, M.L., Chervenak, F., McCollough, L.B. *et al.* (1993) Should all pregnant patients be offered prenatal diagnosis regardless of age? *Obstet Gynecol* **81**, 615–18

Fuchs, F. and Riis, P. (1956) Antenatal sex determination. *Nature* **177**, 330

Haddow, J.E., Palomaki G.E., Knight, G.J. *et al.* (1992) Prenatal screening for Down's syndrome with use of maternal serum markers. *N Engl J Med* **327**, 588–93

Hook, E.B. (1981) Rates of chromosome abnormalities at different maternal ages. *Obstet Gynecol* **58**, 282–5

Hook, E.B. and Hamerton, J.L. (1977) 'The frequency of chromosome abnormalities detected in consecutive newborn studies – Differences between studies – Results by sex and by severity of phenotypic involvement' in E.B. Hook and I.H. Porter (Eds) *Population Cytogenetics: Studies in Humans,* pp.63–80. New York: Academic Press

Jacobson, C.B. and Barter, R.H. (1967) Intrauterine diagnosis and management of genetic defects. *Am J Obstet Gynecol* **99**, 796–807

Macri, J.N. (1978) Maternal serum-alpha-fetoprotein and low birth-weight. *Lancet* **i**, 660

Makowski, E.L., Prem, D.A. and Kaiser, I.H. (1956) Detection of sex of fetuses by the incidence of sex chromatin body in nuclei of cells in amniotic fluid. *Science* **123**, 542–3

Merkatz, I.R., Nitowsky, H.M., Macri, J.N. *et al.* (1984) An association between low maternal serum alpha-fetoprotein and fetal chromosomal abnormalities. *Am J Obstet Gynecol* **148**, 886–94

Nadler, H.L. (1967) Presentation at The American Society of Human Genetics, Toronto, Canada

Nadler, H.L. and Gerbie, A.B. (1970) Role of amniocentesis in the interauterine detection of genetic disorders. *N Engl J Med* **282**, 596–9

Nadler, H.L. and Messina, A.M. (1969) In utero detection of type-II glycogenosis (Pompe's disease). *Lancet* **ii**, 1277–8

Nadler H.L. and Simpson, J.L. (1979a) Maternal serum alpha-fetoprotein screening: promise not yet fulfilled. *Obstet Gynecol* **54**, 333–4

Nadler, H.L. and Simpson, J.L. (1979b) Maternal serum alpha-fetoprotein screening: promise not yet fulfilled. *Am J Obstet Gynecol* **135**, 1–2

National Academy of Sciences (1975) *Genetics Screening: Programs, Principles and Research.* Washington, DC: National Academy of Sciences

NICHD National Registry for Amniocentesis Study Group. (1976) Mid-trimester amniocentesis for prenatal diagnosis. *JAMA* **236**, 1471

Phillips, O.P., Elias, S., Shulman, L.P. *et al.* (1992) Maternal serum screening for fetal Down syndrome in women less than 35 years of age using alpha fetoprotein, hCG, and unconjugated estriol: a prospective 2-year study. *Obstet Gynecol* **80**, 353–8

Serr, D.M., Sachs, L. and Danon, M. (1955) Diagnosis of sex before birth using cells from the amniotic fluid. *Bull Res Counc Isr* **58**, 137

Sicherman, N., Bombard, A.T. and Rappoport, P. (1995) Current maternal age recommendations for prenatal diagnosis: a reappraisal using the expected utility theory. *Fetal Diagn Ther* **10**, 157–66

Simpson, J.L. (1990) Incidence and timing of pregnancy losses: relevance to evaluating safety of early prenatal diagnosis. *Am J Med Genet* **35**, 165–73

Simpson, J.L. and Nadler, H.L. (1987) Maternal serum alpha-fetoprotein screening in 1987. *Obstet Gynecol* **69**, 134–5

Simpson, J.L., Baum, L.D., Marder, R. *et al.* (1986) Maternal serum alpha-fetoprotein (MSAFP) screening: low and high values for detection of genetic abnormalities. *Am J Obstet Gynecol* **155**, 593–7

Simpson, J.L., Mill, J.L, Holmes, L.B. *et al.* (1987) Low fetal loss rates after ultrasound-proved viability in early pregnancy. *JAMA* **258**, 2555–7

Simpson, N.E., Dallaire, L., Miller, J.R. *et al.* (1976) Prenatal diagnosis of genetic disease in Canada: report of a collaborative study. *Can Med Assoc J* **115**, 739–48

Steele, M.W. and Breg, W.R. Jr (1966) Chromosome analysis of human amniotic-fluid cells. *Lancet* **i**, 383–5

Tabor, A., Madsen, M., Obel, E. *et al.* (1986) Randomized controlled trial of genetic amniocentesis in 4606 low risk women. *Lancet* **i**, 1287–93

Tjio, J.H. and Levan, A. (1956) The chromosome number of man. *Hereditas* **42**, 1–6

UK Collaborative Study on Alpha-fetoprotein in Relation to Neural Tube Defects (1977) Maternal serum-alpha-fetoprotein measurement in antenatal screening for anencephaly and spina bifida in early pregnancy. *Lancet* **i**, 1323–32

United States President's Commission for the Study of Ethical Problems in Medicine and Biomedical and Behavioral Research: Screening and Counseling for Genetic Conditions (1983) *A Report on the Ethical, Social and Legal Implications of Genetic Screening.* Counseling and Education Programs. Washington: Government Printing Office

Chapter 11

Consequences from second trimester screening

Discussion

Whittle: Could I ask Professor Chard about the term 'effectiveness of screening'. There is a great deal of confusion in people's minds about what we mean by effectiveness. We talked yesterday about the ability of a test to detect Down syndrome. Is that what people mean by effectiveness? Or is it the application of a screening programme to produce a reduction in the live births of conditions such as Down syndrome? Those two issues need to be separated, because there clearly would be confusion in that area. We have talked a great deal about the ability of tests to detect things, but we really need to consider whether that ability will ultimately have an effect which will be presumably what people want, namely a reduction in the number of Down syndrome babies born.

There is a thread running through this now, about what is right for an individual and what is right for the population. That is another component.

Chard: I used the term 'effectiveness' rather loosely, but if anything, implicitly, according to your last definition, in a rather simplistic view of detection rates versus false positive rates. You want to pick up as many cases as possible for as little trauma as possible. That was what I meant by effective, but I take your point totally about the extra dimensions to the use of that term.

Cuckle: In the current context, if we compare first trimester and second trimester, then we must start off by doing this in a purely theoretical way, looking at theoretical detection rates and false positive rates, and then factoring in differential acceptability rates – although I do not think there is any evidence of differential acceptability for first and second trimesters. In coming up with policy decisions there, that distinction may not be a problem.

I have just realised that what I have just said was not quite right because ultrasound is a bigger player in the first trimester than in the second. We do have evidence that ultrasound is more acceptable than biochemistry, and has a higher uptake rate.

Whittle: There is an important need to distinguish first and second trimester effectiveness in that way because, in the first trimester, we are dealing with Down syndrome and let us say that 50% will not make it through spontaneously to term. Later in pregnancy, we know that that number is less. When we are looking at the final result of screening, which will be how many live born babies with that condition appear, that is when the importance in comparing effectiveness comes about.

Cuckle: That is already taken care of in the detection rate estimates, or it should be. You are right to say that there is a problem there, but the first trimester detection rate should take account of that extra fetal loss. Perhaps there are insufficient data to do that, but that should be the aim in any event.

Chard: Perhaps Professor Whittle's problem is the old one of whether we are detecting the same cases with the same prognosis in the first as in the second trimester.

Marteau: I would like to comment on the rather provocative sections in Professor Chard's chapter concerning the use of the term 'counselling' and ask him where his evidence comes from for an increase in counselling, and then go on to comment a little on national policies in the area of screening.

Counselling is a highly skilled activity and counselling skills are neither appropriate nor indeed feasible for routine obstetric practice. This is quite contentious and I am aware of that. It would neither be desirable nor possible to train obstetricians and midwives to become fully fledged counsellors. We are really talking about people in obstetric care who are presenting these tests having general consultation skills, and, in particular, skills in giving complex information effectively. It would be much more realistic to focus on that. When we start to use the term 'counselling', it is vague and slightly mystifying and it engenders a deal of scepticism.

Professor Chard suggests that the amount of counselling going on in antenatal clinics in this area is rising exponentially. I do not know where his evidence for that comes from. There is certainly a good deal more chat about tests in clinics, and much of this chat concerns the fact that there are lots of tests, how much they cost and where they can be obtained, but I do not have any evidence to show that the amount of good quality information and the effectiveness of the transmission of that information has risen over the last 10, 15 or 20 years.

This leads me into my final comment. You were talking about national or regional screening policies – this is a UK issue – in this area. You suggest that this goes against political tides for the way the NHS is organised, but that is not the explanation as to why we do not have national screening policies in the area of prenatal screening. We do have national screening programmes for breast cancer and cervical screening, as well as neonatal screening programmes. One of the reasons why we do not have a national policy in this area is because, politically, it is deemed to be inappropriate to have a screening policy where there is no treatment and all that can be offered is termination of pregnancy. That political sensitivity means that there is not a will to have a national screening policy, certainly in the UK.

I would, however, argue that we do need to have a national policy on the provision of information in this area – not in providing the screening, but the way in which it is to be conducted. Without that, we have a *laissez-faire* system which is basically a jumble, and we are not conducting our screening appropriately. A national policy, just in that specific area, might be very helpful.

Chard: I do not disagree with anything Professor Marteau says. My slide [shown during my presentation] showed a personal estimate of the rapid increase in counselling activities over the period 1970–1990. Most people involved would agree that there has indeed been a substantial increase in the actual time spent on this activity. My diagram showed a further major increase between 1990 and 2000. I believe that to be true, though obviously it is an extrapolation.

The great contribution that you make to this whole topic – you and others like you working in this particular area, and why it must obviously be continued – is to indicate the minimum set of an amount of counselling that is acceptable within the limits of the resources and the time available. That is clearly hugely important. I put up that picture as a provocation deliberately for you. Let this be the challenge to stop a process and to bring some rationality to this process. There is an opposite extreme, and to the degree that I went to an extreme, it was to provoke exactly the perfectly reasonable response which you have made.

National versus regional policies. I think you finished up almost agreeing with me. On the one hand you saw that you could not really disagree – there really are not too many national and regional policies in this country, and the majority of action is at the district level. At the same time you suggested that was a pity, because it would be nice to have national and regional policies. I am not disagreeing that we should have national and regional policies. I think we should, but I am saying that the reality at this time is that we do not, and we do not look like getting them.

Marteau: I am saying that when we are talking about screening, it is possible to have national policies, and that is different.

Chard: It is possible. And the other examples you give – I do not disagree that it is possible to have a policy – but I am just saying that for Down syndrome screening we do not.

Cuckle: The reason we have counselling in breast cancer screening is because the Government is paying. That is the only reason – otherwise we would not have a national breast screening programme. I cannot see the Government paying for any antenatal screening. As has been pointed out, it is moving further and further away from central Government paying, and towards GPs – it is moving away even from district policy.

Simpson: I have a comment on the counselling issue. I am not sure I would agree with the amount of time increasing. At least, in the States, it certainly is not, and arguably it is becoming worse. It is becoming worse because physicians are seeing figures and graphs pointing out that their productivity needs to increase by about 50% over the next 5–7 years if their income flow is to remain the same. So, if anything, they are seeing more patients in a shorter period of time. *De facto*, with the introduction of various technologies, the patients are increasingly being given brochures and that is the counselling: 'Look at this.'

Getting back to your statement about directive versus non-directive, again, that is a myth, because if you look at individual practices, a physician's patients will either have 90% acceptance of the screening technique, or 10% acceptance. Obviously, the way in which it has been presented has forced that patient into one pathway or the other. In the US, increasingly counselling only occurs after you have had a positive test and then everybody is educated in a hurry, physician and patient alike. Until then, there has been only arguably properly informed consent.

Aitken: Could I ask how Professor Marteau measures the effectiveness of counselling? I am sure I have heard somewhere that, in the context of screening for Down syndrome, if proper counselling is given, then the uptake of screening goes down. At the moment, the uptake is really too high because people do not know what they are getting into. What is the optimum level of uptake which we should look for?

Marteau: That is two separate questions. In answer to your first question about counselling, I go back to my earlier comments. I do not actually use the term 'counselling'. It would depend on what stage of the process we are talking about. If we are talking about the stage of presenting the test to people, we are talking about giving people information. That will obviously involve a certain number of communication skills. In terms of giving information I would go for looking at what people have understood about the test – that is what my outcome measure there would comprise.

As to your question about what is the optimal uptake, I think you know. If the purpose of offering tests is to allow people to make informed decisions, one needs first of all to have an operational definition of what an informed decision is, and therefore the outcome measure will be the proportion of people offered the test who have made an informed decision. The uptake rate then becomes irrelevant.

Grudzinskas: Could I ask Professor Chard to develop his conclusion a little further? His conclusion was that the introduction of screening into the first trimester will be far more difficult in the first trimester than in the second trimester. We should explore that for a moment.

Chard: Just to expand on what I said, I do not think I said *far* more – I just said more difficult, or something like that, because nothing is that extreme. I would raise two particular points – one of which I have already covered and another which I did not.

The point I have already raised is that there is at least the option or possibility – indeed, probability in some cases – of parallel running of two tests of approximately similar specification. That, frankly, is not easy unless people are prepared to make an abrupt change from one to the other. I say that with all due respect to those who might feel differently, but nevertheless, most of us would not be in a position necessarily to make an overnight change of that type.

That did not exist when we introduced second trimester testing. That was a 'green field' situation. We had a test, albeit at that time not a good test, but definitely considerably better than that which had been made available before, i.e. AFP in combination with maternal age was better than maternal age alone.

The other point I would make about first trimester testing goes back to one of the points I made earlier. Remember, second trimester testing was the natural successor to the old NTD testing. All the customers were already being lined up at 15–18 weeks for a blood test. Indeed, as Professor Simpson emphasised, it was the same blood test and it was very easy – you merely adjusted your analytical programme a little to accommodate Down syndrome. At this time, however, we do not have a population of clients who regularly expect to attend in that 9–12 week window in quite the same way that they are being educated to in the particular case of NTD screening.

You could go back into the 1970s and in the experience of that time one of the earliest of our own papers described exactly that process, whereby when we started in the 15–18 week window in 1973 we actually had relatively few takers, but it went up as a result of experience, practice and education, into the 1980s and 1990s. So I am not pessimistic that we cannot achieve this in the first trimester, but it is not in place at present.

Whittle: One of the major practical problems with introducing first trimester screening of any sort would be that of getting patients along at an appropriate time. A survey which has just been finished through the Royal College of Obstetricians and Gynaecologists and Royal College of Radiologists indicates that probably most women book at around 14 weeks, and that would set them up very nicely for second trimester screening. The system alone, even if their GP refers them, has a kind of turgidity that does not allow them to appear, presumably, until 13 or 14 weeks. One could imagine a major practical issue there about getting people along at an appropriate time, and this is an educational problem.

Nicolaides: That is why you have to look at Down syndrome screening in relation to the whole of antenatal care and the changes in antenatal care. In the past we did not have anything useful to offer women in early pregnancy and therefore they did not present early because we did not ask them to come before 16 weeks. If there is a new method of screening that requests them to come earlier, there is extremely good evidence that they would do so.

The evidence for that is based on two things. First of all, women know when they become pregnant on the basis of amenorrhoea and positive pregnancy test. Second, they do visit their general practitioners almost immediately they get pregnant. It is we who did not want them to come to the hospitals, it is not the women not realising what the signs and symptoms of pregnancy were that failed to present early.

The second part of the evidence is that in the centres that have introduced first trimester screening the uptake has been more than 80% and they did turn up. There was a reason for them to go. The whole system managed that quite well.

Simpson: I was going to say much the same thing. I would only add that the availability of home pregnancy tests is quite widespread, at least in the United States and I suspect here too. It is extremely popular and in most private practice settings, and in many non-private practice settings, it is unusual for a patient to come in asking whether she is pregnant: she is telling you that she is pregnant and she is ready to start her prenatal care.

Macintosh: I would like to add the point about the training of people who will perform the invasive testing in the first trimester. We are clearly not prepared for that in our speciality at the moment. For me, that is one of the most practical issues.

Nicolaides: I would like to add to the comment made by Professor Simpson. Contrary to what you believe, the risk of amniocentesis causing miscarriage is not less than one in 100. Actually, there is evidence from confidential surveys showing that the risk of amniocentesis causing miscarriage is in the region of 3–4% in some district general hospitals. Therefore, there is pressure to introduce systems as in Denmark which almost centralise the whole country into one centre. The so-called routine, safe techniques such as amniocentesis are not really safe at all, and even for these procedures you would require specialist centres.

Dr Macintosh's point that in the first trimester we would need CVS and therefore we would properly need trained people, is absolutely right, but to me, and I think Professor Whittle agrees, it must also be true for the second trimester. Amniocentesis in the second trimester must be done by fetal medicine experts who would also know how to carry out CVS.

Macri: In my experience of speaking with both clinicians and parents groups throughout the States, the views I receive are very clear that, if the figures hold up – and the figures certainly seem to be saying that what we can do in the first trimester is at present as good if not better than what we can do in the second – then the patients and clinicians will demand the service. There is no question about that.

Grudzinskas: I would make a brief point to address the concerns that Professor Whittle has raised and Professor Nicolaides has emphasised. There is a changing face to the sort of care that obstetricians provide, certainly at a national policy level in this country. Our focus will very much be on the first half of pregnancy, much earlier than is currently the case.

Professor Chard has some experience of the introduction of screening in the first trimester at an anecdotal level. He is aware of how turgid the whole system is in relation to shifting the provision of care from the second trimester to the first trimester. We should not indulge in too much anecdote, but perhaps Professor Chard would like to comment.

Chard: I would only say yes, and add that a paper is presently in press, describing our experience of 4000 cases at the Homerton Hospital which could be regarded as a typical, slightly upmarket, district level hospital. Our uptake is probably now well in excess of 50% of all the people coming through, but rising rapidly because we are in the early phase of it.

Alberman: It is time someone asked about the cost of bringing the screening process forward. I did not agree with most of what Professor Chard said, but I wanted to point out that the decision making is not so much at the obstetric level but at the purchaser level. I know our purchasers are changing, but we shall have to persuade the purchasers that any change is worthwhile, because they will ask what else we will not do in order to pay for any inevitable increase in cost. A little discussion about costs would be appropriate.

Cuckle: I agree with that entirely. In the five years I have been in Yorkshire I have been trying to persuade purchasers to purchase even basic second trimester screening. They simply refuse on the basis of costs. Perhaps you could bring some data to this.

Nicolaides: I fully agree with everything Professor Chard has said. I agree that the introduction of first trimester screening would be much more difficult largely because of public health planning requiring evidence-based medicine to justify decisions to pay for new services. Since this will be difficult to fund or to have the evidence accepted as adequate, the introduction of first trimester screening will be difficult. That is the main issue.

In terms of economics, first trimester screening will be much cheaper. This is mainly because, with second trimester biochemistry, we deliberately did not include the real costs which are ultrasound and counselling. Those are the real costs of serum biochemistry in the first, second or third trimester. If, as part of the appropriate introduction of serum biochemistry, either in the first or in the second trimester, you have ultrasound scanning as part of the package, then you are already paying for the vast majority of the costs of introducing earlier screening, and you are not actually increasing the costs.

Wald: It is not as specific as that. The main determinant of whether there should be a shift from second trimester to first trimester screening should be efficacy and safety which has to be determined quantitatively and against consistent standards, for example, detection rate being the birth detection rate and not the variable detection rate obtained during pregnancy.

Much of that judgement will have to depend on the quantitative assessment of that evidence, which we clearly have not yet done. We may do at the end of this meeting, but I suspect that we will not because I do not believe at the moment that there are sufficient data to say whether first is sufficiently better than second trimester to warrant the shift. We must wait and see. But that is what should drive the issue, and I think it will.

The secondary factor will be if first trimester is more effective and safe than second trimester screening, what is the relative cost-effectiveness? If it is a comparable cost, then clearly one should shift to earlier screening. If it is better but more expensive there will be a dilemma. If is it not better and it is more expensive, there will be no dilemma and we will stay with 15 week screening. The issue has to be determined on efficacy, safety, and cost – anything else is simply opinion.

Cuckle: That is a very good point at which to end this session. That is a point which I fully endorse.

I would like to make one last Chairman's comment. There are two aspects to the history of the introduction of both NTD screening and Down screening. One is that it has been rather drawn out, so that every new development has taken ten years to get into real practice. It has also been marred by unnecessary controversy. Many of the people who have been involved in the controversy over second trimester screening, both for NTDs and for Down syndrome are in this room now. If we can use this meeting to come to some kind of consensus then we will be able to move more rapidly into the first trimester with a good policy statement from us than would have been the case without this meeting.

SECTION 4

BIOCHEMICAL TESTS IN FIRST TRIMESTER SCREENING

Chapter 12

hCG and its subunits in first trimester Down syndrome screening

Kevin Spencer

The biology of hCG

hCG is a 39.5 kDa dimeric glycoprotein consisting of two different subunits, α (15 kDa) and β (23 kDa). The α subunit is identical to that of the other pituitary glycoprotein hormones, luteinising hormone (LH), follicle stimulating hormone (FSH) and thyroid stimulating hormone (TSH), whilst the β subunits of each hormone are distinct and confer biological activity on the intact hormone. Approximately 80% sequence homology occurs between the β subunit of LH and that of hCG. Only the intact dimeric hormone has biological activity although there is some evidence for the existence of a receptor for the free β subunit (Gillott *et al.* 1996). The synthesis of hCG by the syncytiotrophoblast involves an independent translation of the respective mRNAs for the α and β subunits. At least six genes (on chromosome 19) are known to code for the β subunit with only two of these being transcribed and expressed in the placenta. One gene (on chromosome 6), expressed in both the pituitary and the placenta , codes for the α subunit. Post-translational glycosylation of the subunits occurs before the subunits are released in the form of free α (α-hCG) or free β (β-hCG), along with the combined form of intact hCG.

Regulation of the synthesis of hCG is poorly understood, although it is considered that the production of the β subunit is the rate-limiting step in the formation of intact hCG. Cyclic AMP, insulin, calcium, interleukin-1, fibroblast growth factor, placental derived gonadotrophin releasing hormone and epidermal growth factor are all know to have a positive effect on β subunit production, whereas prolactin, progesterone and inhibin all have a negative effect. More detailed descriptions of the biology, structure and nomenclature of hCG can be found in Ren and Braunstein (1992), Bellet and Bidart (1989) and Stenman *et al.* (1993).

Second trimester screening for Down syndrome

The observation by Merkatz *et al.* (1984) of an association between low levels of maternal serum α-fetoprotein (AFP) and pregnancies affected by fetal chromosomal abnormalities was the beginning of a decade of research into finding more specific biochemical markers for screening for Down syndrome. Although AFP was not a particularly specific marker for Down syndrome (Spencer and Carpenter 1985), the identification of an association between high levels of maternal serum intact hCG and Down syndrome by Bogart *et al.* (1987), the demonstration of an association between lower levels of maternal serum unconjugated oestriol and Down syndrome by Canick *et al.* (1988), the development of multi-analyte screening procedures (Wald *et al.* 1988) and the identification of a more specific association between high levels of maternal serum free β-hCG and Down syndrome (Macri *et al.*1990; Spencer 1991; Spencer *et al.* 1992a) are perhaps significant milestones along this path. Many other analytes have been investigated in the second trimester and their individual performance can be assessed by comparing the Mahalanobis distance (Reynolds 1994), such that the larger the distance the more discriminatory is the marker. Table 12.1 summarises the best estimates to date for the marker Mahalanobis distances in the second trimester. This shows the pre-eminent position of free β-hCG in the discrimination between unaffected and Down syndrome affected pregnancies in the second trimester, and when used in combination with AFP, has led to prospective detection rates within the range 65–75% at a 5% false positive rate (Spencer 1994a; Macri *et al.* 1994). This simple two analyte protocol is now used by over 40% of laboratories screening in the UK with those using a three analyte protocol (including unconjugated oestriol along with AFP, total-hCG (or free β-hCG)) being less than 20% (Cuckle *et al.* 1995b).

Table 12.1.   Mahalanobis distances for various biochemical markers in the second trimester

Marker	Mahalanobis distance
Urea-resistant neutrophil alkaline phosphatase (URNAP)	1.80 (based only on one published study)
Free β-hCG	1.66
Urine free β-hCG	1.47
Urine β-core	1.40
Total or intact hCG	1.36
Dimeric inhibin A	1.04
Free α-hCG	0.98
uE$_3$	0.92
Total immunoreactive inhibin	0.85
AFP	0.71
SP1	0.35
PAPP-A	0.25
CA125	0.16

Table 12.2. Studies of intact or total hCG in cases of Down syndrome in the first trimester

Study	Median MoM	No. of cases
Cuckle *et al.* (1988)	1.10	22
Brock *et al.* (1990)	1.43	21
Johnson *et al.* (1991)	0.91	11
Kratzner *et al.* (1991)	1.23	17
Hogdall *et al.* (1992)	1.10	14
Van Lith (1992)	1.19	24
Aitken *et al.* (1993)	0.97	16
Crandall *et al.* (1993)	1.73	11
Iles *et al.* (1993)	1.35	25
Macintosh *et al.* (1994)	1.40	20
Kellner *et al.* (1994)	0.90	5
Brizot *et al.* (1995)	1.50	41
Wald *et al.* (1996)	1.23	77
Total	1.25 (95% CI 1.08–1.42)	304

Intact or total hCG in the first trimester

In the first trimester there have been some 12 studies in which intact or total hCG has been measured in cases of Down syndrome and the levels compared against an unaffected control population. Table 12.2 summarises the results of these studies and shows on average, that in the first trimester, unlike the second trimester, levels of intact or total hCG are raised to only a very small extent. The size of this elevation when measured against the standard deviation of the distribution produces a small Mahalanobis distance of 0.21 and therefore offers poor discrimination between affected and unaffected populations.

Free α-hCG in the first trimester

In the second trimester, studies with free α-hCG have been somewhat conflicting with evidence for either no increase in the median MoM in Down syndrome pregnancies (Spencer 1993), evidence suggesting levels are twice that in unaffected pregnancies (Bogart *et al.* 1987; Kratzner *et al.* 1991) and evidence suggesting a much more subtle increase to approximately 1.25 MoM (Ryall *et al.* 1992; Spencer 1994b; Wald *et al.* 1994). Despite the more recent data, a substantive case for the use of free α-hCG in screening for Down syndrome in the second trimester has not been established. In the first trimester, data similarly show near-normal values of free α-hCG in pregnancies affected by Down syndrome (Table 12.3), suggesting that this marker will be of little value at this time.

Table 12.3.   Studies of free α-hCG in cases of Down syndrome in the first trimester

Study	Median MoM	No. of cases
Ozturk *et al.* 1990	1.29[a]	9
Kratzner *et al.* 1991	0.77	17
Iles *et al.* 1993	1.00	25
Macintosh *et al.* 1994	1.06	22
Wald *et al.* 1996	0.86	77
Total	0.94 (95% C I 0.52–1.07)	150

[a] Calculated from data presented in the paper.

Free β-hCG in the first trimester

Median levels of free β-hCG in the first trimester

In the first trimester values of free β-hCG reach a peak at around 64 days with values then declining in an almost linear fashion by 1 IU/l (1ng/ml) per day (Berry *et al.* 1995; Spencer *et al.* 1997b; Wald *et al.* 1996; Krantz *et al.* 1996). Typical values observed for these free-β medians are: 9 weeks, 73.3 IU/l; 10 weeks, 62.6 IU/l; 11 weeks, 48.7 IU/l; 12 weeks, 36.3 IU/l; 13 weeks, 26.7 IU/l.

Population parameters and detection rates

Spencer *et al.* (1992b) were the first group to make an association between raised levels (1.85 MoM) of free β-hCG in the maternal serum of pregnancies complicated by Down syndrome in the first trimester. Ozturk *et al.* (1990) some two years earlier had measured both free α- and free β-hCG and the free subunit ratios in a range of pregnancies complicated by either trisomy 18 (eight cases) or trisomy 21 (nine cases). Although they observed low ratios due to low levels of free β-hCG in trisomy 18 cases, despite observing a median MoM for the ratio of 1.68 in the trisomy 21 cases (and a free β-hCG MoM calculated from their data of 1.62), they concluded that, 'no consistent changes in α- or β-subunit ratios were observed in trisomy 21 or other chromosomal abnormalities'.

The initial study by Spencer *et al.* (1992b) was extended in a further study of 25 additional cases, when the median MoM was found to be 2.34 (Macri *et al.* 1993). Since 1993 a number of studies (Table 12.4) have confirmed the initial observation of increased levels of free β-hCG in the first trimester, and the median value from this large world series is now very similar to the elevated levels observed in the second trimester (Macri *et al.* 1994; Cuckle 1995). In addition to providing median data, a number of the larger studies have also provided data on the standard deviation of the distribution of free β-hCG in unaffected and/or Down syndrome cases and from the actual raw MoM results presented in other studies it is possible to obtain some consensus estimates of population parameters in the first trimester (Table 12.5). The consensus estimate would seem to indicate that the $\log_{10}$ SD distribution in both unaffected and Down populations is approximately

Table 12.4.   Studies of free β-hCG in cases of Down syndrome in the first trimester

Study	Median MoM	No. of cases
Ozturk *et al.* 1990	1.62 [a]	9
Spencer *et al.* 1992b	1.85	13
Macri *et al.* 1993	2.34	25
Iles *et al.* 1993	1.52	25
Pescia *et al.* 1993	2.03	5
Macintosh *et al.* 1994	2.10	21
Brambati *et al.* 1994	1.13	13
Kellner *et al.* 1994	2.20	5
Brizot *et al.* 1995	2.00	41
Spencer (unpublished)	2.21	13
Biagiotti *et al.* 1995	2.00	41
Noble *et al.* 1995	2.13	61
Krantz *et al.* 1996	2.09	22
Wald *et al.* 1996	1.79	77
Spencer *et al.* 1997b	1.72	22
Berry *et al.* 1997	1.99	54
Total	1.94 (95% C I 1.68–2.09)	447

[a] Calculated from data presented in the paper.

Table 12.5.   Studies of free β-hCG in the first trimester providing SD information or from which SD information can be derived

Study	Population	No. of cases	SD	Stated/derived
Ozturk *et al.* (1990), Macri *et al.* (1993), Kellner *et al.* (1994), Brambati *et al.* (1994)	Down	52	0.2636	Derived
Macintosh *et al.* (1994)	Down	21	0.3868	Derived
Noble *et al.* (1995)	Down	102	0.2953	Derived
Spencer *et al.* (1994a)	Unaffected	320	0.2950	Stated
	Down	21	0.1669	Stated
Biagiotti *et al.* (1995)	Unaffected	246	0.2208	Stated
	Down	41	0.2294	Stated
Berry *et al.* (1995)	Unaffected	8600	0.288	Stated
Berry *et al.* (1996)	Unaffected	10600 [a]	0.289	Stated
	Down	54	0.306	Stated
Krantz *et al.* (1996)	Unaffected	483	0.1737	Stated
	Down	22	0.2910	Stated
Spencer *et al.* (1997b)	Unaffected	373	0.2642	Stated
	Down	22	0.3732	Stated
Wald *et al.* (1996)	Unaffected	385	0.2833	Stated
	Down	77	0.2870	Stated

[a] An extension of the Berry *et al.* (1995) study.

0.29 and that the $\log_{10}$ mean of the Down population from the world-wide series is 0.2878. Both of these figures are similar to those observed in second trimester (Spencer *et al.* 1992a), with the suggestion that the median value of free β in first trimester Down cases may be about 20% lower than in the second trimester. On the basis of these best estimates of the population parameters, free β-hCG alone, at a 5% false positive rate, would identify 27% of Down syndrome cases – a figure which is approximately 15% less than in second trimester (Spencer *et al.* 1992a). When the free β-hCG distribution is modelled together with the maternal age distribution of pregnancies in England and Wales with a univariate gaussian algorithm, using free β-hCG and maternal age in the first trimester would achieve detection rates in the order of 45% at a 5% false positive rate. This has now been confirmed in a number of practical studies (Biagiotti *et al.* 1995; Krantz *et al.* 1996; Berry *et al.* 1997). This figure of 45% compares with the 54% achieved in the second trimester (Spencer *et al.* 1992a). Similarly, pregnancy associated plasma protein A (PAPP-A), particularly when measured in early first trimester (before 12 weeks), appears to offer similar levels of detection and when both are combined together with maternal age the prospects of a 60–65% detection rate at a 5% false positive rate may be observed (Krantz *et al.* 1996; Wald *et al.* 1996; Berry *et al.* 1997), which is close to the 62% being achieved by use of AFP + total hCG + unconjugated oestriol + maternal age (triple test) and close to the 75% achieved by use of AFP + free β-hCG + maternal age during second trimester screening (Macri and Spencer 1996).

Within pregnancy biological variability between first and second trimester

In any consideration in moving screening from second trimester to first trimester, one important question that we will need to have some answers to relates to the relationship between marker levels in the first and second trimester, particularly for free β-hCG which is a marker that has a universal application across both trimesters. Furthermore, we would want to be sure that high first trimester levels of this marker were not just identifying those cases of trisomy 21 which were destined to abort spontaneously before the end of the first or early second trimester. To answer some of these issues we have investigated the within person biological variability of the marker across the two trimesters and obtained information on how the marker levels vary across both trimesters in cases of Down syndrome which reach second trimester or even term. Some preliminary information on these questions is already available albeit with relatively small numbers of cases of Down syndrome. Spencer *et al.* (1994b) published 12 cases of Down syndrome with data in both first and second trimester and showed that median free β-hCG MoMs were fractionally lower in the first trimester than in the second trimester (2.04 versus 2.07). A further nine cases collected as part of further studies (Macri *et al.* 1993; Spencer 1995, unpublished results) showed an even wider difference of 2.06 in first trimester and 2.56 in the second trimester. Data from the large series of 45 cases in the study by Berry *et al.* (1997) showed a similar pattern of lower values in first trimester (1.99 versus 2.79). When all these data are combined together the 66 sample series shows a first trimester median of 2.06 and a second trimester median of 2.61. Figure 12.1 shows a plot of the individual results. More data exist for the unaffected population, which tends to show a greater correlation of free β MoM between the two trimesters. Figure 12.2

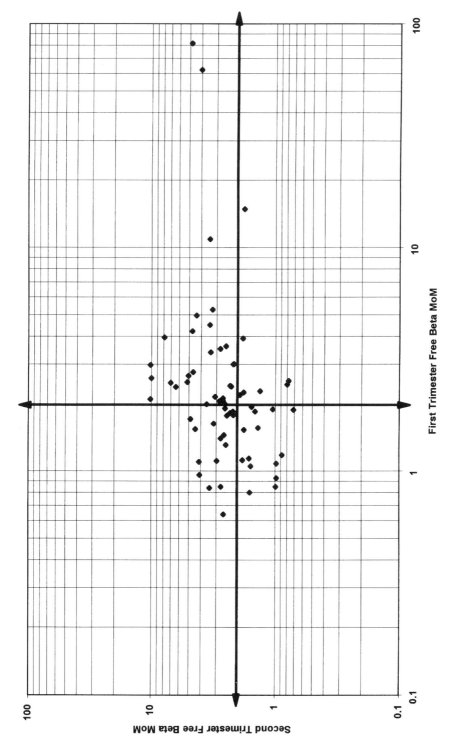

Fig. 12.1. Free β-hCG MoMs in 66 Down syndrome pregnancies in both the first and second trimester. (The bold arrowed line indicates an arbitrary 2.00 MoM cut off.)

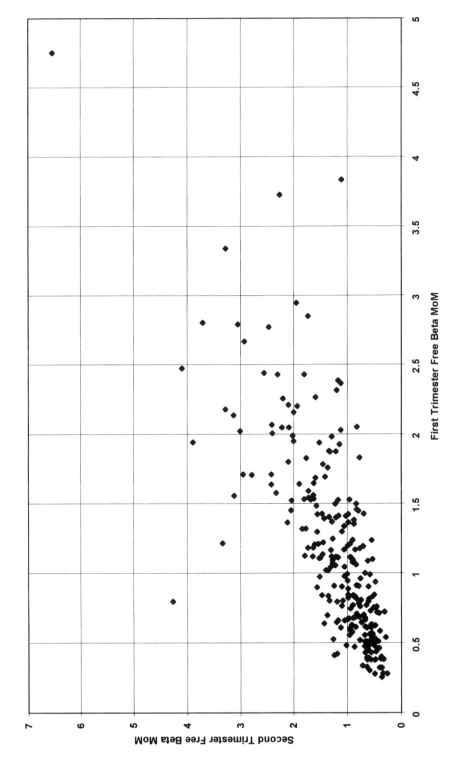

Fig. 12.2.   Free β-hCG MoMs in 300 unaffected pregnancies in the first and second trimester.

shows a typical plot of series of some 300 cases in which the correlation coefficient was 0.729 with a slope of 0.841 and an intercept of 0.245. On the whole, the degree of correlation in either group would suggest that, in the main, a significant proportion of those cases identified in second trimester with raised free β-hCG are likely also to have raised levels in the first trimester, but with a lower overall median MoM. This would support the fact that the world series data in first trimester suggest a smaller Mahalanobis distance (1.1), hence leading to a slightly poorer detection rate performance than observed for free β-hCG in the second trimester.

Multiple pregnancy

In twin pregnancies in the second trimester median values of free β-hCG are approximately twice that found in singleton pregnancies. The median MoM observed in published second trimester series (Spencer *et al.* 1994b; Wald *et al.* 1994; Barnabei *et al.* 1995) containing some 844 cases is 2.06. In those pregnancies in which one twin is affected by Down syndrome, the median MoM in a second trimester series of eight cases was 3.34 (Spencer *et al.* 1994b) and using AFP, free β-hCG and maternal age it was suggested that 50% of twin cases could be identified. In the first trimester values in twins are also increased with the median MoM in 48 unaffected twin pregnancies being 1.73 (Spencer *et al.* 1996, un-published results) but somewhat lower than observed in the second trimester, although data from a much larger series of 136 normal twins showed a median MoM of 1.94, suggesting that it may not be that different from the situation in second trimester (Noble *et al.* 1997). When cases of twins concordant ($n=2$) or discordant ($n=10$) for trisomy 21 were examined in the first trimester (Noble *et al.* 1997), this group found the median MoM in the 12 cases to be 3.10 although they could not achieve the same level of discrimination that had been observed by Spencer *et al.* (1994b) in the second trimester.

Trisomy 18

In cases of trisomy 18 levels of free β-hCG are low in the second trimester and a large series of 52 cases showed the median MoM to be 0.37 in cases not com-plicated by an open neural tube defect or ventral wall defect (Spencer *et al.* 1993). In the first trimester to date there have been some four reports (Ozturk *et al.* 1990; Spencer *et al.* 1992b, 1997b; Brizot *et al.* 1995) containing cases of trisomy 18 with a total number of 39 cases giving a median MoM of 0.31. This again shows very close similarity with the situation in second trimester.

Turner's syndrome

In cases of Turner's syndrome, second trimester levels of free β-hCG are increased to around 4.00 MoM (Laundon *et al.* 1996). Limited data are available in first trimester but a study including eight cases (Spencer *et al.* 1997b) with a median MoM of 1.82 suggests that, as in the second trimester, free β-hCG is also elevated but perhaps not quite to the same level.

Filter paper spot measurement of serum free β-hCG

Macri *et al.* (1996) demonstrated the advantages to be gained in screening for neural tube defects and Down syndrome using maternal blood samples collected from a finger stick onto filter paper as blood spots. These advantages include ease of sample collection, elimination of transport tube breakage, improved biological hazard control, reduced specimen degradation or haemolysis during transport delays, minimisation of the effect of specimen mishandling or the influence of extremes of temperature, ease of transport through conventional mailing and improvement in screening detection efficiency or reduced false positive rates. Although this technique is tried and tested in the area of newborn screening, there has been little application to Down syndrome screening. The study by Macri *et al.* (1996) showed the feasibility of the technique in second trimester screening and found it to reduce the false positive rates for NTD risk and Down risk while still maintaining the same detection efficiency as achieved in liquid based screening procedures. The population variance of the two markers (AFP and free β-hCG) was also lower than in published studies from liquid based procedures. Macri *et al.* (1995) have also shown that such a procedure is applicable to screening in the first trimester and this technique offers considerable advantages, particularly if screening at this time takes place in the community rather than in the hospital or clinic environment.

Urine free β-hCG

The major metabolic route for the removal of intact hCG and free β-hCG involves excretion in urine. In urine the major metabolic excretion product of intact hCG involves the renal parenchymal cell breakdown of the β-subunit to a small molecular weight component of 10 kDa, referred to as β-core or urinary gonadotrophin peptide (UGP). Over 90% of the immunoreactive hCG in urine is in this form (Kato and Braunstein 1988). Free β-hCG, because of its small molecular weight, has a high renal clearance rate and is cleared from the circulation and excreted some 10–24 times more rapidly than those subunits combined as intact hCG (Wehmann and Nisula 1979; Cole 1988). Over the last two years considerable attention has been given to urine as a possible vehicle for screening for Down syndrome, particularly in the second trimester with the marker β-core. Cuckle *et al.* (1994) showed in a study of seven cases of Down syndrome that the median MoM was 6.24. In a follow-up study of 24 cases the same group (Cuckle *et al.* 1995a) found a median MoM of 6.02 and predicted detection rates of 80%. Canick *et al.* (1995), using a commercial β-core assay and 14 cases of Down syndrome, observed median levels of 5.34 and also predicted detection rates of 80%. However, Spencer *et al.* (1997b), using the same commercial assay in a study of 29 Down cases, only observed a median of 2.35 and predicted only a 41% detection rate. The lower values for β-core have also been seen in three other studies, one using an assay with poor specificity for β-core (Hayashi and Kozu 1995) which found a median MoM of 1.33 in three cases and two using specific β-core assays when medians of 1.90 in 30 cases (Muller *et al.* 1996, personal communication) and close to 4 in 13 cases (Cole 1996, personal communication) were obtained.

Where free β-hCG has been examined in urine in the second trimester, levels similar to those found in maternal serum (Macri *et al.* 1994) and amniotic fluid (Spencer *et al.* 1997a) have been observed in maternal urine from pregnancies affected by Down syndrome (Spencer *et al.* 1996; Muller *et al.* 1996, personal communication; Cole 1996, personal communication; Hayashi *et al.* 1996). Spencer *et al.* (1996) found levels of 2.47 MoM in a study of 29 Down syndrome cases, Muller *et al.* (1996, personal communication), similarly found levels of 2.86 MoM in a study of 30 Down syndrome cases. Hayashi *et al.* (1996) found levels of 3.52 MoM in a small study of three Down syndrome cases, and Cole (1996, personal communication) found levels of 3.9 MoM in a study of 13 Down syndrome cases. In three of these studies detection rates of 54–58% have been suggested (Spencer *et al.* 1996; Cole 1996, personal communication; Muller *et al.* 1996, personal communication).

In the first trimester, levels of urine free β-hCG and β-core are increased in Down syndrome (Spencer *et al.* 1997b), with average MoMs of 1.87 and 2.91, respectively, although the spread of results in the control and Down populations for both markers is twice that seen in the second trimester, with $\log_{10}$ SDs in the range of 0.53 for free β-hCG and 0.90 for β-core. The ability of both markers to discriminate affected and unaffected cases is considerably poorer than that reported by Spencer *et al.* (1996) in the second trimester. Detection rates for urine free β-hCG and maternal age was 36% at a 5% false positive rate and 34% using β-core, compared with 44% for serum free β-hCG and 82% for nuchal translucency. When combined together, maternal age, nuchal translucency and urine free β-hCG gave a 85% detection rate compared with 87% when serum free β-hCG was used.

It would appear unlikely that any of the urine markers will be of value in first trimester screening and that optimal first trimester screening programmes will develop around the use of nuchal translucency, serum free β-hCG and possibly PAPP-A.

Biochemistry and biophysical markers

Of the markers evaluated to date for use in screening for trisomy 21 in the first trimester, nuchal translucency measured under standardised conditions by trained staff has clearly been demonstrated in a number of centres as the marker offering greatest potential. By combining biochemical markers with biophysical measurements further smaller gains in detection rate over the 80% demonstrated with nuchal translucency (Noble *et al.* 1995) will be achievable, providing the individual markers are independent measures of the risk of Down syndrome. Estimates of the correlation of nuchal translucency particularly with serum free β-hCG have already been established in samples taken in the first trimester and show correlation coefficients close to zero in both unaffected and Down syndrome groups (*r*(Down)=−0.151 *r*(unaffected)=0.010 (Brizot *et al.* 1995); *r*(Down) =0.13 *r*(unaffected)=−0.04 (Noble *et al.* 1995); *r*(Down)=0.000 *r*(unaffected) =0.097 (Spencer *et al.* 1997b)). Although these studies have been carried out in preselected populations derived from women referred to a tertiary referral centre as a result of either increased nuchal translucency or who presented as a result of advance maternal age or previous family history, evidence from an ongoing study of an unselected population suggests that the correlation in unaffected cases is of the same magnitude (*r*(unaffected)=0.007 (Spencer *et al.* 1996, unpublished observations)). Similarly, correlation of nuchal translucency with serum free β-hCG in samples taken in the second trimester is small (r(unaffected)=0.014 (Spencer *et al.* 1996, unpublished observations)). Modelled detection rates using maternal age, serum free β-hCG and nuchal translucency have shown that rates of 85–90% could be achieved at 5% false positive rates with this approach (Noble *et al.* 1995; Spencer *et al.* 1997b).

The future direction

The direction for the future clearly involves the use of nuchal translucency in first trimester screening. Whether the promise that this technique holds can be reproduced in all routine obstetric ultrasound departments remains to be thoroughly tested. Other questions that also require consideration involve the choice of biochemical marker(s). It is likely that because of its universal applicability across both first and second trimester, free β-hCG would be the marker of choice, but if nuchal translucency detection rates of 50–60% are more likely to be the norm, then in order to achieve 80–90% detection rates PAPP-A would also be required. There are some logistical issues around sample timing since preliminary studies have shown that optimal detection using PAPP-A occurs at around 10 weeks of gestation (Bersinger *et al.* 1994; Berry *et al.* 1997; Wald *et al.* 1996). One possible solution might revolve around blood being collected from or by the patient in the community, say by filter paper collection technique, at around the 8–10 or 9–11 week window. This sample would be sent to the laboratory for analysis prior to the patient being seen in the ultrasound department for dating and nuchal translucency scan. When the patient arrived at the clinic for the ultrasound, the biochemical result (in concentration terms) would be available at the clinic and once the patient had been scanned for dates the results could be converted into MoMs and a combined risk calculated incorporating the nuchal translucency,

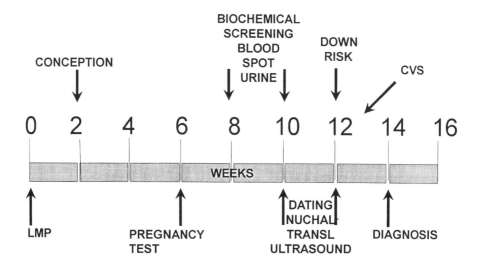

Fig. 12.3.   One possible scenario for a first trimester Down syndrome screening programme.

maternal age and the biochemical measurements. Thus, this would allow for screening to be completed by week 12 and for CVS to be offered and a result confirmed in those cases requiring follow up, prior to week 14 (Figure 12.3).

Although the science for this new development is almost in place, the challenge for the next few years will be to overcome the logistical issues in bringing such a scheme as this into routine service.

References

Aitken, D.A., McCaw, G., Crossley, J.A. *et al.* (1993) First trimester biochemical screening for fetal chromosome abnormalities and neural tube defects. *Prenat Diagn* **13**, 681–9

Barnabei, V.M., Krantz, D.A., Macri, J.N. and Larsen, J.W. (1995) Enhanced twin pregnancy detection within an open neural tube defect and Down syndrome screening protocol using free beta-hCG and AFP. *Prenat Diagn* **15**, 1131–4

Bellet, D. and Bidart, J.-M. (1989) *Structure–Function Relationship of Gonadotrophins.* New York: Raven Press

Berry, E., Aitken, D.A., Crossley, J.A., Macri, J.N. and Connor, J.M. (1995) Analysis of maternal serum alpha-fetoprotein and free beta human chorionic gonadotrophin in the first trimester: implications for Down syndrome screening. *Prenat Diagn* **15**, 555–65

Berry, E., Aitken, D.A., Crossley, J.A., Macri, J.N. and Connor, J.M. (1997) Screening for Down syndrome: changes in marker levels and detection rates between first and second trimesters. *Br J Obstet Gynaecol* (in press)

Bersinger, N.A., Brizot, M.L., Johnson, A. *et al* (1994) First trimester maternal serum PAPP-A and SP1 in fetal trisomies. *Br J Obstet Gynaecol* **101**, 970–4

Biagiotti, R., Cariati, E., Brizzi, L. and D'Agata, A. (1995) Maternal serum screening for Down syndrome in the first trimester of pregnancy. *Br J Obstet Gynaecol* **102**, 660–2

Bogart, M.H., Pandian, M.R. and Jones, O.W. (1987) Abnormal maternal serum chorionic gonadotropin levels in pregnancies with fetal chromosome abnormalities. *Prenat Diagn* **7**, 623–30

Brambati, B., Tului, L., Bonacchi, I., Shrimanker, K., Suzuki, Y. and Grudzinskas, J.G. (1994) Serum PAPP-A and free beta-hCG are first trimester screening markers of Down syndrome. *Prenat Diagn* **14**, 1043–7

Brizot, M.L., Snijders, R.J.M., Butler, J., Bersinger, N.A. and Nicolaides, K.H. (1995) Maternal serum-hCG and fetal nuchal translucency thickness for the prediction of fetal trisomies in the first trimester of pregnancy. *Br J Obstet Gynaecol* **102**, 127–32

Brock, D.J.H., Barron, L., Hollway, S., Liston, W.A., Hillier, S.G. and Seppala, M. (1990) First trimester maternal serum biochemical indicators in Down syndrome. *Prenat Diagn* **10**, 245–51

Canick, J.A., Knight, G.J., Palomaki, G.E., Haddow, J.E., Cuckle, H.S. and Wald, N.J. (1988) Low second trimester maternal serum unconjugated oestriol in pregnancies with Down syndrome. *Br J Obstet Gynaecol* **95**, 330–3

Canick, J.A., Kellner, L.H., Saller, D.N., Palomaki, G.E., Walker, R.P. and Osathanondh, R. (1995) Second trimester levels of maternal urinary gonadotropin peptide in Down syndrome pregnancy. *Prenat Diagn* **15**, 739–44

Cole, L.A. (1988) 'Occurrence and properties of glycoprotein hormone free subunits' in H. Grotjan and B. Keel (Eds) *Microheterogeneity of Glycoprotein Hormones.* Boca Raton, Fl: CRC Press

Crandall, B.F., Hanson, F.W., Keener, S., Matsumoto, M. and Miller, W. (1993) Maternal serum screening for AFP, UE3 and hCG between 11 and 15 weeks of pregnancy to detect fetal chromosomal abnormalities. *Am J Obstet Gynecol* **168**, 1864–9

Cuckle, H. (1995) Improved parameters for risk estimation in Down syndrome screening. *Prenat Diagn* **15**, 1057–65

Cuckle, H.S., Wald, N.J., Barkai, G. *et al.* (1988) First trimester biochemical screening for Down syndrome. *Lancet* **ii**, 851–2

Cuckle, H.S., Iles, R.K. and Chard, T. (1994) Urinary beta core human chorionic gonadotrophin: a new approach to Down syndrome screening. *Prenat Diagn* **14**, 953–8

Cuckle, H.S., Iles, R.K., Sehmi, I.K., Oakey, R.E., Davies, S. and Ind, T. (1995a) Urinary multiple marker screening for Down syndrome. *Prenat Diagn* **15**, 745–51

Cuckle, H.S., Ellis, A.R. and Seth, J. (1995b) Provision of screening for Down syndrome. *BMJ* **311**, 512

Gillott, D.J., Iles, R.K. and Chard, T. (1996) The effects of beta human chorionic gonadotrophin on the in vivo growth of bladder cancer cell lines. *Br J Cancer* **73**, 323–6

Hayashi, M. and Kozu, H. (1995) Maternal urinary beta core fragment of hCG/creatinine ratios and fetal chromosomal abnormalities in the second trimester of pregnancy. *Prenat Diagn* **15**, 11–16

Hayashi, M., Kozu, H. and Takei, H. (1996) Maternal urinary free beta subunit of human chorionic gonadotrophin:creatinine ratios and fetal chromosomal abnormalities in the second trimester of pregnancy. *Br J Obstet Gynaecol* **103**, 577–80

Hogdall, C.K., Hogdall, E.V.S., Arends, J., Nørgaard-Pedersen, B., Smidt-Jensen, S. and Larsen, S.O. (1992) CA125 is a maternal serum marker for Down syndrome in the first and second trimester. *Prenat Diagn* **12**, 223–7

Iles, R.K., Sharma, K., Wathen, N.C. *et al.* (1993) hCG, free subunit and PAPP-A composition of maternal serum in normal and Down syndrome pregnancies. Fourth Conference: Endocrinology and Metabolism in Human Reproduction, London, May (Abstract) p. 32

Johnson, A., Cowchock, F.S., Darby, M., Wapner, R. and Jackson, L.G. (1991) First trimester maternal serum alpha fetoprotein and chorionic gonadotropin as a marker of fetal chromosomal disorders. *Prenat Diagn* **11**, 443–50

Kato, Y. and Braunstein, G.D. (1988) Beta core fragment is a major form of immunoreactive urinary gonadotropin in human pregnancy. *J Clin Endocrinol Metab* **66**, 1197–201

Kellner, L.H., Weiss, R.R., Weiner, Z., Neur, M. and Martin, G. (1994) Early first trimester maternal serum AFP, UE3, hCG and free beta-hCG measurements in unaffected and affected pregnancies with fetal Down syndrome. *Am J Hum Genet* **55**, A281

Krantz, D.A., Larsen, J.W., Buchanan, P.D. and Macri, J.N. (1996) First trimester Down syndrome screening: free beta human chorionic gonadotropin and pregnancy associated plasma protein A. *Am J Obstet Gynecol* **174**, 612–16

Kratzner, P.G., Globus, M.S., Monroe, S.E., Finkelstein, D.E. and Taylor, R.N. (1991) First trimester aneuploidy screening using serum human chorionic gonadotropin. *Prenat Diagn* **11**, 751–63

Laundon, C.H., Spencer, K., Macri, J.N., Anderson, R.W. and Buchanan, P.D. (1996) Free beta-hCG screening of hydropic and nonhydropic Turner's syndrome pregnancies. *Prenat Diagn* **16**, 853–6

Macri, J.N. and Spencer, K. (1996) Toward the optimal protocol for Down syndrome screening. *Am J Obstet Gynecol* **174**, 1668–9

Macri, J.N., Kasturi, R.V., Krantz, D.A. *et al.* (1990) Maternal serum Down syndrome screening: free beta protein is a more effective marker than human chorionic gonadotropin. *Am J Obstet Gynecol* **163**, 1248–53

Macri, J.N., Spencer, K., Aitken, D.A. *et al.* (1993) First trimester free beta-hCG screening for Down syndrome. *Prenat Diagn* **13**, 557–62

Macri, J.N., Spencer, K., Garver, K. *et al.* (1994) Maternal serum free beta-hCG screening: results of studies including 480 cases of Down syndrome. *Prenat Diagn* **14**, 97–103

Macri, J.N., Berry, E., Aitken, D. *et al.* (1995) First trimester free beta-hCG in maternal serum and maternal dried whole blood paper spots. *Am J Hum Genet* **56**, A284

Macri, J.N., Anderson, R.W., Krantz, D.A., Larsen, J.W. and Buchanan, P.D. (1996) Prenatal maternal dried blood screening with alpha fetoprotein and free beta human chorionic gonadotropin for open neural tube defect and Down syndrome. *Am J Obstet Gynecol* **174**, 566–72

Merkatz, I.R., Nitowsky, H.M., Macri, J.N. and Johnson, W.E. (1984) An association between low maternal serum alpha fetoprotein and fetal chromosomal abnormalities. *Am J Obstet Gynecol* **148**, 886–94

Macintosh, M.C.M., Iles, R., Teisner, B. *et al.* (1994) Maternal serum-hCG and PAPP-A, markers for fetal Down syndrome at 8–14 weeks. *Prenat Diagn* **14**, 203–8

Noble, P.L., Abraha, H.D., Snijders, R.J.M., Sherwood, R. and Nicolaides, K.H. (1995) Screening for fetal trisomy 21 in the first trimester of pregnancy: maternal serum free beta-hCG and fetal nuchal translucency thickness. *Ultrasound Obstet Gynecol* **6**, 390–5

Noble, P.L., Snijders, R.J.M., Abraha, H., Sherwood, R. and Nicolaides, K.H. (1997) Screening for fetal trisomies in twin pregnancies: maternal serum free beta-hCG and fetal nuchal translucency thickness. *Br J Obstet Gynaecol* (in press)

Ozturk, M., Milunsky, A. Brambati, B., Sachs, E.S., Miller, S.L. and Wands, J.R. (1990) Abnormal maternal levels of hCG subunits in trisomy 18. *Am J Med Genet* **36**, 480–3

Pescia, G., Marguerat, P.H., Weihs, D. *et al.* (1993) First trimester free beta-hCG and SP1 as markers for fetal chromosomal disorders: a prospective study of 250 women undergoing CVS. Fourth Conference: Endocrinology and Metabolism in Human Reproduction, London, May (Abstract) p.45

Ren, S.G. and Braunstein, G.D. (1992) Human chorionic gonadotropin. *Semin Reprod Endocrinol* **10**, 95–105

Reynolds, T.M. (1994) 'Screening by test combination: a statistical overview' in J.G. Grudzinskas, T. Chard, M. Chapman and H. Cuckle (Eds) *Screening for Down Syndrome*, pp.47–71. Cambridge: Cambridge University Press

Ryall, R.G., Staples, A.J., Robertson, E.F. and Pollard, A.C. (1992) Improved performance in a prenatal screening programme for Down syndrome incorporating serum free-hCG subunit analysis. *Prenat Diagn* **12**, 251–61

Spencer, K. (1991) Evaluation of an assay of the free beta subunit of choriogonadotropin and its potential value in screening for Down syndrome. *Clin Chem* **37**, 809–14

Spencer, K. (1993) Free alpha-hCG in Down syndrome. *Am J Obstet Gynecol* **165**, 132–5

Spencer, K. (1994a) Depistage de la trisomie 21 à l'aide de la β-HCG libre: notre experience sur trois ans. *Medecine Foetale et Echographie en Gynecologie* **20**, 67–9

Spencer, K. (1994b) 'The measurement of hCG subunits in screening for Down syndrome' in J.G. Grudzinskas, T. Chard, M. Chapman and H.S. Cuckle (Eds) *Screening for Down Syndrome*, pp.85–100. Cambridge: Cambridge University Press

Spencer, K. and Carpenter, P. (1985) Screening for Down syndrome using serum alpha fetoprotein: a retrospective study indicating caution. *BMJ* **290**, 1940–3

Spencer, K., Coombes, E.J., Mallard, A.S. and Milford Ward, A. (1992a) Free beta human choriogonadotropin in Down syndrome screening: a multicentre study of its role compared with other biochemical markers. *Ann Clin Biochem* **29**, 506–18

Spencer, K., Macri, J.N., Aitken, D.A. and Connor, J.M. (1992b) Free beta hCG as first trimester marker for fetal trisomy. *Lancet* **339**, 1480

Spencer, K., Mallard, A.S., Coombes, E.J. and Macri, J.N. (1993) Prenatal screening for trisomy 18 with free beta human chorionic gonadotrophin as a marker. *BMJ* **307**, 1455–8

Spencer, K., Aitken, D. A., Crossley, J. A. *et al.* (1994a) First-trimester biochemical screening for trisomy 21. The role of free beta-hCG, AFP and pregnancy-associated plasma protein-A. *Ann Clin Biochem* **31**, 447–54

Spencer, K., Salonen, R. and Muller, F. (1994b) Down syndrome screening in multiple pregnancies using alpha-fetoprotein and free beta-hCG. *Prenat Diagn* **14**, 537–42

Spencer, K., Aitken, D.A., Macri, J.N. and Buchanan, P.D. (1996) Urine free beta-hCG and beta core in pregnancies affected by Down syndrome. *Prenat Diagn* **16**, 605–13

Spencer, K., Muller, F. and Aitken, D.A. (1997a) Biochemical markers of trisomy 21 in amniotic fluid. *Prenat Diagn* **17**, 31–7

Spencer, K., Noble, P., Snijders, R.J.M. and Nicolaides, K.H. (1997b) First trimester urine free beta-hCG, beta core and total oestriol in pregnancies affected by Down syndrome: implications for first trimester screening with nuchal translucency and serum free beta-hCG. *Prenat Diagn* (in press)

Stenman, U.-H., Bidart, J.-M., Birken, S., Mann, K., Nisula, B. and O'Connor, J. (1993) Standardization of protein immunoprocedures – choriogonadotropin. *Scand J Clin Lab Invest* **53** (Suppl 216), 42–78

Van Lith, J.M.M. (1992) First trimester maternal serum-hCG as a marker for fetal chromosomal disorders. *Prenat Diagn* **12**, 495–504

Wald, N.J. and Densem, J.W. (1994) Maternal serum free beta human chorionic gonadotrophin levels in twin pregnancies: implications for screening for Down syndrome. *Prenat Diagn* **14**, 321–2

Wald, N.J., Cuckle, H.S., Densem, J.W. *et al.* (1988) Maternal serum screening for Down syndrome in early pregnancy. *BMJ* **297**, 883–7

Wald, N.J., Densem, J.W., Smith, D. and Klee, G.G. (1994) Four marker serum screening for Down syndrome. *Prenat Diagn* **14**, 707–16

Wald, N.J., George, L., Smith, D., Densem, J.W. and Petterson, K. (1996) Serum screening for Down syndrome between 8 and 14 weeks of pregnancy. *Br J Obstet Gynaecol* **103**, 407–12

Wehmann, R.E. and Nisula, B.C. (1979) Metabolic clearance rates of the subunits of human chorionic gondotropin in man. *J Clin Endocrinol Metab* **48**, 753–9

Chapter 13

Measurement of urinary β-core of hCG in Down syndrome

Timothy Chard, Ray Iles and Mary C.M. Macintosh

The single most effective analyte for Down screening in mid-trimester is maternal serum human chorionic gonadotrophin (hCG). In particular, the free β-subunit of this molecule appears to be a better index than does measurement of the intact hormone (see Chapter12).

The principal form of hCG in urine is a metabolite of the free β-subunit known as 'β-core' (Iles and Chard 1993). This consists of amino acids 6–40 and 55–92 of the β-subunit, joined by disulphide bridges. Since there is a relatively greater increase of free β-subunit in Down syndrome pregnancies, it would be expected that this would be reflected in the levels of β-core in urine. Furthermore, this increase should be simpler to detect because free β-subunit constitutes only 1–2% of total hCG in the circulation, whereas β-core constitutes 50% or more of hCG-like molecules in urine.

A number of authors have described assays which are relatively specific for β-core (e.g. Lee et al. 1991). Originally these assays were directed towards measurement of β-core as a potential diagnostic and prognostic marker of pelvic epithelial tumours (Iles and Chard 1991; Carter et al. 1993) However, it is also apparent that such assays would be well-suited to evaluating β-core levels in the urine of women carrying a Down syndrome fetus.

A number of authors have described the results of measurement of urine β-core in Down syndrome pregnancies (Table 13.1). The findings of these studies show wide divergence: from those in which the mean multiple of the median (MoM) was little or no different from that of free β-subunit in the circulation, to those in which the mean MoM was six or greater. The difference in these findings might be attributable to a number of factors, including: (1) differences in assay procedure (Cole 1995; Cole et al.1996). For example, Canick and colleagues (Kellner et al. 1996a) have shown that the median MoM for urine hCG-like material in Down syndrome cases ranges from 2.14 for a kit which measures intact hCG to 5.34 for the Ciba-Corning UGP assay. However, findings at both extremes have been achieved using apparently identical materials (Table 13.1); (2) a difference in the procedures for sample collection and storage; and (3) chance

Table 13.1. Studies on the measurement of urinary fragments of hCG for the detection of Down syndrome. Most authors correct for urine creatinine concentration

Reference	No. of cases Control	Down syndrome	Gestation of Down syndrome (weeks)	Analyte levels in Down syndrome cases as mean MoM	Assay method[a]	Predicted detection rate (%) (5% screen positive)
Spencer *et al.* (1996)	400	29	14–24	2.35	1	41
Hayashi and Kozu (1995)	150	5	15–17	1.66	2	–
Hayashi *et al.* (1996)	160	3	16–17	3.3	3	–
Cuckle *et al.* (1994)	67	7	19–22	6.11	4	–
Canick *et al.* (1995)	91	14	17–21	5.34	1	88
Cuckle *et al.* (1995)	294	24	11–23	6.02	4	79.6
Canick *et al.* (1996)	130	18	14–21	6.18	1	67[b]
Cole *et al.* (1996)	400	29	–	2.8–6.2	5	–

[a] 1, Triton UGP EIA, Ciba Corning; 2, Wakotest; 3, ELISA-free β-hCG, CIS (UK); 4, Barts beta-core; 5, Various.
[b] For an 8.5% false positive rate

differences in the populations studied. Clearly further evidence is required before a final conclusion can be reached. However, if the more optimistic findings can be confirmed, then clearly measurement of β-core in urine would offer a test of exceptional convenience with detection rates comparable to that of present blood tests.

Levels of urinary oestriol (E_3) are also reduced in Down syndrome pregnancies; a combination of β-core and E_3 gives results superior to β-core alone (Kellner *et al.* 1996b, c).

The final and probably the most important question is whether or not measurement of urine β-core performs as effectively in the first trimester as it does in the second trimester. Disappointingly, current evidence suggests that this is not the case. Although levels of urine β-core are undoubtedly elevated in Down syndrome pregnancies at 10–12 weeks of pregnancy, the increase is relatively no greater than that of the free β-subunit in blood at the same period of time. However, the number of subjects studied is still relatively small, and the matter cannot be regarded as finally concluded until further data are available.

References

Canick, J.A., Kellner, L.H., Saller, D.N., Palomaki, G.E., Walker, R.P. and Osathanondh, R. (1995) Second-trimester levels of maternal urinary gonadotropin peptide in Down syndrome pregnancy. *Prenat Diagn* **15**, 739–44

Canick, J.A., Kellner, L.H., Saller, D.N. *et al.* (1996) A second level of evaluation of maternal urinary gonadotropin peptide as a marker for second trimester Down syndrome screening. *Rec Adv Prenat Diagn* Abstract No. P28

Carter, P.G., Iles, R.K., Neven, P., Prys Davies, A., Shepherd, J.H. and Chard, T. (1993) The measurement of urinary beta core fragment in conjunction with serum CA125 does not aid the differentiation of malignant from benign pelvic masses. *Gynecol Oncol,* **51**, 368–71

Cole, L.A. (1995) Down's syndrome screening using urine β-core fragment test: choice of immunoassay. *Prenat Diagn* **15**, 679–80

Cole, I., Isozaki, T., Palomaki, G. *et al.* (1996) Detection of β-core fragment in second trimester Down's syndrome pregnancies. *Rec Adv Prenat Diagn for Aneuploidy* Abstract A16

Cuckle, H.S., Iles, R.K. and Chard, T. (1994) Urinary β-core human chorionic gonadotrophin: a new approach to Down's syndrome screening. *Prenat Diagn* **14**, 953–8

Cuckle, H.S., Iles, R.K., Sehmi, I.K. *et al.* (1995) Urinary multiple marker screening for Down's syndrome. *Prenat Diagn* **15**, 745–51

Hayashi, M. and Kozu, H. (1995) Maternal urinary β-core fragment of hCG/creatinine ratios and fetal chromosomal abnormalities in the second trimester of pregnancy. *Prenat Diagn* **15**, 11–16

Hayashi, M., Kozu, H. and Takei, H. (1996) Maternal urinary free β-subunit of human chorionic gonadotrophin:creatinine ratios and fetal chromosomal abnormalities in the second trimester of pregnancy. *Br J Obstet Gynaecol* **103**, 577–80

Iles, R.K. and Chard, T. (1991) Human chorionic gonadotrophin expression by bladder cancers: biology and clinical potential. *J Urol* **145**, 453–8

Iles, R.K. and Chard, T. (1993) Molecular insights into the structure and function of human chorionic gonadotrophin. *J Mol Endocrinol* **10**, 217–34

Kellner, L.H., Canick, J.A., Palomaki, G.E. *et al.* (1996a) Maternal urine screening for fetal Down syndrome: comparison of beta-core fragment, free-beta subunit and hCG. *Am J Obstet Gynecol* **174**, 446A (Abstract)

Kellner, L.H., Canick, J.A., Palomaki, G.E. *et al.* (1996b) Urinary markers: a new approach to screening for Down syndrome in the second trimester. *Am J Hum Genet* **59**, Abstract 41

Kellner, L.H., Canick, J.A., Saller, D.N. *et al.* (1996c) Second trimester levels of maternal urinary total estriol (TE3) in Down syndrome pregnancy. *Rec Adv Prenat Diagn* Abstract No. A16

Lee, C.L., Shepherd, J.H., Hudson, C.N. and Chard, T. (1991) The purification and development of a radioimmunoassay for beta-core fragment of human chorionic gonadotrophin in urine: application as a marker of gynaecological cancer in premenopausal and postmenopausal women. *J Endocrinol* **130**, 481–9

Spencer, K., Aitken, D.A., Macri, J.N. and Buchanan, P.D. (1996) Urine free beta hCG and beta core in pregnancies affected by Down's syndrome. *Prenat Diagn* **16**, 605–13

Chapter 14

First-trimester fetal aneuploidy screening: maternal serum PAPP-A and free β-hCG

Bruno Brambati, James N. Macri, Lucia Tului,
Terrence W. Hallahan, David A. Krantz and Ezio Alberti

Introduction

The prospect of maternal serum screening for fetal aneuploidy in the first-trimester of pregnancy with subsequent karyotyping of fetal tissues offers distinct advantages to expectant parents and their clinicians. Current protocols, which do not initiate the process of screening and diagnosis until the second trimester, offer little time for decision making and the ominous prospect of late termination of an affected fetus.

Associations between maternal serum markers and fetal aneuploidy in the first trimester have been sought in an effort to provide an earlier alert. This would offer patients valuable time and the option of safer, earlier termination procedures. With the exception of the maternal serum marker free β-hCG, none of the commonly known second trimester markers (α-fetoprotein (AFP), human chorionic gonadotrophin (hCG), α-hCG, unconjugated oestriol and inhibin) are effective in first-trimester screening protocols. One additional biochemical marker, however, has been identified as productive specifically in the first trimester and this marker is pregnancy associated plasma protein-A (PAPP-A).

PAPP-A is a 750–800 kDa dimeric (α_2) macromolecular glycoprotein (Lin et al. 1976; Bischof 1979; Sutcliffe et al. 1980). Each subunit consists of 1547 amino acid residues in a unique sequence and is derived from a larger precursor of placental origin (Kristensen et al. 1994). PAPP-A is a zinc-containing protein (Sinosich et al. 1983) and has been demonstrated to bind reversibly and with high affinity to heparin (Sinosich et al. 1982; Davey et al. 1983). The gene for PAPP-A has been localised to the long arm of chromosome 9, locus 33.1 (Silahtaroglu et al. 1993). PAPP-A isolated from pooled pregnancy serum has been shown to be a disulphide bridged complex with the pro-form of eosinophil major basic protein (Oxvig et al. 1993). Circulating levels are detected from 28 days after conception and increase throughout pregnancy. After delivery, PAPP-A is cleared from the maternal circulation with a half-life of 3–4 days (Lin *et al.* 1976) and remains detectable for 3–4 weeks.

PAPP-A has been localised to the trophoblastic tissue of the placenta (Lin *et al.* 1976; Wahlstrom *et al.* 1981; Tornehave *et al.* 1984) which is considered the main source of circulating PAPP-A in pregnancy. PAPP-A-like material has also been found in the non-pregnant state generating the hypothesis of a dual origin, both from the trophoblast and from the maternal endometrium (Sjoberg *et al.* 1984, 1986). Although the identification of a PAPP-A-like material in tissues other than trophoblast and in the non-pregnant state would more likely be the consequence of poor specificity of the antibody preparations in use, the site of synthesis remains a subject of considerable debate.

The biological function of PAPP-A is still unknown, however, a non-competitive inhibition of human granulocyte elastase has been demonstrated (Sinosich *et al.* 1982) and a possible role in modulating the maternal immune response has been suggested (Bischof *et al.* 1982; Kristensen *et al.* 1994; Smart 1984). The clinical usefulness of PAPP-A seems to be limited to the first trimester of pregnancy. Very low maternal serum PAPP-A values have been observed days or even weeks before fetal demise. This observation has been confirmed in a large number of cases and indicates the high predictive value of PAPP-A for pregnancy failure (Brambati *et al.* 1991; Westergaard *et al.* 1983a, 1985; Masson 1983). Abnormally depressed values have also been reported in a high number of cases of trophoblastic disease (Bischof *et al.* 1981, 1982; Folkersen *et al.* 1981) and extrauterine pregnancy (Riddle *et al.* 1991; Johnson *et al.* 1993). Moreover, PAPP-A may be a specific marker of Cornelia de Lange syndrome where in some cases PAPP-A levels are virtually undetectable (Westergaard *et al.* 1983b). Brambati *et al.* (1991) were the first to describe an association between depressed maternal serum PAPP-A levels and fetal aneuploidy. In recent years a number of studies have confirmed this finding, showing that maternal serum PAPP-A levels may be substantially reduced in pregnancies with a chromosomally abnormal fetus (Brambati *et al.* 1994; Spencer *et al.* 1994; Brizot *et al.* 1994; Bersinger *et al.* 1994; Macintosh *et al.* 1994; Aitken *et al.* 1995; Wald *et al.* 1995; Krantz *et al.* 1996), where its greatest clinical value may be its measurement in the first trimester in screening for Down syndrome and other aneuploidies.

PAPP-A combined with maternal age can detect 40–50% of Down syndrome cases at a 5% false positive and the addition of free β-hCG increases the detection efficiency to 60–70% for the same false positive rate (Brambati *et al.* 1994; Krantz *et al.* 1996; Wald *et al.* 1996). The current study further evaluates first-trimester fetal aneuploidy screening with the combination of the maternal serum markers free β-hCG and PAPP-A.

Materials and methods

Study population

Maternal serum samples from 751 singleton pregnancies with a chromosomally normal fetus, 31 Down syndrome (DS), eight trisomy 18 (T18), three trisomy 13 (T13) and ten other chromosome aberration cases were evaluated. In addition,

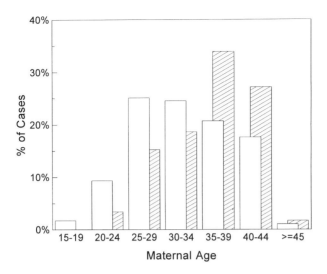

Fig. 14.1. Maternal age distribution in Down syndrome: affected (striped bars) and unaffected pregnancies (solid bars).

samples from 39 normal twin, three twin discordant for trisomy 21 and 17 normal triplet pregnancies were measured. On patients in whom weight and cigarette smoking data were available there were 651 non-smokers and 89 smokers. All samples were collected between eight and 13 weeks' gestation and stored at $-20°C$ until assayed. Gestational age was calculated from last menstrual date and confirmed by ultrasonic measurement. All samples were prospectively collected and maternal blood was drawn immediately prior to CVS. Biochemical analyses were conducted retrospectively in a blind coded protocol. To increase the size and scope of the study, previously reported results (Krantz *et al.* 1996) from 483 unaffected cases and 22 DS cases from 10–13 weeks' gestation were added to the study group, as well as six additional Down syndrome cases from 7–9 weeks, leading to a total of 1234 chromosomally normal and 59 DS cases for study. The mean maternal age in the unaffected pregnancies was 32.6 years ($\pm$6.6) and for the DS affected pregnancies, 35.5 years ($\pm$5.7 years). Fig. 14.1 shows the maternal age distribution in both normal and abnormal groups.

Dried blood spot technology

A prospective study of 444 singleton pregnancies including three cases of DS, two cases of trisomy 18, two cases of triploidy, one case of anencephaly and one chromosome translocation t(3;4) were evaluated using dried blood technology. Seven cases with miscellaneous disorders were eliminated from the study. In addition 96 paired liquid and dried specimens were compared to assess the correlation between the two assay methods.

Liquid specimens were collected by venepuncture without the use of anti-coagulants. For matched dried specimens, five small aliquots (approximately 50 µl each of whole blood) were immediately removed, spotted onto a filter paper collection device (Schleicher and Schuell 903 collection paper) and allowed to dry at room temperature for at least 1 h. The remaining liquid samples were allowed to clot and serum was isolated before transport to the laboratory. Upon receipt in the laboratory, two 5.5 mm disks were punched from each dried specimen directly into the wells of a microtitre plate. Elution buffer was added and blood components were allowed to elute from the filter paper.

Biochemical and statistical analysis

Free β-hCG and PAPP-A levels were determined with in-house microtitre plate enzyme-linked immunosorbent assays previously described (Macri *et al.* 1993; Spencer *et al.* 1994). The intra- and inter-assay coefficients of variability for free β-hCG were 5.3% and 4.7%, respectively, and for PAPP-A were 5.0% and 2.7%, respectively. To calculate MoMs in the blind retrospective samples, gestational week specific medians were calculated for each analyte at 8–13 weeks of gestation. These observed medians were then regressed. The regression formula was then used to determine medians. Interpolation was used to calculate day-specific medians.

Likelihood ratios were calculated for the blind retrospective samples and the previously reported samples separately based on the distributions observed in each group. Down syndrome risks were then calculated using Bayes' rule. False positive rates and detection rates were calculated by modelling the observed likelihood ratios with the distribution of live births as previously described.

To screen for trisomy 18 and other chromosomal abnormalities, atypicality indices were calculated for each patient using Mahalanobis' squared distance (MSD). A cut-off of 9.21, representing the 99th percentile was used. In addition, for a result to be considered atypical both analytes had to be less than 2.0 MoM.

Results

Free β-hCG levels rise between eight and nine weeks' gestation and then gradually decline approximately 20% per week for the remainder of the first trimester (Fig. 14.2a). In contrast, PAPP-A levels steadily increase approximately 30% per week from 8 to 13 weeks' gestation (Fig. 14.2b).

Down syndrome

The free β-hCG and PAPP-A MoM values for the 59 Down syndrome cases are illustrated in Fig. 14.3 (a and b). Free β-hCG is significantly raised in cases of Down syndrome from 7 to 13 weeks' gestation (1.85 median MoM). PAPP-A values in contrast are significantly decreased across the 7–13 week gestational range (0.5 median MoM).

A scatter plot of free β-hCG versus PAPP-A of the Down syndrome cases demonstrates a clustering in the upper left quadrant (Fig. 14.4) with 25/59 cases having a free β-hCG MoM above 2.0 and 28/59 having a PAPP-A MoM less than

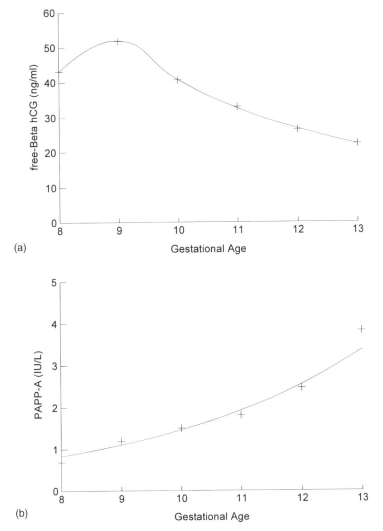

Fig. 14.2. Gestational age specific medians in 751 normal singleton pregnancies. Observed (+) and regressed (——) medians. (a) Free β-hCG; (a) PAPP-A.

0.5. In the 751 samples from the blind study group the standard deviation (natural logs) of the unaffected samples was 0.5470 for PAPP-A and 0.6304 for free β-hCG. These values were lower than observed previously (0.67 for free β-hCG and 0.83 for PAPP-A) (Krantz *et al.* 1996). In the 31 DS cases the SD for PAPP-A was 0.6198 and for free β-hCG 0.5242 as compared to the previously reported 0.64 and 0.40 (Krantz *et al.* 1996).

ROC curves based on the combined study group, using the analytes individually and in combination are illustrated in Fig. 14.5. At a 5% false positive rate the combined analytes detected 61% of the Down syndrome cases. The detection efficiency at various term risk cut off levels is shown in Table 14.1.

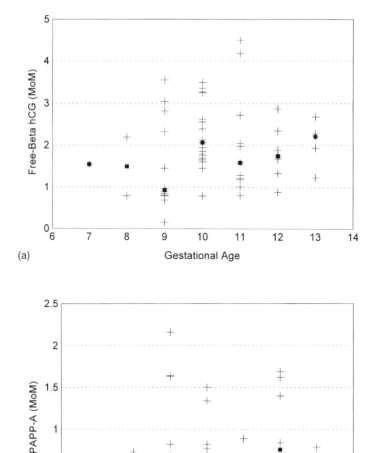

(a)

(b)

Fig. 14. 3.   Multiple of the median values in 59 Down syndrome cases grouped by gestational age. (a) Free β-hCG; (b) PAPP-A. Down syndrome case (+) and gestational age specific medians (■) are shown.

Trisomy 18

The MoM values for the eight trisomy 18 cases are illustrated in a scatter plot in Fig. 14.6. In contrast to Down syndrome cases, the trisomy 18 cases cluster in the lower left quadrant. All eight trisomy 18 cases had a free β-hCG value less than 0.5 MoM (median free β-hCG MoM=0.115) and 6/8 had a PAPP-A value less than 0.5 MoM (median PAPP-A MoM=0.315). Combining the two markers yielded a detection efficiency of 88% at a 0.5% false positive rate.

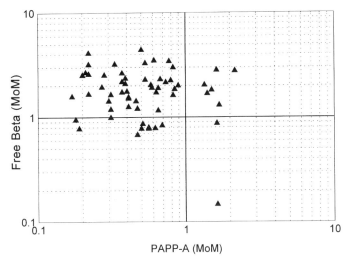

Fig. 14.4. Scatter plot of free β-hCG vs PAPP-A values in 59 cases of Down syndrome.

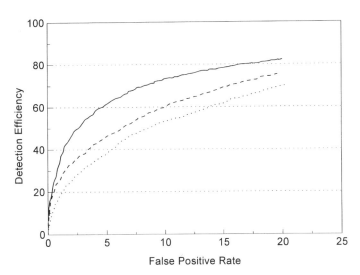

Fig. 14.5. ROC curves using free β-hCG (...), PAPP-A (---) and a combination of the two markers (——)

Trisomy 13 and other aneuploidies

The MoM values for the three trisomy 13 cases and ten other numerical and structural anomalies are listed in Table 14.2. The median MoM values for free β-hCG and PAPP-A in the 13 cases were 0.82 and 0.82, respectively. However, significantly low values for both markers are obtained if only autosomal aneuploidy and triploidy cases were considered (free β-hCG MoM=0.19 and PAPP-A MoM=0.55).

Table 14.1.   Detection efficiencies at various term cut-off values

Cut off	5% FP		1/250		1/380	
Analyte(s)	FP	DE	FP	DE	FP	DE
Free β-hCG	5%	38%	4.6%	37%	9.0%	51%
PAPP-A	5%	46%	4.0%	43%	7.1%	52%
Combined	5%	61%	4.4%	60%	7.5%	69%

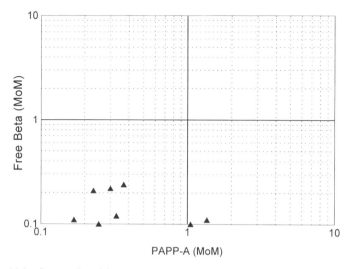

Fig. 14.6.   Scatter plot of free β-hCG vs PAPP-A values in eight cases of trisomy 18.

Table 14.2.   Free β-hCG and PAPP-A MoM values in 17 other cases of fetal aneuploidy

Condition	Free β MoM	PAPP-A MoM
Trisomy 13	0.13	0.55
Trisomy 13	0.54	0.67
Trisomy 13	0.19	1.08
47,XXX	1.06	0.31
47,XXY	0.94	0.82
47,XXY	0.95	1.36
46,XX,-6P	3.84	1.27
46,XY,-t(21;21)	0.69	0.36
46,XY,t(3;18)	1.69	0.85
46,XX,-t(1;18)de novo	0.82	1.61
69,XXY	0.14	0.30
48,XXY,+18	0.36	0.54
48,XXXY	0.90	1.73

Table 14.3. Free β and PAPP-A MoM values in cases of multiple pregnancy

Multiple #	n	free-β (MoM)	PAPP-A (MoM)
Twins (dichorionic)	35	1.96	1.50
Twins (monochorionic)	4	1.62	1.53
Twins (total)	39	1.94	1.50
Twins (1 Down syndrome)	3	2.48	1.03
Triplets	17	2.77	2.22

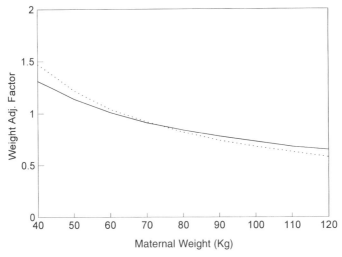

Fig. 14.7. Maternal weight adjustment for free β-hCG (——) and PAPP-A (⋯). Adjustment formulas developed were: Free β-$=$EXP($-0.6439 \times$Log$_e$(wt) $+ 2.6466$), $r=-0.143$. PAPP-A$=$EXP($-0.08390 \times$Log$_e$(wt) $+ 3.4771$), $r=-0.221$.

Multiple pregnancies

Both free β-hCG and PAPP-A levels rise approximately in proportion with increasing multiplicity (Table 14.3). Furthermore, in the three twin pregnancies discordant for Down syndrome the maternal serum level for free β-hCG and PAPP-A changed significantly as expected from the experience in singletons (free β-hCG and PAPP-A MoM values in the three cases were 2.48 and 0.75; 3.24 and 1.03; 1.49 and 4.32).

Maternal factors

Neither free β-hCG nor PAPP-A correlate with maternal age ($r=-0.016$ and $r=0.063$, respectively). However, both analytes demonstrated a small but significant negative correlation with maternal weight (free β-hCG, $r=-0.143$ and PAPP-A, $r=-0.221$). Fig. 14.7 illustrates the change in analyte levels with maternal weight.

Table 14.4.   Effect of maternal smoking on free β-hCG and PAPP-A analyte levels

| | | MOM values | |
| | | Non-smokers ($n=651$) | Smokers ($n=89$) |
Analyte	Weight adjustment		
Free β-hCG	No	0.99	0.95
	Yes	0.97	0.93
PAPP-A	No	1.01	0.98
	Yes	1.01	0.97

Maternal cigarette smoking does not appear to have a significant impact on first-trimester maternal serum screening. Differences in the median analyte levels in smokers and non-smokers both before and after weight adjustment are given in Table 14.4.

Dried blood technology

Biochemical results from dried blood assays correlated well with those derived from matched liquid serum assays ($r=0.951$ and 0.884 for free β-hCG and PAPP-A, respectively). In the prospective sample set of 444 dried specimens, the overall false positive rate was 5.8% (25/428) for Down syndrome and 0.7% (3/428) for trisomy 18. There were three cases of Down syndrome which were all detected. In addition one case of trisomy 18, two cases of 69,XXX, one case of anencephaly and one translocation t(3;4) were detected using an atypicality index. One case of trisomy 18 was not detected. The standard deviation (natural logs) of the unaffected cases in this sample group was 0.5337 and 0.5368 for free β-hCG and PAPP-A.

Discussion

The detection rate for DS cases achieved in the present study (61%) is comparable to the results reported in the few previous reports ranging between 62% and 79% (Brambati *et al.* 1995; Krantz *et al.* 1996; Wald *et al.* 1996). These screening parameters are similar to most second trimester screening protocols with the significant advantage of much earlier detection.

Serum free β-hCG and PAPP-A levels are significantly reduced in cases of trisomy 18 and combined achieve a detection efficiency of 88% at a 0.5% false positive rate. Although more cases are required to confirm these results this level of detection exceeds that seen in second-trimester screening of this very serious condition. Moreover, from this preliminary experience it appears that biochemical screening in the first trimester might also be efficient in detecting other autosomal aneuploidies as well as some chromosomal translocations, whereas poor sensitivity has been observed for sex chromosome aberrations. It is also noteworthy that normal biochemical levels have been observed in the presence of confined placental anomaly (unpublished data), suggesting first trimester serum testing may be a potentially helpful discriminating tool when chromosomal anomalies are suspected to be confined to the placenta. The proportionality observed in normal multiple pregnancies indicates that with the establishment of reference values an atypicality index may be used for prenatal screening. However, as in second-trimester screening, more data from multiple pregnancies discordant for Down syndrome would be required to determine Down syndrome detection efficiency in first trimester screening of multiple pregnancies.

Maternal factors such as age and cigarette smoking do not appear to have a significant effect on first-trimester biochemical screening markers. However, maternal weight adjustment does offer a small improvement. This data set comprised predominantly Caucasian patients therefore ethnic variation could not be evaluated. However, ethnic variation in second trimester screening is well documented and is likely to play a role in first-trimester screening as well.

First-trimester screening utilising dried blood sampling correlated very well with liquid sampling and can achieve comparable detection efficiencies. The advantages of dried blood technology include; ease of sample collection, elimination of transport tube breakage, improved biohazard control, reduced haemolysis and specimen degradation during transport delays and minimisation of the effects of specimen mishandling and the extremes of temperature.

Any discussion of policy for first-trimester screening for fetal anomalies should take into account the recent advances in sonography. Currently available data suggest that effective screening can also be achieved by measuring fetal nuchal translucency (NT) between 10 and 13 weeks (Brambati *et al.* 1995; Snijders *et al.* 1996). Although results on the efficacy of the sonographic marker are still controversial (Brambati *et al.* 1996), a relationship between abnormal NT thickness and fetal aneuploidy is clearly established. Moreover, studies examining the relationship between PAPP-A, free β-hCG and NT have demonstrated that there is no significant association between the biochemical and sonographic markers (Brizot *et al.* 1994, 1995; Brambati, unpublished data). Therefore, it is expected that the combination of all three indicators could further enhance the efficacy of screening fetal chromosomal anomalies in the late first trimester.

References

Aitken, D.A., Ireland, M., Berry, E. and Macri, J.N. (1995) Pregnancy associated plasma protein A (PAPP-A) in maternal serum from pregnancies with Cornelia de Lange syndrome. *Proc Assoc Clin Biochem Natl Meeting,* pp. 84–5 (A70)

Bersinger, N.A., Brizot, M.L., Johnson, A. *et al.* (1994) First trimester maternal serum pregnancy associated plasma protein-A and pregnancy specific beta 1-glycoprotein in fetal trisomies. *Br J Obstet Gynaecol* **101**, 970–4

Bischof, P. (1979) Purification and characterisation of PAPP-A. *Arch Gynecol* **227**, 315–26

Bischof, P., Rapin, C.H., Weil, A. and Herrmann, W. (1981) Is PAPP-A a tumor marker? *Am J Obstet Gynecol* **143**, 379–81

Bischof, P., DuBerg, S. and Schindler, A.M. (1982) Is pregnancy associated plasma protein-A an immunomodulator during human pregnancy? *Placenta* **4** Suppl, 93–102

Brambati, B., Lanzani, A. and Tului, L. (1991) 'Ultrasound and biochemical assessment of first trimester pregnancy' in M. Chapman, G. Grudzinskas and T. Chard (Eds) *The Embryo: Normal and Abnormal Development and Growth*, pp. 181–94. New York: Springer-Verlag

Brambati, B., Tului, L., Bonacchi, I., Shrimanker, K., Suzuki, Y. and Grudzinskas, J.G. (1994) First trimester free Beta hCG and PAPP-A in pregnancies with aneuploid fetuses. *Prenat Diagn* **14**, 1043–7

Brambati, B., Cislaghi, C., Tului, L. e*t al.* (1995) First trimester Down's syndrome screening using nuchal translucency: a prospective study in patients undergoing chorionic villus sampling. *Ultrasound Obstet Gynecol* **5**, 9–14

Brambati, B., Tului, L. and Alberti, E. (1996) Sonography in the first trimester screening of trisomy 21 and other fetal aneuploidies. *Early Preg Biol Med* **2,** 155–67

Brizot, M.L., Snijders, R.J.M., Bersinger, N.A., Kuhn, P. and Nicholaides, K.H. (1994) Maternal serum pregnancy associated plasma protein-A and fetal nuchal translucency thickness for the prediction of fetal trisomies in early pregnancy. *Obstet Gynecol* **84**, 918–22

Brizot, M.L., Snijders, R.J.M., Butler, J., Bersinger, N.A. and Nicolaides, K.H. (1995) Maternal serum hCG and fetal nuchal translucency thickness for the prediction of fetal trisomies in the first trimester of pregnancy. *Br J Obstet Gynaecol* **102**, 127–32

Davey, M.W., Teisner, B., Sinosich, M. and Grudzinskas, J.G. (1983) Interaction between heparin and human PAPP-A: a simple purification procedure. *Anal Biochem* **131**, 18–24

Folkersen, J., Grudzinskas, J.G., Hinderson, P., Teisner, B. and Westergaard, J.G. (1981) Pregnancy-associated plasma protein-A: circulation levels during normal pregnancy. *Am J Obstet Gynecol* **139**, 910–14

Johnson, M.R., Riddle, A.F., Grudzinskas, J.G. *et al.* (1993) Endocrinology of IVF pregnancies during the first trimester. *Hum Reprod* **8**, 316–22

Krantz, D.A., Larsen, J.W., Buchanan, P.D. and Macri, J.N. (1996) First-trimester Down syndrome screening: free β-human chorionic gonadotropin and pregnancy-associated plasma protein A. *Am J Obstet Gynecol* **174**, 612–16

Kristensen, T., Oxvig, C., Sand, O., Moller, N.P.H. and Sottrup-Jensen, L. (1994) Amino acid sequence of pregnancy associated plasma protein-A derived from cloned cDNA. *Biochemistry* **33**, 1592–8

Lin, T.M., Halbert, S.P., Spellacy, W.N. and Gall, S. (1976) Human pregnancy-associated plasma proteins during the postpartum period. *Am J Obstet Gynecol* **124**, 382–7

Macintosh, M.C.M., Iles, R., Teisner, B. *et al.* (1994) Maternal serum human chorionic gonadotropin and pregnancy-associated plasma protein A: markers for fetal Down syndrome at 8–14 weeks. *Prenatal Diagn* **14**, 203–8

Macri, J.N., Spencer, K., Anderson, R.W. and Cook, E.J. (1993) Free beta chorionic gonadotropin: a cross reactivity study of two immunometric assays used in prenatal maternal serum screening for Down syndrome. *Ann Clin Biochem* **30**, 94–8

Masson, G.M., Anthony, F. and Wilson, M.S. (1983) Value of Schwangerschaftsprotein 1 (SP1) and pregnancy-associated plasma protein-A (PAPP-A) in the clinical management of threatened abortion. *Br J Obstet Gynaecol* **90**, 146–9

Oxvig, C., Sand, O., Kristensen, T., Gleich, G.J. and Sottrup-Jensen, L. (1993) Circulating human pregnancy-associated plasma protein-A is disulphide-bridged to the proform of eosinophil major basic protein. *J Biol Chem* **17**, 12243–6

Riddle, A.F., Johnson, M.R., Sharma,V., Nicolaides, K.H. and Grudzinskas, J.G. (1991) Ovarian and placental hormones in ectopic pregnancy following IVF: the predictive value of hCG, SP-1, PAPP-A, estriol and progesterone. Presented at The British Congress of Obstetrics and Gynaecology, June, Manchester, Abstr. 207

Silahtaroglu, A.N., Tumer, Z., Kristensen, T., Sottrup-Jensen, L. and Tommerup, N. (1993) Assignment of the gene for pregnancy-associated plasma protein-A (PAPP-A) to 9q33.1 by fluorescence *in situ* hybridization to mitotic and meiotic chromosomes. *Cytogenet Cell Genet* **62**, 214–16

Sinosich, M.J., Davey, M. W., Ghosh, P. and Grudzinskas, J.G. (1982) Specific inhibition of human granulocyte elastase by human pregnancy-associated plasma protein-A. *Biochem Int* **5**, 777–86

Sinosich, M.J., Teisner, B., Folkersen, J., Saunders, D.M. and Grudzinskas, J.G. (1983) Comparative studies of pregnancy-associated plasma protein-A and alpha 2 macroglobulin using metal chelate chromatography. *Biochem Int* **7**, 33–42

Sjoberg, J., Wahlstrom, T. and Seppala, M. (1984) Pregnancy associated plasma protein A in the human endometrium is dependent on the effect of progesterone. *J Clin Endocrinol Metab* **58**, 359–62

Sjoberg, J., Wahlstrom, T., Grudzinskas, J.G. and Sinosich, M.J. (1986) Demonstration of pregnancy associated plasma protein-A (PAPP-A)-like material in the fallopian tube. *Fertil Steril* **45**, 517–21

Smart, Y.C. (1984) Pregnancy-associated plasma protein-A (PAPP-A): an immunosuppressor in pregnancy? *Fertil Steril* **41**, 508–10

Snijders, R.J.M., Johnson, S., Sebire, N.J., Noble, P.L. and Nicolaides, K.H. (1996) First-trimester ultrasound screening for chromosomal defects. *Ultrasound Obstet Gynecol* **7**, 216–26

Spencer, K., Aitken, D.A., Crossley, J.A. *et al.* (1994) First-trimester biochemical screening for trisomy 21: the role of free-beta hCG, alpha-fetoprotein and pregnancy associated plasma protein-A. *Ann Clin Biochem* **34**, 447–54

Sutcliffe, R.G., Kukulska-Langlands, B.M., Coggins, J.R., Hunter, J.B. and Gore, G.H. (1980) Studies on human pregnancy associated plasma protein-A. Purification by affinity chromatography and structural comparison with alpha 2-macroglobulin. *Biochem J* **191**, 799–809

Tornehave, D., Cheminitz, J., Teisner, B., Folkersen, J. and Westergaard, J.G. (1984) Immunohistochemical demonstration of pregnancy associated plasma protein-A (PAPP-A) in the syncytiotrophoblast of the normal placenta at different gestational ages. *Placenta* **5**, 427–32

Wahlstrom, T., Teisner, B. and Folkersen, J. (1981) Tissue localization of pregnancy associated plasma protein-A (PAPP-A) in normal placenta. *Placenta* **2**, 253–8

Wald, N.J., Kennard, A. and Hackshaw, A.K. (1995) First trimester serum screening for Down syndrome. *Prenat Diagn* **15**, 1227–40

Wald, N.J., George, L., Smith, D., Densem, J.W. and Petterson, K. (1996) Serum screening for Down syndrome between 8 and 14 weeks of pregnancy. *Br J Obstet Gynaecol* **103**, 407–12

Westergaard, J.G., Sinosich, M.J., Bugge, M., Madsen, L.T., Teisner, B. and Grudzinskas, J.G. (1983a) Pregnancy-associated plasma protein-A in prediction of early pregnancy failure. *Am J Obstet Gynecol* **145**, 67–9

Westergaard, J.G., Chemnitz, J., Teisner, B. *et al.* (1983b) Pregnancy associated plasma protein-A: a possible marker in the classification and prenatal diagnosis of Cornelia de Lange syndrome. *Prenat Diagn* **3**, 225–32

Westergaard, J.G., Teisner, B., Sinosich, M.J., Madsen, L.T. and Grudzinskas, J.G. (1985) Does ultrasound examination render biochemical tests obsolete in the prediction of early pregnancy failure? *Br J Obstet Gynaecol* **92**, 77–83

Chapter 15

Maternal serum screening for Down syndrome in first trimester using Schwangerschaftsprotein 1, PAPP-A/proMBP-complex and the proform of eosinophil major basic protein as markers

Michael Christiansen and Bent Nørgaard-Pedersen

Introduction

As described in the Royal College of Obstetricians and Gynaecologists (RCOG) report from April 1993 (RCOG 1993) second trimester maternal serum screening for Down syndrome (DS) and severe fetal malformations, using the markers alpha-fetoprotein (AFP), human chorionic gonadotrophin (hCG) and un-conjugated estriol (uE$_3$) ('triple screening'), can detect about two-thirds of affected pregnancies with a false positive rate of about 5%. Such screening is now being carried out in many countries and the addition of new markers for DS such as free β- and free α-hCG, inhibin and β-core hCG may increase the detection rate for DS to 70–80%. Therefore maternal serum screening at 16–18 weeks of pregnancy is certainly an alternative or supplement to invasive diagnostics such as amniocentesis (AC) and chorionic villus sampling (CVS).

However, a major disadvantage of all techniques currently in clinical use is that results will be available rather late in pregnancy so that termination of pregnancy normally cannot be performed before week 13–15 (CVS or early AC) or week 18–21 (triple screening and/or AC).

Recently, however, first trimester biochemical screening at about 10 weeks has seemed feasible (Brock *et al.* 1990; Cuckle *et al.* 1992; Aitken *et al.* 1993; Brambati *et al.* 1993; Muller *et al.* 1993; Wald and Voller 1993; Wald *et al.* 1996; Van Lith 1994). Several markers have been suggested, such as AFP, uE$_3$, free β-hCG, α-hCG, β-core hCG, cancer antigen-125 (CA-125), inhibin, dimeric inhibin A, progesterone and pregnancy-associated plasma protein-A (PAPP-A). Retrospective studies seem to indicate that it should be possible to reach a screening performance in first trimester comparable to that of second trimester screening, especially by the use of free β-hCG and PAPP-A (Wald *et al.* 1996).

Furthermore, a new technique, measurement of nuchal translucency by ultrasound in week 10–13, has shown such promising results that it should be considered an alternative or supplement to other diagnostic or screening procedures in centres that are able to perform it (Szabo and Gellen 1990; Nicolaides *et al.* 1992; Schulte-Vallentin and Schindler 1992; Kornman *et al.* 1996).

This chapter reviews three markers – Schwangerschaftsprotein 1 (SP₁), pregnancy associated plasma protein-A/proform of eosinophil major basic protein-complex (PAPP-A/proMBP-complex) and proMBP – as first trimester DS screening markers. The evaluation will include each marker separately and in combination with other markers, especially free β-hCG.

Schwangerschaftsprotein 1 (SP₁)

SP₁, also known as pregnancy-specific glycoprotein, is a family of glycoproteins, synthesised by placental syncytiotrophoblast (Bohn 1979), belonging to the immunoglobulin superfamily and exhibiting strong homology with carcino-embryonic antigen (CEA) and N-CAM (Zheng *et al.* 1990; Leslie *et al.* 1990; Streydio *et al.* 1990; Barnett *et al.* 1990). SP₁ is a major synthetic product of the placenta and is found in elevated concentrations in maternal serum from gestational week 2–3. The concentration increases exponentially during the first trimester (Sørensen *et al.* 1995) and continues to increase, but with a decreasing slope, during the second and third trimesters to reach a level of 200–300 mg/l or around 100 IU/l at term (Bischof 1992; Lin *et al.* 1974). Several fetal or placental disorders (fetal death, fetal growth retardation, placenta insufficiency, pre-eclampsia, diabetes, ectopic pregnancy and threatened abortion) (Gordon *et al.* 1977; Chapman *et al.* 1981; Wurz *et al.* 1981; Hertz and Schultz-Larsen 1983; Tamsen *et al.* 1983; Grudzinskas *et al.* 1983; Masson *et al.* 1983; MacDonald *et al.* 1983; Sterzick *et al.* 1986, 1989; Briese and Glockner 1991; Mantzavinos *et al.* 1991; Silver *et al.* 1993) have been associated with a decrease in maternal serum concentration of SP₁. Elevated serum SP₁ levels may also be found in trophoblastic disease (Sørensen 1982). The function of SP₁ is not known, but from the homology with adhesion molecules, a tentative hypothesis might be, that SP₁ is involved in maintaining the integrity of the placenta.

SP₁ can be measured by numerous immunochemical methods (Schultz-Larsen *et al.* 1979; Bischof 1992). Enzyme-linked immunosorbent assays (ELISA), radio-immunoassay (RIA) or time-resolved fluorescent assays (TrIFMA) are very suitable for analysis early in pregnancy. As SP₁ is a heterogeneous mixture of glycoproteins and aggregation may affect quantitation (Teisner *et al.* 1979; Pala *et al.* 1992), it is probably sensible to rely on a polyclonal antibody for immunodetection. For standardisation an international reference preparation made from freeze-dried third trimester serum, WHO IRP 78/610 (WHO International Laboratory, Statens Serum Institut, Denmark), is available. The content of SP₁ is expressed in international units (IU), the WHO IRP 78/610 having a concentration of 100 IU/l when reconstituted (Bohn *et al.* 1980).

SP₁ was initially found in elevated concentrations in second trimester in women with a DS fetus (Bartels and Lindemann 1988) and this finding was confirmed in several subsequent studies with larger patient numbers (Wald *et al.* 1989; Knight *et al.* 1989; Bartels *et al.* 1990, 1994; Petrocik *et al.* 1990; Graham *et al.* 1992).

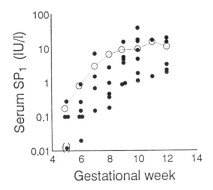

Fig. 15.1. Maternal serum SP_1 concentrations in 39 DS pregnancies in first trimester (●). The empirical median based on 306 normal control pregnancies (○). The point in parentheses had an undetectable SP_1 concentration.

However, the clinical importance of this finding should not be overestimated, as attempts to calculate the increase in sensitivity by addition of SP_1 as a marker (Wald *et al.* 1989; Bartels *et al.* 1994) have shown, that this increase is marginal when hCG is also determined.

In first trimester, several studies with few DS pregnancies have shown a conflicting pattern as some studies indicate SP_1 to be reduced in DS pregnancies (Brock *et al.* 1990; Brambati *et al.* 1992; Macintosh *et al.* 1993; Bersinger *et al.* 1994), whereas others have not been able to confirm this (Spencer 1991; Macintosh *et al.* 1993). One reason for this discrepancy may, as suggested by Macintosh (1994), be differences in the gestational age distribution of first trimester samples analysed. A recent meta-analysis on SP_1 (Cuckle 1994) found, that the median SP_1 MoM of DS pregnancies analysed before 15 weeks was 0.60 ($n=35$) and 1.46 ($n=261$) in pregnancies analysed after week 15. This was confirmed (Qin *et al.* 1997) in a study of 39 DS pregnancies from weeks 5 to 12, where the median MoM in weeks 5–9 was 0.27 (95% confidence interval: 0.11–0.59) ($n=25$), significantly lower than in normal controls, and increasing to 0.89 (0.20–2.09) ($n=14$) in weeks 10–12, not significantly different from normal controls, and further increasing to 1.28 (1.11–1.49) in weeks 14–20 ($n=117$) (Fig. 15.1). The use of SP_1 as a first trimester marker for DS thus seems to be very dependent on the gestational period chosen for screening and use after week 9 is probably not sensible. We have found the sensitivity in weeks 5–9 by ROC analysis to be *c.* 35 % for a false positive rate of 5 %.

However, the use of SP_1 in screening for DS should, as well as the precise definition of optimal diagnostic windows, await further prospective studies.

In our 39 DS pregnancies (Qin *et al.* 1997) no difference in MoM was found between first trimester samples from pregnancies terminated after diagnosis of a DS pregnancy by CVS or AC ($n=32$) and pregnancies where the diagnosis was made at birth ($n=7$), so it is not likely that the DS pregnancies found by SP_1 are the ones destined for abortion, even though SP_1 is often reduced in pathological pregnancies, as described above. This matter, which is of major importance for the evaluation of the efficacy of screening in early first trimester, must await further studies with larger patient numbers.

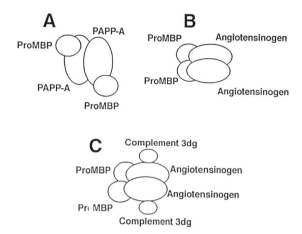

Fig. 15.2. Schematic representation of proMBP-complexes described in serum from pregnant women. (**A**) PAPP-A/proMDP-complex, (**B**) ProMDP-angiotensinogen-complex, (**C**) ProMBP-angiotensinogen-complement 3dg-complex (Oxvig *et al.* 1993, 1994). These drawings are purely schematic and the precise structure of these complexes is unknown at present.

In conclusion, SP$_1$ – used as a single marker – is promising as an adjunct to other screening parameters, particularly in early first trimester (weeks 5–9), but more data should be collected before its role can be finally addressed.

PAPP-A/proMBP-complex

Pregnancy associated protein-A (PAPP-A) was described in 1974 (Lin *et al.* 1974) as a high-molecular-weight constituent of pregnant serum. PAPP-A was found to have an apparent molecular weight of 750–820 kDa and an α-2-electrophoretic mobility. From cDNA sequencing, PAPP-A was found to consist of 1547 amino acids and to show homology with metalloproteinases (Kristensen *et al.* 1994). As described below, PAPP-A has recently been found to exist in maternal serum complexed 2:2 with the proform of eosinophil major basic protein (Oxvig *et al.* 1993, 1994) (Fig. 15.2).

Using polyclonal antibodies and gel precipitation techniques (Folkersen *et al.* 1981), the concentration of PAPP-A was found to increase throughout pregnancy. The major site of synthesis was suggested to be the syncytiotrophoblast (Lin and Halbert 1976). Low or undetectable PAPP-A in maternal serum has been associated with Cornelia de Lange syndrome (Westergaard *et al.* 1983) and several pregnancy complications. In none of the latter, however, has determination of PAPP-A led to clinical usage (Stabile *et al.* 1988; Bischof 1992). A clinical application was proposed when it was observed that maternal serum PAPP-A concentrations were reduced in first trimester in DS pregnancies (Brambati *et al.* 1991), a finding confirmed in several subsequent studies (Wald *et al.* 1992, 1996; Muller *et al.* 1993; Hurley *et al.* 1993; Macintosh 1994; Brambati *et al.* 1993; Qin *et al.* 1996a). In these studies the median PAPP-A MoMs varied from 0.23 to 0.57 with DS pregnancies from week 6 to 14. By contrast in the second trimester,

PAPP-A levels were only marginally reduced (Cuckle *et al.* 1992) or normal (Knight *et al.* 1993; Wald and Voller 1993).

Initially, PAPP-A concentrations were measured using gel precipitation techniques: radial immunodiffusion (sensitivity: 19 IU/l), antigen antibody crossed immuno-electrophoresis (sensitivity: 18 IU/l), rocket immunoelectrophoresis (sensitivity: 5–10 IU/l), radiorocket line electrophoresis (sensitivity: 19 mIU/l) (Westergaard 1987). Apart from the latter technique which is difficult and costly, none of these assays have the sensitivity necessary for quantification of PAPP-A in the first trimester. This became possible with the development of radioimmunoassays (Bischof *et al.* 1981; Sinosich *et al.* 1982; Anthony *et al.* 1983; Pinto-Furtado *et al.* 1984), where a sensitivity of 3–20 µg/l (≈ 6–40 mIU/l) was attained. However, these RIAs employ purified and labelled PAPP-A which only has a shelf life of approximately three weeks (Bersinger *et al.* 1995). Furthermore, as the RIA technique depends on the similarity between analyte and tracer for the specificity of the measurement, the use of partly modified – by radio-labelling/degradation – tracer may give specificity problems.

Also ELISAs were developed, all (Bersinger *et al.* 1995; Pledger and Belfield 1983) employing polyclonal antibodies, apart from one study using a monoclonal antibody (Mowles *et al.* 1986). For calibration, the pregnancy serum protein standard WHO 78/610 is available, as mentioned above with SP_1, but many studies have used purified PAPP-A for calibration.

The specificity of the polyclonal antibodies used both for measurements of PAPP-A in body fluids and for immunohistochemical localisation has been a source of controversies for more than a decade (Bischof and Meisser 1989; Chemnitz *et al.* 1986; Bischof 1992). The most used commercial polyclonal

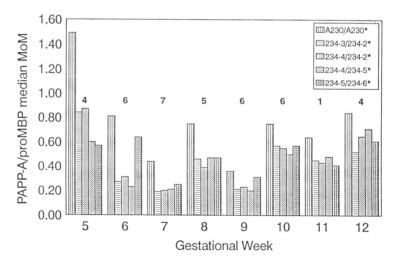

Fig. 15.3. Comparison of different sandwich immunoassays for PAPP-A/proMBP with respect to the median MoMs obtained in the same DS pregnancies in first trimester. The number of DS pregnancies in each gestational week is shown above the columns. A230 denotes the DAKO polyclonal (unabsorbed) antiserum and it is clearly seen, that the MoMs are higher with this antibody than with the monoclonal combinations. Antibodies denoted 234-X are from Statens Serum Institut, Copenhagen.

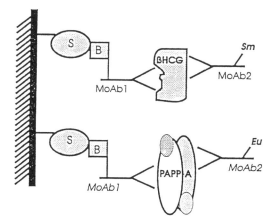

Fig. 15.4. The design of a dual label time resolved immunofluorescent assay for PAPP-A/proMBP-complex and free β-hCG using monoclonal antibodies. S, streptavidin; B, biotin; Sm, Sm^{3+}-chelate; Eu, Eu^{3+}-chelate.

antibody aganist PAPP-A, DAKO A230, has been shown to cross-react with SP_1 (Bersinger *et al.* 1995), recombinant proMBP (Oxvig *et al.* 1993) and haptoglobin (Bueler and Bersinger 1989) in different assay systems. We developed a sandwich immunofluorescent assay for PAPP-A using the DAKO antibody and only found a detection rate of 9% for a false positive rate of 5% in 7–12 weeks (Qin *et al.* 1996a), with a median MoM in 29 affected pregnancies of 0.57 (95% confidence interval: 0.47–0.99). Furthermore, we developed and characterised ten monoclonal antibodies against PAPP-A/proMBP-complex of which eight reacted with the PAPP-A-part of the complex (Qin *et al.* 1996b). In a comparison of sandwich assays either based on two monoclonal antibodies (both reactive with the PAPP-A part of the PAPP-A/proMBP-complex) or a double polyclonal assay the MoMs of DS pregnancies were significantly lower using the double monoclonal assays (Qin *et al.* 1996c) (Fig. 15.3). The same was found when comparing the MoMs obtained with double monoclonal assays with a polyclonal–monoclonal assay (Pettersson *et al.* 1993; Wald *et al.* 1996) in nine DS pregnancies and 67 controls (Qin *et al.* 1996b). From the low MoMs obtained using an absorbed polyclonal antibody (Bersinger *et al.* 1995), it would seem as though the difference in performance could be due to cross-reactivity on the part of the polyclonal antibody. As absorbing-out cross-reactivities from an antiserum is complicated and difficult to do reproducibly, the emergence of commercially available assays based on well characterised monoclonal antibodies will represent an important advance.

A recent methodological advance is the construction of a time-resolved dual-label assay for PAPP-A/proMBP-complex and free β-hCG (Fig. 15.4), enabling the simultaneous determination of both of these analytes in one microtitre well (K. Pettersson, personal communication). With the excellent performance data of this assay (Fig. 15.5), and the reduction in variation obtainable both by performing one combined measurement instead of two and the possibility of automation, it should be possible to reduce the analytical source of reduced performance using the markers PAPP-A/proMBP and free β-hCG.

As different levels of PAPP-A/proMBP complex are seen, depending on the

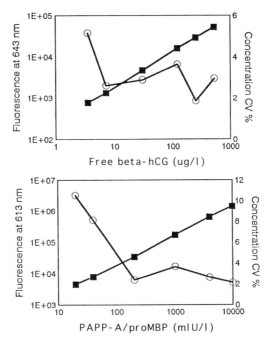

Fig. 15.5. Standard curves and precision profiles for the dual label assay detailed in Fig. 15.4. CV, intra-assay coefficient of variation.

choice of antibodies (Qin *et al.* 1996c), particularly in first trimester, it is very important to establish normal medians with the assay that is going to be used to assay samples and as long as the precise reason for this phenomenon (micro-heterogeneous variants, conformers or cross-reactive neoantigens) has not been established, it is wise for each laboratory to establish normal medians on their own representative normal samples.

In conclusion, PAPP-A/proMBP complex (formerly 'PAPP-A') is an important first trimester serum marker with a well documented performance in retrospective studies. The assay technology is close to being available for all interested centres.

The proform of eosinophil major basic protein

Material with an immunoreactivity similar to that of eosinophil major basic protein (MBP), the most abundant constituent of the specific granules of the eosinophil leucocyte (Gleich and Adolphson 1986), has been found in high concentrations in plasma of pregnant women (Maddox *et al.* 1983) and immuno-histochemically in X cells and giant cells of the placenta (Maddox *et al.* 1984). These and other studies (Wasmoen *et al.* 1989) indicate that the MBP found in pregnancy is not synthesised by eosinophils and is either bound to macro-molecules or synthesised as a form larger than the normal MBP.

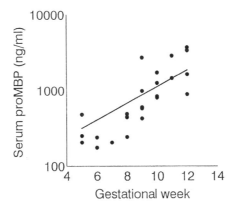

Fig. 15.6.   Maternal serum proMBP concentrations in DS pregnancies (points). The line shows the log-regressed median of normal pregnancies.

The proform of eosinophil major basic protein (proMBP) was found to be complex-bound to PAPP-A (Oxvig *et al.* 1993, 1994) and angiotensinogen, complement C3dg and possibly other proteins (Oxvig *et al.* 1995) in pregnancy serum (Fig. 15.2). The MBP immunoreactivity described in pregnant serum before the discovery of the proMBP complexes is well explained by the presence of these complexes (Oxvig 1995). ProMBP mRNA has been located in placenta X cells by *in situ* hybridisation, whereas PAPP-A mRNA was found both in X cells and syncytiotrophoblast (Bonno *et al.* 1994). The serum level of proMBP has been shown to correlate with the number of septa, septal cysts and subchorial cysts in placenta (Wasmoen *et al.* 1991). In our study a correlation was found between serum proMBP and placenta weight (Wagner *et al.* 1993). The serum level of proMBP rises exponentially from week 5 to reach a plateau around week 20 (Wasmoen *et al.* 1987; Wagner *et al.* 1993) and rises in serum level in late third trimester have been shown to correlate with the onset of spontaneous labour (Wasmoen *et al.* 1987). However, there does not seem to be a clearcut relation between preterm labour and a rise in serum proMBP (Wagner *et al.* 1993).

Table 15.1.   Spearman rank correlation of log MoM values for each marker in two intervals of first trimester. Rs is given for DS pregnancies and controls (parentheses)

	PAPP-A/ proMBP	ProMBP	AFP	Free β-hCG	Intact hCG
SP1					
4-8 week	0.44 (0.72)	0.51 (0.56)	0.26 (0.27)	0.23 (0.64)	0.55 (0.85)
9-12 week	0.30 (0.60)	0.60 (0.49)	0.21 (0.25)	0.19 (0.28)	0.46 (0.47)
PAPP-A/proMBP					
4-8 week	–	0.53 (0.70)	0.36 (0.28)	−0.15 (0.55)	0.23 (0.67)
9–12 week	–	0.70 (0.65)	0.19 (0.32)	0.36 (0.22)	0.25 (0.26)
ProMBP					
4-8 week	–	–	0.66 (0.23)	0.01 (0.47)	0.49 (0.56)
9–12 week	–	–	0.25 (0.10)	0.18 (0.40)	0.14 (0.23)

Preliminary data on the use of proMBP as a marker for DS pregnancy in first trimester have been presented (Christiansen *et al.* 1996) (Fig. 15.6), and it seems as though serum proMBP is reduced very early (< week 10) in first trimester of DS pregnancies. In a comparison of the discriminatory potential of different combinations of serum markers proMBP was found to be low in weeks 7–9 and elevated in weeks 15–19 and the correlation between log MoM values for PAPP-A/proMBP complex (determined with a double polyclonal sandwich immunoassay) was very clear (Table 15.1). ProMBP and its complexes are also important as potential cross-reactants in assays for PAPP-A/proMBP-complex, as described above.

Presently, the technique required to measure proMBP (or pregnancy MBP immunoreactivity) is only available in a few laboratories and due to the denaturation step (Wagner *et al.* 1993) required to release proMBP from its complexes it may be difficult to design assay systems suitable for large scale analysis.

In conclusion, the potential role of proMBP in first trimester DS screening must await the appearance of more data, but it seems to be an interesting marker for biochemical screening very early in first trimester, if the technical problems associated with its determination can be solved.

Simultaneous use of several serum markers

Other serum markers than SP_1, PAPP-A/proMBP-complex and proMBP are important in first trimester screening for DS, especially free β-hCG. In order to estimate the effect of a screening procedure it is necessary to evaluate the effect of several markers used simultaneously. This may be done in several ways, either by modelling each marker (or a transformed derivative) by a normal distribution and based on these distributions and the covariation between markers establish di- or trivariate normal risk distributions ('likelihood ratio-method') or by discriminant analysis of 'risk-indices', i.e. functions containing all risk markers. In both methods it is customary to use logarithmic MoM values. However, both methods require large patient materials, rarely available for retrospective studies in first trimester screening, to give accurate estimates. We have recently evaluated different combinations of these four markers together with AFP and intact hCG on a panel of 156 sera from DS pregnancies with 39 DS cases from weeks 4 to 12 and 546 control samples with 306 from weeks 4 to 12. An initial screening of the data showed that proMBP, PAPP-A/proMBP-complex and SP_1 were clearly low in DS pregnancies in weeks 7–9 and that free β-hCG was high and SP_1 low in DS pregnancies in weeks 10–12, whereas free β-hCG, intact hCG and proMBP were high and AFP low in DS pregnancies from week 15 to 19. As the material was not very large we estimated the discriminatory potential of combinations of markers by calculating the Mahalanobis distance ($D=(m_d - m_n)/ \sqrt{(s_d^2 + s_n^2)/2}$), where m_d and m_n are means of log MoM in DS pregancies and controls, respectively and s^2 denotes the variance in the same groups. The larger the Mahalanobis distance the better the discrimination between DS pregnancies and controls. Based on the data screening the following indices were constructed: index A=log MoM proMBP + log MoM SP_1 + log MoM PAPP-A/proMBP; index B=2×log MoM free β-hCG – log MoM SP_1 and index C=log MoM free β-hCG + log MoM proMBP – log MoM AFP. In weeks 7–9 index A had a D=1.32, in weeks 10–12 index B had a D=1.29 and index C had a D of 1.43 in weeks 15–19. Thus, index A and B in weeks 7–9 and 10–12, respectively, had a Mahalanobis distance comparable to that of the second trimester index, with the consequence that biochemical screening with several markers seems as promising in first trimester as in second trimester. Table 15.1 shows correlation coefficients between markers in first trimester. In spite of correlations between markers, the use of several markers may confer increased sensitivity to a screening programme.

Problems in early screening for DS

Before introducing first trimester screening for DS there are several aspects which should be considered. First, it is known that about half of all DS pregnancies abort spontaneously from week 10 of gestation until term with about half of these miscarriages occurring before week 16 (Macintosh *et al.* 1995). Therefore, some of the affected pregnancies detected in first trimester would go on to abort spontaneously. However, this is also the case for those pregnant women who are offered an invasive test such as CVS in first trimester. Secondly, serum AFP screening for neural tube defect (NTD) cannot be performed in first trimester. Therefore, a malformation screening should be offered either as a serum AFP screening at 16–18 weeks of pregnancy or a malformation scan at about 18 weeks. Thirdly, ultrasound scanning should be carried out especially in pregnancies with uncertainty about last menstrual period and a measurement of nuchal trans- lucency (NT) should be carried out at 10–13 weeks and used as an independent risk parameter. Biochemical markers may be used before, during and after the optimal window for NT in the hands of experienced clinicians, so the use of biochemical screening is more flexible than NT. Furthermore, the dissipation into clinical practice of the technique of using NT for screening for DS seems to be difficult (Kornman *et al.* 1996). Lastly, it is important that strict quality control criteria are defined, both for the analysis of markers but also for the whole operation of the screening programme, including logistics, technical performance, normal medians, false positives and other aspects of the risk calculation.

It should be taken into account that retrospective studies using frozen samples cannot obviate the need for careful ongoing monitoring of a screening programme.

Conclusions and recommendations

In our opinion there are now sufficient data for starting closely monitored prospective intervention trials on a combined biochemical and ultrasound screen- ing for DS at 10–13 weeks of pregnancy. The risk parameters in such intervention trials should be free β-hCG, PAPP-A/proMBP-complex, nuchal translucency and maternal age. Serum and urine samples should be taken in both the first and second trimesters and all pregnant women included in the trial should be offered malformation screening by serum AFP at 16–18 weeks and/or a malformation scan at 18 weeks of pregnancy.

References

Aitken, D.A., Mccaw, G., Crossley, J.A. *et al.* (1993) First trimester biochemical screening for fetal chromosome abnormalities and neural tube defects. *Prenat Diagn* **13**, 681–9

Anthony, F., Masson, G.M. and Wood, P.J. (1983) Development of a radioimmuno-assay for pregnancy-associated plasma protein-A and establishment of normal levels in the first trimester of pregnancy. *Ann Clin Biochem* **20**, 26–30

Barnett, T.R., Pickle, W. and Elting, J.J. (1990) Characterization of two new members of the pregnancy-specific beta 1-glycoprotein family from the myeloid cell line KG-1 and suggestion of two distinct classes of transcription unit. *Biochemistry* **29**, 10213–18

Bartels, I. and Lindemann, A. (1988) Maternal levels of pregnancy-specific β_1-glycoprotein (SP-1) are elevated in pregnancies affected by Down's syndrome. *Hum Genet* **80**, 46–8

Bartels, I., Thiele, M. and Bogart M.H. (1990) Maternal serum hCG and SP$_1$ in pregnancies with fetal aneuploidy. *Am J Med Genet* **37**, 261–4

Bartels, I., Bockel, B., Caesar, J. *et al.* (1994) Risk of fetal Down syndrome based on maternal age and varying combinations of maternal serum markers. *Arch Gynecol Obstet* **255**, 57–64

Bersinger, N.A., Keller, P.J., Naiem, A. *et al.* (1987) Pregnancy-specific and pregnancy-associated proteins in threatened abortion. *Gynecol Endocrinol* **1**, 379–84

Bersinger, N.A., Brizot, M.L., Johnson, A. *et al.* (1994) First trimester maternal serum pregnancy-associated plasma protein A and pregnancy-specific β1-glycoprotein in fetal trisomies. *Br J Obstet Gynaecol* **101**, 970–4

Bersinger, N.A., Zakher, A., Huber, U. *et al.* (1995) A sensitive enzyme immunoassay for pregnancy-associated plasma protein A (PAPP-A): a possible first trimester method of screening for Down syndrome and other trisomies. *Arch Gynecol Obstet* **256**, 185–92

Bischof, P. (1992) 'Pathological aspects of the different proteins produced by the placenta during the evolution of pregnancy' in J.R. Pasqualini and R. Scholler (Eds) *Hormones and Fetal Pathophysiology*, pp.277–341. New York: Marcel Dekker

Bischof, P. and Meisser, A. (1989) Immunological heterogeneity of pregnancy-associated plasma protein-A (PAPP-A). Effects on the radioimmunoassay of PAPP-A. *Br J Obstet Gynaecol* **96**, 870–5

Bischof, P., Haenggeli, L., Sizonenko, M.T. *et al.* (1981) Radioimmuno-assay for the measurement of pregnancy associated plasma protein A (PAPP-A) in humans. *Biol Reprod* **24**, 1076–81

Bohn, H. (1979) 'Placental and pregnancy proteins' in F.G. Lehmann (Ed.) *Carcino-embryonic Proteins*, vol. 1, pp.289–99. Amsterdam: Elsevier

Bohn, H., Chard, T., Grudzinskas, J.G. *et al.* (1980) Reference preparation for assays of some pregnancy and cancer associated proteins. *Lancet* **ii**, 796

Bonno, M., Oxvig, C., Kephart, G.M. *et al.* (1994) Localization of pregnancy-associated plasma protein-A and colocalization of pregnancy-associated plasma protein-A messenger ribonucleic acid and eosinophil granule major basic protein messenger ribonucleic acid in placenta. *Lab Invest* **71**, 560–6

Brambati, B., Lanzani, A. and Tului, L. (1991) 'Ultrasound and biochemical assessment of first trimester pregnancy' in M. Chapman, G. Grudzinskas and T. Chard (Eds) *The Embryo*, pp.181–94. London: Springer-Verlag

Brambati, B., Chard, T., Grudzinskas, J.G. *et al.* (1992) Potential first trimester biochemical screening tests for chromosome anomalies. *Prenat Diagn* **12** (Suppl), S4

Brambati, B., Macintosh, M.C., Teisner, B. *et al.* (1993) Low maternal serum levels of pregnancy-associated plasma protein A (PAPP-A) in the first trimester in association with abnormal fetal karyotype. *Br J Obstet Gynaecol* **100**, 324–6

Briese, V. and Glockner, E. (1991) Placental function test, clinical and biochemical parameters in diabetic pregnancy complicated by retinopathy. *Zentralbl Gynakol* **113**, 1033–41

Brock, D.J., Barron, L., Holloway, S. *et al.* (1990) First-trimester maternal serum biochemical indicators in Down syndrome. *Prenat Diagn* **10**, 245–51

Bueler, M.R. and Bersinger, N.A. (1989) Antiserum to pregnancy associated plasma protein A (PAPP-A) recognises human haptoglobin. *Br J Obstet Gynaecol* **96**, 867–9

Chan, W.Y., Zheng, Q.X., McMahon, J. and Tease, L.A. (1991) Characterization of new members of the pregnancy-specific beta 1-glycoprotein family. *Mol Cell Biochem* **106**, 161–70

Chapman, M.G., O'Shea, R.T., Jones, W.R. and Hillier, R. (1981) Pregnancy specific β1 glycoprotein as a screening test for risk pregnancies. *Am J Obstet Gynecol* **141**, 499–502

Chemnitz, J., Folkersen, J., Teisner, B. *et al.* (1986) Comparison of different antibody preparations against pregnancy-associated plasma protein-A (PAPP-A) for use in localisation and immunoassay studies. *Br J Obstet Gynaecol* **93**, 916–23

Christiansen, M., Oxvig, C., Wagner, J.M. *et al.* (1995) 'The proform of eosinophilic major basic protein: a new maternal serum marker for Down's syndrome in first trimester' in *Screening for Down's Syndrome in the First Trimester of Pregnancy*. Sixth International Conference, Endocrinology and Metabolism in Human Reproduction, 11–13 October. Abstract

Cuckle, H. (1994) 'Screening at 11–14 weeks of gestation: the role of established markers and PAPP-A' in J.G. Grudzinskas, T. Chard, M. Chapman and H. Cuckle. (Eds) *Screening for Down's Syndrome*, pp.311–24. Cambridge: Cambridge University Press

Cuckle, H., Lilford, R.J., Teisner, B. *et al.* (1992) Pregnancy-associated plasma protein A in Down syndrome. *Br Med J* **305**, 425

Folkersen, J., Grudzinskas, J.G., Hindersson, P. *et al.* (1981) Pregnancy-associated plasma protein-A: circulating levels during normal pregnancy. *Am J Obstet Gynecol* **139**, 910–14

Gleich, G.J. and Adolphson, C.R. (1986) The eosinophil leukocyte: structure and function. *Adv Immunol* **39**, 177–253

Gordon, Y.B., Grudzinskas, J.G., Jeffrey, D. and Chard, T. (1977) Concentrations of pregnancy specific β1 glycoprotein in maternal blood in normal pregnancy and in intrauterine growth retardation. *Lancet* **i**, 331–5

Graham, G.W., Crossley, J.A., Aitken, D.A. and Connor, J.M. (1992) Variation in the levels of pregnancy-specific β-1-glycoprotein in maternal serum from chromosomally abnormal pregnancies. *Prenat Diagn* **12**, 505–12

Grudzinskas, J.G., Gordon, Y.B., Menabawey, M. *et al.* (1983) Identification of high risk pregnancy by the routine measurement of pregnancy specific β1 glycoprotein. *Am J Obstet Gynecol* **147**, 10–12

Hertz, J.B. and Schultz-Larsen, P. (1983) Human placental lactogen, pregnancy specific β1 glycoprotein and alpha-fetoprotein in serum in threatened abortion. *Int J Gynaecol Obstet* **21**, 111–17

Hughes, G., Bischof, P., Wilson, G. *et al.* (1980) Tests of fetal well-being in the third trimester of pregnancy. *Br J Obstet Gynaecol* **87**, 650–6

Hurley, P.A., Ward, R.H., Teisner, B. *et al.* (1993) Serum PAPP-A measurements in first trimester screening for Down's syndrome. *Prenat Diagn* **13**, 903–8

Knight, G.J., Palomaki, G.E., Haddow, J.E. *et al.* (1989) Maternal serum levels of the placental products hCG, hPL, SP1 and progesterone are all elevated in cases of fetal Down syndrome. *Am J Hum Genet* **45**, A263

Knight, G.J., Palomaki, G.E., Haddow, J.E. *et al.* (1993) Pregnancy-associated plasma protein A as a marker for Down's syndrome in the second trimester of pregnancy. *Prenat Diagn* **13**, 222–3

Kornman, L., Morssink, L.P., Beekhuis, J. R., De Wolf, T.H.M. *et al.* (1996) Nuchal translucency cannot be used as a screening test for chromosomal abnormalities in the first trimester of pregnancy in a routine ultrasound practice. *Prenat Diagn* **16**, 797–805

Kristensen, T., Oxvig, C., Sand, O. *et al.* (1994) Amino acid sequence of human pregnancy-associated plasma protein-A derived from cloned cDNA. *Biochemistry* **33**, 1592–8

Larsen, S.O., Christiansen, M., Qin, Q.P. and Nørgaard-Pedersen B. (1997) Six maternal serum markers in screening for Down's syndrome. Discriminatory potential in the first and second trimester. (submitted)

Leslie, K.K., Watanabe, S., Lei, K.J. *et al.* (1990) Linkage of two human pregnancy-specific beta 1-glycoprotein genes: one is associated with hydatidiform mole. *Proc Natl Acad Sci USA* **87**, 5822–6

Lin, T.M. and Halbert, S.P. (1976) Placental localization of human pregnancy-associated plasma proteins. *Science* **193**, 1249–52

Lin, T.M., Halbert, S.P., Kiefer, D. *et al.* (1974) Characterization of four human pregnancy-associated plasma proteins. *Am J Obstet Gynecol* **118**, 223–36

MacDonald, D.H., Scott, J.M., Gemmell, R.S. and Mack, D.S. (1983) A prospective study of three biochemical fetoplacental tests: serum human placental lactogen, pregnancy specific β_1 glycoprotein, and urinary estrogens, and their relationship to placental insufficiency. *Am J Obstet Gynecol* **147**, 430–6

Macintosh, M.C.M. (1994) 'Schwangerschaftsprotein 1 (SP₁) and biochemical screening for Down's syndrome' in J.G. Grudzinskas, T. Chard, M. Chapman and H. Cuckle (Eds) *Screening for Down's Syndrome*, pp.171–80. Cambridge: Cambridge University Press

Macintosh, M.C.M., Brambati, B., Chard, T. and Grudzinskas, J.G. (1993) First trimester maternal serum schwangerschaftsprotein 1 (SP₁) in pregnancies associated with chromosomal anomalies. *Prenat Diagn* **13**, 563–8

Macintosh, M.C.M., Wald, N.J., Chard, T. *et al.* (1995) The selective miscarriage of Down's syndrome from 10 weeks of pregnancy. *Br J Obstet Gynaecol* **102**, 798–801

Maddox, D.E., Butterfield, J.H., Ackerman, S.J. *et al.* (1983) Elevated serum levels in human pregnancy of a molecule immunochemically similar to eosinophil granule major basic protein. *J Exp Med* **158**, 1211–26

Maddox, D.E., Kephart, G.M., Coulam, C.B. *et al.* (1984) Localization of a molecule immuno-chemically similar to eosinophil major basic protein in human placenta. *J Exp Med* **160**, 29–41

Mantzavinos, T., Phocas, I., Chrelias, H. *et al.* (1991) Serum levels of steroid and placental protein hormones in ectopic pregnancy. *Eur J Obstet Gynecol Reprod Biol* **39**, 117–22

Masson, G.M., Anthony, F. and Wilson, M.S. (1983) Value of Schwanger-schaftsprotein 1 (SP₁) and pregnancy-associated plasma protein-A (PAPP-A) in the clinical management of threatened abortion. *Br J Obstet Gynaecol* **90**, 146–9

Mowles, E.A., Pinto-Furtado, L.G. and Bolton, A.E. (1986) A two-site immuno-radiometric assay for human pregnancy-associated plasma protein A (PAPP-A) using monoclonal antibodies. *J Immunol Meth* **95**, 129–33

Muller, F., Cuckle, H., Teisner, B. and Grudzinskas, J.G. (1993) Serum PAPP-A levels are depressed in women with fetal Down's syndrome in early pregnancy. *Prenat Diagn* **13**, 633–6

Nicolaides, K.H., Azar, G., Byrne, D. *et al.* (1992) Fetal nuchal translucency: ultrasound screening for chromosomal defects in the first trimester of pregnancy. *Br Med J* **304**, 867–9

Nicolaides, K.H., Brizot, M.I. and Snijders, R.J.M. (1994) Fetal nuchal translucency: ultrasound screening for fetal trisomy in the first trimester of pregnancy. *Br J Obstet Gynaecol* **101**, 782–6

Oxvig, C. (1995) Two pregnancy proteins and their mutual complex: pregnancy-associated plasma protein-A and proform of eosinophil major basic protein. PhD thesis. University of Aarhus

Oxvig, C., Sand, O., Kristensen, T. *et al.* (1993) Circulating human pregnancy-associated plasma protein-A is disulfide-bridged to the proform of eosinophil major basic protein. *J Biol Chem* **268**, 12243–6

Oxvig, C., Sand, O., Kristensen, L. and Sottrup-Jensen, L. (1994) Isolation and characterization of circulating complex between human pregnancy-associated protein-A and proform of eosinophil major basic protein. *Biochim Biophys Acta* **1201**, 415–23

Oxvig, C., Haaning, J., Kristensen, L. *et al.* (1995) Identification of angiotensinogen and complement C3dg as novel proteins binding proform of eosinophil major basic protein in human pregnancy serum and plasma. *J Biol Chem* **270**, 13645–51

Pala, A., Di-Ruzza, A., Rossetto, G. *et al.* (1992) Distribution of SP₁ immuno-reactivity among different plasma proteins: real molecular heterogeneity or adsorption of SP₁-beta to other plasma proteins? *Clin Chim Acta* **207**, 87–97

Petrocik, E., Wassman, E.R., Lee, J.J. and Kelly, J.C. (1990) Second trimester maternal serum pregnancy specific beta-1 glycoprotein (SP-1) levels in normal and Down's syndrome preg-nancies. *Am J Med Genet* **37**, 114–18

Pettersson, K., Nørgaard-Pedersen, B., Stenman, U. and Stigbrand, T. (1993) 'Optimisation of immunometric assays for the measurement of PAPP-A first trimester samples from normal and trisomy 21 pregnancies' in *Screening for Down's Syndrome*, Royal College of Obstetricians and Gynaecologists, 24–26 May, Abstract no. 35

Pettersson, K., Qin, Q.P., Jones, M. *et al.* (1996) Rapid, sensitive and robust two-site Delfia assay for the specific determination of pregnancy-associated plasma protein A (PAPP-A) in serum. Recent Advances in Prenatal Diagnosis for Aneuploidy. Amsterdam, 30 April–3 May. Abstract

Pinto-Furtado, L.G., Bolton, A.E., Grudzinskas, J.G. *et al.* (1984) The development and validation of a radioimmunoassay for pregnancy-associated plasma protein-A (PAPP-A). *Arch Gynecol* **236**, 83–91

Pledger, D.R. and Belfield, A. (1983) An ELISA for pregnancy-associated plasma protein A. *Ann Clin Biochem* **20**, 236–40

Qin, Q.P., Nguyen, T.H., Christiansen, M., Larsen, S.O., Nørgaard-Pedersen, B. (1996a) Time-resolved immunofluorometric assay of pregnancy-associated plasma protein-A in maternal serum screening for Down's syndrome in first trimester of pregnancy. *Clin Chim Acta* **253**, 113–29

Qin, Q.P., Christiansen, M., Oxvig, C. *et al.* (1996b) Monoclonal antibodies against the complex of human pregnancy-associated plasma protein-A and the proform of eosinophil major basic protein (PAPP-A/proMBP-complex): Production, characterization, epitope analysis and application in immunochemical assays for PAPP-A/proMBP-complex. Recent Advances in Prenatal Diagnosis for Aneuploidy, Amsterdam, 30 April–3 May. Abstract

Qin, Q.P., Christiansen, M., Oxvig, C., Petterson, K., Koch, C. and Nørgaard-Pedersen, B. (1996c) Comparison of four double monoclonal time-resolved immunofluorometric assays for PAPP-A/proMBP-complex with respect to first trimester maternal serum screening for Down's syndrome. Recent Advances in Prenatal Diagnosis for Aneuploidy, Amsterdam, 30 April–3 May. Abstract.

Qin, Q.P., Christiansen, M., Nguyen, T.H. *et al.* (1997) Schwangerschaftsprotein 1 (SP₁) as maternal serum marker for Down's syndrome in first and second trimester. *Prenat Diagn* **17**, 101–8

Royal College of Obstetricians and Gynaecologists (1993) *Report of the RCOG Working Party on Biochemical Markers and the Detection of Down's Syndrome.* London: Royal College of Obstetricians and Gynaecologists

Schindler, A.M., Bordignon, P. and Bischof, P. (1984) Immunohistochemical localisation of pregnancy-associated plasma protein A in decidua and trophoblast: comparison with human chorionic gonadotrophin and fibrin. *Placenta* **5**, 227–35

Schulte-Vallentin, M. and Schindler, H. (1992) Non-echogenic nuchal oedema as a marker in trisomy 21 screening. *Lancet* **339**, 1053

Schultz-Larsen, P., Lyngbye, J., Westergaard, J.G. and Teisner, B. (1979) Pregnancy-specific β₁-glycoprotein (SP₁) determined by means of electroimmuno-assay, radial immunodiffusion and nephelometry. *Clin Chim Acta* **99**, 59–69

Silver, R.M., Heyborne, K.D. and Leslie, K.K. (1993) Pregnancy specific β₁ glycoprotein (SP-1) in maternal serum and amniotic fluid; preeclampsia, small for gestational age fetus and fetal distress. *Placenta* **14**, 583–9

Sinosich, M.J., Teisner, B., Folkersen, J. *et al.* (1982) Radioimmunoassay for pregnancy-associated plasma protein A (PAPP-A). *Clin Chem* **28**, 50–3

Sørensen, S. (1982) Pregnancy-'specific' β₁-glycoprotein (SP₁): purification, characterization, quantification and clinical application in malignancies (A review). *Tumour Biol* **5**, 275–302

Sørensen, S., Momsen, G., Ruge, S. and Pedersen, J.F. (1995) Differential increase in the maternal serum concentrations of the placenta proteins human chorionic gonadotrophin, pregnancy-specific beta 1-glycoprotein, human placental lactogen and pregnancy-associated plasma protein A during the first half of normal pregnancy, elucidated by means of a mathematical model. *Hum Reprod* **10**, 453–8

Spencer, K. (1991) Pregnancy specific beta 1 glycoprotein in Down's syndrome screening: does it have any value ? Proceedings of the ACB Meeting. *Ann Clin Biochem* **C46**, 108

Stabile, I., Grudzinskas, J.G. and Chard, T. (1988) Clinical applications of pregnancy protein estimations with particular reference to pregnancy-associated plasma protein A (PAPP-A). *Obstet Gynecol Surv* **43**, 73–82

Sterzick, K., Wenske, C., Rossmanith, W. and Benz, R. (1986) Beta 1 glycoprotein determination in normal and disturbed pregnancy. *Int J Gynecol Obstet* **24**, 65–8

Sterzick, K., Rosenbusch, B. and Benz, R. (1989) Serum specific protein 1 and β concentrations in patients with suspected ectopic pregnancies. *Int J Gynecol Obstet* **28**, 253–6

Streydio, C., Swillens, S., Georges, M. *et al.* (1990) Structure, evolution and chromosomal localization of the human pregnancy-specific beta 1-glycoprotein gene family. *Genomics* **7**, 661–2

Szabo, J. and Gellen, J. (1990) Nuchal fluid accumulation in trisomy-21 detected by vagino-sonography in first trimester. *Lancet* **336**, 1133

Tamsen, L., Johansson, S.G.O. and Axelsson, O. (1983) Pregnancy specific beta 1 glycoprotein (SP-1) in serum from women with pregnancies complicated by intrauterine growth retardation. *J Perinat Med* **11**, 19–25

Teisner, B., Grudzinskas, J.G., Hindersson, P., Al-Ani, A.T.M., Westergaard, J.G. and Chard, T.

(1979) Molecular heterogeneity of pregnant specific β₁ glycoprotein: the effect on measurement by radioimmunoassay and electroimmunoassay. *J Immunol Meth* **31**, 141–9

Van Lith, J.M. (1994) First-trimester maternal serum alpha-fetoprotein as a marker for fetal chromosomal disorders. Dutch Working Party on Prenatal Diagnosis. *Prenat Diagn* **14**, 963–7

Wagner, J.M., Bartemes, K., Vernof, K.K. *et al.* (1993) Analysis of pregnancy-associated major basic protein levels throughout gestation. *Placenta* **14**, 671–81

Wald, N.J. and Voller, A. (1993) Pregnancy associated plasma protein A in Down's syndrome. *BMJ* **305**, 425

Wald, N.J., Cuckle, H.S. and Densem, J.W. (1989) Maternal serum specific β1-glycoprotein in pregnancies associated with Down's syndrome. *Lancet* **2**, 450

Wald, N., Stone, R., Cuckle, H.S. *et al.* (1992) First trimester concentrations of pregnancy-associated plasma protein A and placental protein 14 in Down's syndrome. *BMJ* **305**, 28

Wald, N.J., George, L., Smith, D. *et al.* (1996) Serum screening for Down's syndrome between 8 and 14 weeks of pregnancy. *Br J Obstet Gynaecol* **103**, 407–12

Wasmoen, T.L., Coulam, C.B., Leiferman, K.M. and Gleich, G.J. (1987) Increases of plasma eosinophil major basic protein levels late in pregnancy predict onset of labor. *Proc Natl Acad Sci USA* **84**, 3029–32

Wasmoen, T.L., McKean, D.J., Benirschke, K. *et al.* (1989) Evidence of eosinophil granule major basic protein in human placenta. *J Exp Med* **170**, 2051–63

Wasmoen, T.L., Coulam, C.R., Benirschke, K. and Gleich, G.J. (1991) Association of immuno-reactive eosinophil major basic protein with placental septa and cysts. *Am J Obstet Gynecol* **165**, 416–20

Westergaard, J.G., Chemnitz, J., Teisner, B. *et al.* (1983) Pregnancy-associated plasma protein-A: a possible marker in the classification and prenatal diagnosis of Cornelia de Lange syndrome. *Prenat Diagn* **3**, 225–32

Westergaard, J.G. (1987) Studies on pregnancy associated plasma protein-A (PAPP-A) in normal and abnormal pregnancy. Thesis. University of Odense, Denmark

Westergaard, J.G., Sinosich, M.J., Bugge, M. *et al.* (1983) Pregnancy-associated placenta protein A in the prediction of early pregnancy failure. *Am J Obstet Gynecol* **145**, 67–9

Wurz, H., Geiger, W., Kunzig, H.J. *et al.* (1981) Radioimmunoassay of SP-1 in maternal blood and in amniotic fluid in normal and pathological pregnancies. *J Perinat Med* **2**, 67–78

Zheng, Q.X., Tease, L.A., Shupert, W.L. and Chan, W.Y. (1990) Characterization of cDNAs of the human pregnancy-specific beta 1-glycoprotein family, a new subfamily of the immuno-globulin gene superfamily. *Biochemistry* **29**, 2845–52

Chapter 16

Maternal serum markers for aneuploidy in early pregnancy

Jan M.M. Van Lith

Introduction

Maternal serum screening has been introduced to identify those pregnancies at highest risk for Down syndrome to offer invasive prenatal diagnostic procedures. The risk is estimated based on maternal age and the measurements of several biochemical analytes in the second trimester of pregnancy. Prospective studies have confirmed the detection rates and false-positive rates as predicted from the models (Cuckle 1996). Moving maternal serum screening forward to the first trimester appears to be logical and studies have shown it to be feasible (Van Lith 1994a).

In this chapter, an overview of all published biochemical markers for Down syndrome before 15 weeks will be given, except PAPP-A and free β-hCG which are described in other chapters.

Method

The literature was reviewed on biochemical markers for Down syndrome before 15 weeks of gestation. A search in *Medline* was performed and references from published articles were examined to find articles on this subject. Care was taken to avoid duplication of results.

Publications were available for 13 serum markers, of which PAPP-A and free β-hCG were excluded: α-fetoprotein (AFP), hCG, free α-hCG, unconjugated estriol (uE₃), cancer antigen 125 (CA125), immunoreactive inhibin, dimeric inhibin A, placental alkaline phosphatase (PLAP), β-1 glycoprotein (SP-1), progesterone and placental protein 14 (PP-14). The results of the markers are given in multiples of the median (MoM) and the marker levels had an approximately Gaussian distribution. All studies were examined to obtain information on the distribution of gestational ages and the parameters of the marker distributions in normal and Down syndrome pregnancies, being the mean marker level in the latter and the standard deviation in both. The mean level in the normal pregnancies is 1 MoM. The mean was estimated by the median and the standard deviation was estimated from the 10th–90th centile range divided by 2.563 after log transformation.

The estimated parameters from the studies were entered into a meta-analysis to derive weighted overall parameters. Multivariate Gaussian distributions with the parameters from the meta-analysis were used for statistical modelling. The maternal age distribution of England and Wales in 1989–1993 was used. Based on this model the detection and false-positive rates were estimated.

Results

Thirteen maternal serum markers for Down syndrome have been evaluated before 15 weeks of gestation, of which PAPP-A and free β-hCG were excluded. AFP, uE$_3$, and SP-1 are related with Down syndrome (Tables 16.1–16.3). The estimated

Table 16.1. Maternal serum levels of alpha-fetoprotein in unaffected and Down syndrome pregnancies before 15 weeks of gestation[a]

Study	Unaffected pregnancy		Down syndrome pregnancy			
	n	SD	n	MoM	Mean	SD
Brambati et al. 1986	–	–	8	0.75	–	–
Barkai et al. 1987	–	–	2	0.65	–	–
Cuckle et al. 1988	110	?	22	0.72	−0.1427	0.1376
Milunsky et al. 1988	500	0.2399	10	0.81	−0.0706	0.2316
Mantingh et al. 1989	183	0.2352	5	0.7	−0.1871	0.2042
Brock et al. 1990	63	0.4185	21	0.71	−0.1487	0.3727
Nebiolo et al. 1990	–	–	9	0.70	–	–
Wenger et al. 1990	–	–	10	0.90	–	–
Crandall et al. 1991	1364	0.1502	10	0.75	−0.1249	0.1306
Johnson et al. 1991	145	0.2246	11	0.67	−0.1739	0.3135
Van Lith et al. 1991	–	–	9	0.71	–	–
Hogdall et al. 1992	61	0.191	14	0.91	−0.039	0.239
Fuhrmann et al. 1993	2337	0.1827	18	0.97	−0.0410	0.1207
Crandall et al. 1993	836	0.1814	11	0.74	−0.1308	0.1348
Aitken et al. 1993	–	–	16	0.65	–	–
Van Lith et al. 1994b	2404	0.19	32	0.83	−0.0809	0.2198
Spencer et al. 1994	320	0.2756	21	0.80	−0.17031	0.26236
Biagiotti et al. 1995	246	0.2087	41	0.74	−0.1308	0.2158
Brizot et al. 1995	342	0.2069	35	0.86	−0.0757	0.2827
Forest et al. 1995	500	0.1559	12	0.87	−0.060	0.2658
Wald et al.1995	383	?	77	0.87	−0.0655	?
Zimmermann et al. 1996	300	0.1980	4	0.65	−0.1870	0.2948

[a] The studies without mean and SD are omitted from the meta-analysis.

Table 16.2. Maternal serum levels of unconjugated oestriol in unaffected and Down syndrome pregnancies before 15 weeks of gestation[a]

Study	Unaffected pregnancy		Down syndrome pregnancy			
	n	SD	n	MoM	Mean	SD
Cuckle *et al.* 1988	110	?	17	0.35	−0.1938	0.2236
Brock *et al.* 1990	63	0.2201	21	0.67	−0.1739	0.3906
Crandall *et al.* 1991	1364	0.1674	10	0.73	−0.1367	0.2000
Crandall *et al.* 1993	836	0.1876	11	0.64	−0.1938	0.2629
Aitken *et al.* 1993	–	–	16	0.67	–	–
Spencer *et al.* 1994	320	0.1775	21	0.67	−0.27805	0.34324
Biagiotti *et al.* 1995	246	0.1998	41	0.64	−0.1938	0.2236
Forest *et al.* 1995	500	0.1697	12	0.86	−0.0655	0.2628
Wald *et al.* 1995	383	?	77	0.96	−0.0177	?

[a] The studies without mean and SD are omitted from the meta-analysis.

Table 16.3. Maternal serum levels of β-1 glycoprotein (SP-1) in unaffected and Down syndrome pregnancies before 15 weeks of gestation

Study	Unaffected pregnancy		Down syndrome pregnancy			
	n	SD	n	MoM	Mean	SD
Brock *et al.* 1990	40	0.3597	19	0.79	−0.1024	0.4068
Macintosh *et al.* 1993	662	0.63	14	0.40	−0.3979	0.4248
Bersinger *et al.* 1994	210	0.1874	29	0.91	−0.0410	0.2613

Table 16.4. Distribution parameters of AFP, uE$_3$, hCG and SP-1 in unaffected and Down syndrome pregnancies before 15 weeks of gestation

Marker	Unaffected pregnancy		Down syndrome pregnancy		
	n	SD	n	Mean	SD
AFP	9232	0.19	326	−0.10	0.24
uE$_3$	3329	0.18	210	−0.13	0.28
SP-1	912	0.55	62	−0.14	0.72

population parameters for normal and Down syndrome pregnancies of AFP and uE$_3$ are shown in Table 16.4. The other markers show no or no clear relation with Down syndrome before 15 weeks of gestation (Tables 16.5 and 16.6).

There appears to be no correlation of maternal serum markers with maternal age. The correlation coefficients for AFP and uE$_3$ in normal and Down syndrome pregnancies are 0.21 and 0.18, respectively. The correlation coefficients between AFP and SP-1 in normal and Down syndrome pregnancies are 0.03 and −0.04, respectively. As no data are available for the correlation between uE$_3$ and SP-1, the assumption was made that no correlation existed. The detection rates for a fixed false-positive rate of 5% using the individual markers combined with maternal age and a combination of these markers are given in Table 16.7.

Table 16.5. Maternal serum levels of total and alpha human chorionic gonadotrophin in unaffected and Down syndrome pregnancies before 15 weeks of gestation

Study	Unaffected pregnancy		Down syndrome pregnancy			
	n	SD	*n*	MoM	Mean	SD
Total hCG						
Cuckle *et al.* 1988	110	0.2643	22	1.1	0.0414	0.2469
Bogart *et al.* 1989	247	0.1510	6	1.17	0.0682	0.1228
Brock *et al.* 1990	63	0.2090	21	1.43	0.1553	0.2018
Johnson *et al.* 1991	145	0.1356	11	0.91	−0.0410	0.3944
Kratzer *et al.* 1991	112	0.1875	17	1.23	0.0899	0.1166
Van Lith *et al.* 1992	1348	0.1904	24	1.19	0.0767	0.2429
Hogdall *et al.* 1992	61	0.160	14	1.10	0.053	0.188
Aitken *et al.* 1993	320	?	16	0.97	−0.0132	0.3139
Crandall *et al.* 1993	836	0.1876	11	1.73	0.2380	0.0592
Macintosh *et al.* 1994	258	0.2897	23	1.4	0.1461	0.4517
Brizot *et al.* 1995	394	0.2891	41	1.5	0.1761	0.2275
Biagiotti *et al.* 1995	246	0.2458	41	1.12	0.0492	0.2555
Forest *et al.* 1995	500	0.1663	12	1.83	0.2625	0.2653
Wald *et al.* 1995	383	?	77	1.23	0.0864	?
Alpha hCG						
Ozturk *et al.* 1990	666	?	9	1.29	0.1106	0.3244
Kratzer *et al.* 1991	112	0.2142	17	0.77	−0.1135	0.2520
Macintosh *et al.* 1994	258	0.1785	23	1.06	0	0.2204
Forest *et al.* 1995	500	0.1628	12	1.32	0.1206	?
Wald *et al.* 1995	383	?	77	0.86	−0.0655	?

Table 16.6. Maternal serum levels of CA 125, immunoreactive and dimeric A inhibin, PLAP, progesterone and PP-14 in Down syndrome pregnancies before 15 weeks of gestation

Marker	Study	*n*	MoM
CA 125	Van Lith *et al.* 1991	9	0.45
	Norton and Golbus 1992	15	0.93
	Hogdall *et al.* 1992	14	?
	Van Lith *et al.* 1993	20	0.97
Inhibin Immunoreactive	Van Lith *et al.* 1994b	23	1.3
	Wallace *et al.* 1994	11	1.21
	Wallace *et al.* 1994	11	1.18
Inhibin Dimeric A	Wallace *et al.* 1995	23	2.46
	Wald *et al.* 1995	75	1.19
PLAP	Brock *et al.* 1990	21	0.92
Progesterone	Kratzer *et al.* 1991	17	0.93
PP-14	Wald *et al.* 1992	11	0.93

Table 16.7. Estimated detection rates of Down syndrome pregnancies before 15 weeks of gestation using a combination of maternal age with AFP, uE$_3$ or SP-1 at a 5% false-positive rate

	Detection rate (%)
Age + AFP	33
Age + uE$_3$	44
Age + SP-1	31
Age + AFP + uE$_3$	52
Age + AFP + SP-1	40
Age + uE$_3$ + SP-1	53
Age + AFP + uE$_3$ + SP-1	56

Discussion

Several biochemical markers in maternal serum are related to Down syndrome pregnancies before 15 weeks of gestation. Using them to screen for Down syndrome in early pregnancy is feasible. The most strongly related biochemical marker for Down syndrome in early pregnancy is PAPP-A. In a model based on a meta-analysis the detection rate of PAPP-A was 46% at a 5% false-positive rate (Van Lith 1996). Free β-hCG is also clearly related to Down syndrome in early pregnancy. These two biochemical markers are described in other chapters. The overview presented in this chapter shows that of eleven biochemical markers described in the literature, only AFP, uE$_3$ and SP-1 are related to Down syndrome. Question marks can be put at dimeric inhibin A, which will need further evaluation. When uE$_3$ is used in a model to estimate detection rates for Down syndrome before 15 weeks of gestation it reaches 44% at a 5% false-positive rate. This rate is comparable to the detection rates of PAPP-A. It seems advisable to study in detail the possibilities of uE$_3$ as an early marker, especially the technical problem of measuring low concentrations. AFP and SP-1 may be useful in screening programmes based on a combination of markers maybe adding a few percentage points to the detection rate (or decreasing the false-positive rate).

Nuchal translucency measurement as a marker for aneuploidy may have detection rates of 80% when combined with maternal age (Pandya *et al.* 1995). The combination of nuchal translucency measurement with PAPP-A and free β-hCG showed the highest detection rate of 87% in a model (Van Lith 1996).

In the near future, early screening for Down syndrome may be feasible in routine clinical practice. Aspects of antenatal care organisation, miscarriage rate and acceptability need to be evaluated.

Acknowledgement. Most of this work was performed at the Centre of Reproduction, Growth and Development, University of Leeds. I would like to thank Professor Howard Cuckle for his help with the analysis of the data.

References

Aitken, D.A., McCaw, G., Crossley, J.A. *et al.* (1993) First trimester biochemical screening for fetal chromosomal abnormalities and neural tube defects. *Prenat Diagn* **13**, 681–9

Barkai, G., Shaki, R., Pariente, C. and Goldman, B. (1987) First trimester alpha-fetoprotein levels in normal and chromosomally abnormal pregnancies. *Lancet* **ii**, 165

Bersinger, N.A., Brizot, M.L., Johnson, A. *et al.* (1994) First trimester maternal serum pregnancy associated plasma protein A and pregnancy specific β1-glycoprotein in fetal trisomies. *Br J Obstet Gynaecol* **101**, 970–4

Biagiotti, R., Cariate, E., Brizzi, L. and D'Agata, A. (1995) Maternal serum screening for Down syndrome in the first trimester of pregnancy. *Br J Obstet Gynaecol* **102**, 660–2

Bogart, M.H., Golbus, M.S., Sorg, N.D. and Jones, O.W. (1989) Human chorionic gonadotrophin levels in pregnancies with aneuploid fetuses. *Prenat Diagn* **9**, 379–84

Brambati, B., Simoni, G., Bonacchi, I. and Piceni, L. (1986) Fetal chromosomal aneuploidies and maternal serum alpha-fetoprotein levels in first trimester. *Lancet* **ii**, 165–6

Brizot, M.L., Snijders, R.J.M., Butler, J., Bersinger, N.A. and Nicolaides, K.H. (1995) Maternal serum hCg and fetal nuchal translucency thickness for the prediction of fetal trisomies in the first trimester of pregnancy. *Br J Obstet Gynaecol* **102**, 127–32

Brock, D.J.H., Barron, L., Holloway, S., Liston, W.A., Hillier, S.G. and Seppala, M. (1990) First-trimester maternal serum indicators in Down syndrome. *Prenat Diagn* **10**, 245–51

Crandall, B.F., Golbus, M.S., Goldberg, J.D. and Matsumoto, M. (1991) First-trimester maternal serum unconjugated oestriol and alpha-fetoprotein in fetal Down's syndrome. *Prenat Diagn* **11**, 377–80

Crandall, B.F., Hanson, F.W., Keener, M.S., Matsumoto, M. and Miller, W. (1993) Maternal serum screening for alpha-fetoprotein, unconjugated estriol and human chorionic gonadotropin between 11 and 15 weeks of pregnancy to detect fetal chromosome abnormalities. *Am J Obstet Gynecol* **168**, 1864–9

Cuckle, H.S. (1996) Established markers in second trimester maternal serum. *Early Hum Dev* **47**, S27–9

Cuckle, H.S., Wald, N.J., Barkai, G. *et al.* (1988) First trimester biochemical screening for Down syndrome. *Lancet* **ii**, 851–2

Forest, J., Masse, J., Rousseau, F., Moutquin, J., Brideau, N. and Belanger, M. (1995) Screening for Down syndrome during the first and second trimesters: impact of risk estimation parameters. *Clin Biochem* **28**, 443–9

Fuhrmann, W., Altland, K., Jovanovic, V. *et al.* (1993) First-trimester alpha-fetoprotein screening for Down syndrome. *Prenat Diagn* **13**, 215–18

Hogdall, C.K., Hogdall, E.V.S., Arends, J., Nørgaard-Pedersen, B., Smidt-Jensen, S. and Larsen, S.O. (1992) CA-125 as a maternal serum marker for Down's syndrome in the first and second trimesters. *Prenat Diagn* **12**, 223–7

Johnson, A., Cowchock, F.S., Darby, M., Wapner, R. and Jackson, L.G. (1991) First-trimester maternal serum alpha-fetoprotein and chorionic gonadotropin in aneuploid pregnancies. *Prenat Diagn* **11**, 443–50

Kratzer, P.G., Golbus, M.S., Monroe, S.E., Finkelstein, D.E. and Taylor, R.N. (1991) First trimester aneuploidy screening using serum human chorionic gonadotropin, free alpha-hCG and progesterone. *Prenat Diagn* **11**, 751–65

Macintosh, M.C.M., Brambati, B., Chard, T. and Grudzinskas, J.G. (1993) First-trimester maternal serum schwangerschafts protein 1 (SP1) in pregnancies associated with chromosomal anomalies. *Prenat Diagn* **13**, 563–8

Macintosh, M.C.M., Iles, R., Teisner, B. *et al.* (1994) Maternal serum human chorionic gonadotrophin and pregnancy associated plasma protein A, markers for fetal Down syndrome at 8–14 weeks. *Prenat Diagn* **14**, 203–8

Mantingh, A., Marrink, J., De Wolf, B., Breed, A.S.P.M., Beekhuis, J.R. and Visser, G.H.A. (1989) Low maternal serum alpha-fetoprotein at 10 weeks gestation and fetal Down's syndrome. *Br J Obstet Gynaecol* **96**, 499–500

Milunsky, A., Wands, J., Brambati, B., Bonacchi, I. and Currie, K. (1988) First-trimester maternal serum alpha-fetoprotein screening for chromosome defects. *Am J Obstet Gynecol* **159**, 1209–13

Nebiolo, L., Ozturk, M., Brambati, B., Miller, S., Wands, J. and Milunsky, A. (1990) First-trimester maternal serum alpha-fetoprotein and human chorionic gonadotropin screening for chromosome defects. *Prenat Diagn* **10**, 575–581

Norton, M.E. and Golbus, M.S. (1992) Maternal serum CA 125 for aneuploidy detection in early pregnancy. *Prenat Diagn* **12**, 779–81

Ozturk, M., Milunsky, A., Brambati, B., Sachs, E.S., Miller, S.L. and Wands, J. (1990) Abnormal maternal serum levels of human chorionic gonadotrophin free subunits in trisomy 18. *Am J Med Genet* **36**, 480–3

Pandya, P.P., Snijders, R.J.M., Johnson, S.P., Brizot, M.L. and Nicolaides, K.H. (1995) Screening for fetal trisomies by maternal age and fetal nuchal translucency thickness at 10 to 14 weeks of gestation. *Br J Obstet Gynaecol* **102**, 957–62

Spencer, K., Aitken, D.A., Crossley, J.A. *et al.* (1994) First trimester biochemical screening for trisomy 21: the role of free beta hCG, alpha fetoprotein and pregnancy associated plasma protein A. *Ann Clin Biochem* **31**, 447–54

Van Lith, J.M.M. (1991) First-trimester screening for fetal chromosomal abnormalities. Preliminary results. *Prenat Diagn* **11**, 621–4

Van Lith J.M.M. (1992) First trimester maternal serum human chrorionic gonadotrophin as a marker for fetal chromosomal disorders. *Prenat Diagn* **12**, 495–504

Van Lith, J.M.M. (1994a) *First Trimester Screening for Down's Syndrome.* Amsterdam: Rodopi

Van Lith, J.M.M. (1994b) First trimester maternal serum alpha-fetoprotein as a marker for fetal chromosomal disorders. *Prenat Diagn* **14**, 963–71

Van Lith, J.M.M. (1996) Early biochemical screening for aneuploidy. *Early Hum Dev* **47**, S105–9

Van Lith, J.M.M., Mantingh, A., Beekhuis, J.R., De Bruijn, H.W.A. and Breed, A.S.P.M. (1991) First trimester CA 125 and Down's syndrome. *Br J Obstet Gynaecol* **98**, 493–4

Van Lith, J.M.M., Mantingh, A. and De Bruijn, H.W.A. (1993) Maternal serum CA 125 levels in pregnancies with chromosomally normal and abnormal fetuses. *Prenat Diagn* **13**, 1123–31

Van Lith, J.M.M., Mantingh, A. and Pratt, J.J. (1994) First trimester maternal serum immunoreactive inhibin in chromosomally normal and abnormal pregnancies. *Obstet Gynecol* **83**, 661–4

Wald N.J., Stone, R., Cuckle, H.S. *et al.* (1992) First trimester concentrations of pregnancy associated plasma protein A and placental protein 14 in Down's syndrome. *BMJ* **305**, 28

Wald, N.J., Kennard, A. and Hackshaw, A.K. (1995) First trimester screening for Down's syndrome. *Prenat Diagn* **15**, 1227–40

Wallace, E.M., Harkness, L.M., Burns, S. and Liston, W.A. (1994) Evaluation of maternal serum immunoreactive inhibin as a first trimester marker of Down syndrome. *Clin Endocrinol* **41**, 483–6

Wallace, E.M., Grant, V.E., Swanston, I.A. and Groome, N.P. (1995) Evaluation of maternal serum dimeric inhibin A as a first trimester marker for Down syndrome. *Prenat Diagn* **15**, 359–62

Wenger, D., Miny, P., Holzgreve, W., Fuhrmann, W. and Altland, K. (1990) First trimester maternal serum alpha-fetoprotein screening for Down syndrome and other aneuploidies. *Am J Med Genet* **7** (Suppl.), 89–90

Zimmermann, R., Hucha, A., Salvodelli, G., Binkert, F., Achermann, J. and Grudzinskas, J.G. (1996) Serum parameters and nuchal translucency in first trimester screening for fetal chromosomal abnormalities. *Br J Obstet Gynaecol* **103**, 1009–14

Chapter 17

Biochemical tests in first trimester screening

Discussion

Simpson: Does it make biological sense that there would be no correlation with free urinary β-core, given that there is with serum free β-hCG?

Chard: No.

Adinolfi: You mention that only two out of the six β-chain hCG genes are expressed in the placenta. Are these the only two genes whose expression is affected in Down syndrome? Is the transcription of the maternal hCG affected as well? And if this is the case, what are the factors released by the Down syndrome fetus?

Chard: The genes are all identical. Any of them, theoretically, will produce the β-core as I illustrated. The two active genes will both produce it.

Adinolfi: The pseudo-genes are expressed?

Chard: There is one pseudo-gene in the group, and all the rest are apparently normal, but not typically expressed in the placenta.

Adinolfi: Is there a change in the expression of these genes?

Chard: We assume that there is a quantitative change in the expression. This question was addressed to Dr Spencer, but there has been no work at this time at the level which you are asking about.

Spencer: There is the beginnings of work, looking at messenger RNA levels for these in the free α and the free β-subunits in placenta, and that is largely from a study in which the Harris Birthright group has been involved. But in terms of answering the question whether there is a substantial change in either one of these two genes that may be involved in the β beta production, there is no evidence. I am not aware of any studies that are moving in that direction.

Cuckle: Going back to urinary β-core hCG, just a couple of points of information. First, there is another second trimester study from Canick which has been published in abstract form (Canick *et al.* 1996), with 18 additional Down syndrome cases yielding a MoM in the five to six range. In another first trimester paper (Cuckle *et al.* 1996) which has eleven cases of Down syndrome confirmed, there is a MoM of around two rather than six in the first trimester.

All these things have been presented in MoM terms, and that is not a fair comparison between markers because β-core hCG has a wider spread than serum hCG, serum free β, for example, and we need to take that into account. It may have a narrower spread in the first trimester, but that is another issue. So, just looking at MoMs by themselves is not the best way of comparing the data – although I think you showed Mahalonobis distance as well.

Chard: And low detection rates.

Cuckle: There are cases of all sorts.

Spencer: Was I correct in hearing you suggest that it was a narrower standard deviation in the first trimester compared with the second trimester for β-core?

Cuckle: I do not know. It is variable between different assays and different times. Another point I wanted to make is that the assays that are being used at present require a 15,000–20,000-fold dilution. Manufacturers are developing assays with no dilution required and one can expect that a substantial part of the spread will be reduced. It may be that we will have to change the story – we do not know the answer yet.

Spencer: It was certainly our experience with the Harris Birthright dataset that the spread of the standard deviation both in terms of free β-hCG and also β-core hCG was about twice that which we would see in the second trimester.

Cuckle: That is not our experience. It is controversial, we all agree with the conclusion that it is still a new technology that has not been fully developed yet and there are no answers yet.

I was also going to mention urine versus serum here. There may be other markers in urine and even if β-core hCG was only as good as maternal serum-free β, then you would not necessarily throw urine away, because we can certainly already measure oestriol. Both Kellner and ourselves have shown that it is better than maternal serum uE$_3$, so there are two markers already that are at least comparable with serum and we only need a further one or two.

Hicks: You showed us a slide looking at the variations in serum hCG levels with gestational age and showed the very rapid changes at around 8–10 weeks in international units per litre per day. How does that translate into risk prediction? What does a small difference in estimates of gestational age make to an individual's risk prediction, and how accurately can one now estimate gestational age?

Spencer: That is one of the practical problems of moving screening to the first trimester that early. That is certainly one of the negative sides of using free β that early. Any error in gestational dating can have quite a dramatic effect on the median MoM and therefore on the risk. It could be a significant practical problem.

Hicks: And that is down to the gestational age per day.

Spencer: Yes. One needs to be dating on a day basis – one cannot date accurately enough on a week basis.

Davies: We have looked at the issue of how to set medians in the first trimester, and it is not true, from what Dr Spencer says. There is no difference in the discrepancy in the effect of the gestational age in the first trimester as it is in the second – you just need a good mathematical model to fit the data.

Nicolaides: Just for clarification from Professor Brambati, and perhaps also Dr Macri, are the differences between different populations explained by the distribution of the gestational age? How do the combination test data look – is there a difference at eight weeks from 15 weeks?

Brambati: The American experience which Dr Macri presented was carried out between 10 and 13 weeks. It does not seem that the sensitivity of PAPP-A changes between 8 and 13 weeks, as I reported there. Perhaps with a higher number of cases it would be exponential but we should be careful. In terms of population there may be some biological reason to explain the difference.

Macri: I do not have much to add. All of the studies that have been generated to date are sufficiently small so that it is hazardous to make any real conclusions. We have seen some biological variation – for example, in a small study conducted in the south of Italy where we generated Italian medians, there was a small but significant difference between those and our American medians. We certainly need more data before we can draw any conclusions.

Grudzinskas: Is that a height or weight related phenomenon? There are these differences between the north and south for obvious reasons.

Macri: We corrected for that.

Alberman: This is a very interesting point. Can any of the people from the States tell us about any differences between black and white? The mean gestational age of black babies is shorter than that of white babies. Also, in the South of England, to my knowledge the babies are much bigger for their dates than in other populations. If you are looking early, it will have quite a big effect.

Barry-Kinsella: This is very relevant to us in the Republic of Ireland, because we use the reference range from the British populations which obviously are not homogeneous. If there are differences based on population, we need to be clear on that.

Simpson: Perhaps you said this, but I did not hear a statement as to whether SP-1 would increase the detection rate in the first trimester beyond the 62% that would be achieved with age, free β-hCG and PAPP-A. Has that been calculated? Is that a marker which is of additional use?

Nørgaard-Pedersen: In the multi-marker study we showed that SP-1 gives additional information, even in the gestational age window from 10 to 12 weeks of pregnancy.

Grudzinskas: Perhaps we could start the general discussion with the subject of biochemical testing. Are there any particular questions that we need to address in relation to any one of the analytes that has been discussed already this morning.

Reynolds: There is one question for which we need the figures, which is the detection rates for the combination of AFP and free β-hCG in the first trimester. If you take it from the lab's point, why have three different assays, some early and some late, if you can use the same combination all the way through? Women are liable to present in the first trimester, halfway through in the first and second, and in the second trimester. If you use the same assays all the way through, it makes it simpler for the lab. The marginal benefit of using PAPP-A and free β-hCG is quite small. Using just AFP and free β all the way through might be more advantageous in getting first trimester screening.

Grudzinskas: If I understand your question correctly, you would like to know what the detection rate in the first trimester is for free β-hCG and AFP. Doctor Spencer might have that answer.

Spencer: It is about 50%.

Simpson: I would like to go back to Dr Spencer's point, although perhaps Dr Macri should answer it. He stated that with the dry blood spot test the false positive rate was 2.3 or 3.2% – rather lower than we would have expected. Is that due to the assay itself, or is that a reflection of the population that has been studied with, presumably, better dates on ultrasound and more salutary results there?

Macri: I cannot attribute it to the population studied. I have to think that we are looking at a better reflection of *in vivo* values and we have actually just tightened the distribution. We know that things happen to analytes when you remove them from the body, and, depending on the length of time they are out and the conditions they are subjected to, changes occur. Whatever it is about this remarkable filter paper, it seems to impart tremendous stability to the analytes. That is probably where the beneficial aspects come.

Nørgaard-Pedersen: Being responsible for a newborn screening programme in Denmark, we certainly work with filter paper We also know that several analytes are not stable on filter paper. We also know that they are even more stable on filter paper than in liquid. We have not looked into PAPP-A and free β-hCG yet as to whether they are stable, but there is the possibility of enhancing the stability by adding ascorbic acid to the filter paper beforehand because it has some antioxidant effects. Dr Macri may be right that these markers are more stable on filter paper than they are in liquid solution.

I have recently attended the International Newborn Screening Conference in Boston and certainly the cost for filter paper is less than if you had a liquid. However, there are new recommendations by the US Mail that you have to take precautions when you are sending even filter paper – it has to be in a special box – and so the cost is also mounting there.

Macri: We have looked at some of the stability characteristics of both free β-hCG and PAPP-A on dried blood spots. Free β-hCG does rather well. PAPP-A seems to have some problems with stability, even on the dry blood spot, but I do not think that is anything that cannot be worked with.

Macintosh: I would like to make the comment that we are being very loose with our terminology of detection rates. We should make it clear whether we are talking about detection rate at the time of first trimester, or detection rates at birth. That is a most important point which we should not forget.

So far, there are no intervention prospective demonstration projects showing what the effect is on birth. Part of our job should be to consider whether there is enough evidence, whether this can and should be organised.

Grudzinskas: Before Professor Cuckle comes back to that, I would like to ask the speakers from the earlier session to clarify what they meant by detection rates in the material they presented.

Spencer: That was based on term incidence.

Grudzinskas: Does that answer the point you raised with respect of free β-hCG and hCG, Dr Macintosh?

Macintosh: I would prefer to know at what stage we are talking about detection rates for every analyte, basically. We are talking about grading analytes scientifically and we have to be very precise.

Nørgaard-Pedersen: As I showed, some of the results we had in the latest serum material is from those who were born with Down syndrome. Of course, we looked into the difference between the values in this population compared to the serum sample from those being detected by CVS or amniocentesis. For instance, for SP-1 we have not been able to achieve any significance in the level. However, the material is small, and our detection rate is also detection at term.

Chard: The detection rate I quoted was the figures published in the papers to which I made reference, without saying anything else about it. We all sit here saying that of course it is all detection rate at term, but I am not sure that most of these things are detection rate at term. Most of these studies were samples collected from women who were undergoing invasive procedures, diagnosis and termination – how on earth do we know what would happen at term?

Cuckle: This is the point I was going to make. The best estimate we have from term or interrupted pregnancies for any of these markers is based on the usual mixed collection of material and most people would agree that that is a better estimate than simply observing their detection rates from the data because of the biases and the use of selectivity.

The model predicted detection rate for PAPP-A and free β-hCG based on meta-analysis is 67% for a 5% false positive rate. However, the model parameters are based on data from a wide gestational window and perhaps one should be more focused than that. The results may not be as good at the most practical time to do the testing, which is probably 10–12 weeks. We need predicted rates for different first trimester gestations.

Having said this, the missing piece of information from those models is whether the average level of PAPP-A in Down is different in survivable, viable Down from non-viable Down syndrome pregnancies. None of the information which has been presented today has addressed that issue, and I do not think it really can. However, there are some papers which have a mixture of first trimester pre-CVS samples from Down, and second trimester samples – or rather, first trimester samples from Down that did not surface until the second trimester.

For example, Dr Muller's paper on PAPP-A (Muller *et al.* 1993) is based purely on samples that were taken for toxoplasmosis and were not going to be Down until second trimester screening or term. In her paper, the median MoM for PAPP-A in the Down is no different from what you would predict from all the other studies combined. So that is reassuring.

There is also some Harris Birthright data of that nature, which supports that notion too. There is some material which Doctor Aitken mentioned, where he has paired first and second trimester samples. There, presumably, the pregnancy survived into its second trimester, and I think I am right in saying that the PAPP-A and free β in those samples were not very different from other studies, pre-CVS and terminated cases. If that is true, then that is sufficient information not to have to carry out a prospective intervention study before you can put your hand on your heart and say that this is as good as second trimester screening.

Grudzinskas: For the sake of completeness, I would just add that Wald *et al.* (1992) published data based on serum PAPP-A and PP-14 levels in the *British Medical Journal*, on term-ascertained Down syndrome, and they are likely to expand on that. Like many of you, I am included in the *et al.* part of that report, but in general it seems that if one is looking at that particular analyte PAPP-A prior to 13 weeks, the median MoM in the affected pregnancy, whether they are identified and terminated, is no different from those cases which are ascertained at term. There may be other comments.

Wald: Our PAPP-A data were not at term – they were first trimester, or diagnosed shortly thereafter. Even though we produced a paper which produced a 62% for a 5% false positive rate, it is an estimate at first trimester.

There are two problems. One is that quite a few papers that are intervention studies record the number of Down syndrome cases detected at first trimester, say by nuchal translucency, and then the pregnancies continue and, say, the others were missed cases that were determined at birth. So let us say that these are the kind of figures that have been reported. Sixteen are detected at around 11 weeks and four emerge at birth – the missed cases. So there were 20 in all, as people think. Sixteen out of 20 is judged to be an 80% detection rate.

There is a denominator problem here. Of those 16, half might have miscarried.

So really, one has to think in terms of the numerator being not 16 but eight. Then in the denominator, you have the 16 you detected, but you subtract the eight that would have miscarried, leaving eight plus the four you missed. You then have eight over 12, which is 67% rather than 80%, just for allowing for the natural fetal loss during pregnancy. A shift from 80% to 67% is quite an important difference in the sort of figures we have been talking about, and it is simply a numerical error in analysis.

The second problem was raised by Professor Cuckle: is there an additional effect because there may be an association between not so much these markers, be it nuchal translucency, or PAPP-A and miscarriage, but is that effect enhanced in pregnancies with Down syndrome? Is there a preferential effect? He concluded that if it was, it was rather small. We would have to go back over the study together, but it is my conclusion that there is a small effect. There are two main studies I am comparing – and there may be others – one in which Professor Nicolaides, with Hyatt, looked at it in Down; Dr Muller looked in the general population. You find that both of those are associated with, for example, with nuchal translucency and miscarriage.

The point estimate is that it is slightly larger in Professor Nicolaides' Down series, which suggests that there might be a greater tendency for the Down syndrome pregnancies with the big nuchal translucencies to miscarry, compared to the tendency for non-Down syndrome with big nuchal translucency to miscarry. At this stage, however, we are extremely uncertain about that – that is my own view. These are just glimmers of information that are coming through in a few papers, and that does need to be clarified.

Nicolaides: I will present the data on nuchal translucency (NT) later. The good thing for the biochemistry is that there is definitely a relationship between intra-uterine fatality and nuchal translucency – that is very clear. The good news for biochemists is that there is no apparent relationship in the deviation from normality in either free β-hCG or PAPP-A, and the deviation from normality in nuchal translucency. So a baby with an extremely large nuchal translucency is not much more likely to have a very abnormal biochemical result. Since nuchal translucency is related to lethality, that may provide some evidence that biochemical screening may not be.

Cuckle: I think we should put NT aside for this session, and just talk about first trimester biochemistry.

We have sufficient evidence that, theoretically, free β-hCG and PAPP-A in combination, and perhaps a third marker if you like, will give the same kind of detection rate that is achieved with a two or three second trimester marker screen. There is, however, the caveat, that there may be differential lethality, but there is no evidence for differential lethality. That is fairly weak, because there are few data which could address the issue. As to what data there are which could address the issue, however – and I am talking about free β-hCG and PAPP-A and not nuchal translucency – it does not appear that there is anything. Given that there is no effect of free β-hCG in the second trimester – indeed any second trimester marker on second trimester lethality – why should we believe that the first trimester is different?

There are two steps there. First, the model predictions. I do not think anyone would disagree that the model predictions for a two-marker first trimester is giving a similar result for a two or three marker second trimester. With the second step there, the one about lethality, it is a little more tenuous, but it is a two-step argument. No one has yet shown any biochemical marker to be related to lethality in a serious way – differential lethality. Where it has been looked at, nobody has seen a difference in lethality between first and second trimester for these two first trimester markers. I can therefore only draw one conclusion from that, which is that we are ready to go with a first trimester screening test based on two or three markers.

Grudzinskas: Perhaps I could put your first contention to the group to develop further, either in a positive or a negative way. Could you repeat it?

Cuckle: The simple statement is: 'In principle, in theory, based on models, would we agree that a two-marker, free β-hCG, PAPP-A combination in the first trimester is giving similar predicted detection rates for a given false positive rate, compared to a two or three marker second trimester combination?'

Aitken: That should be qualified to the extent that it possibly depends on looking at the data within a particular narrow gestation. That may not be true at seven weeks and at, say 14 or 13 weeks. It may be true at 12 weeks, or something like that.

Cuckle: Then can we re-phrase it to 10–12 weeks? We are talking about 10–12 weeks, are we not? We are not really talking about 6 or 7 weeks, although a PAPP-A is better at 6 or 7 weeks, no doubt. hCG is probably worse, and nobody will really have an intricate model.

Aitken: No doubt women will continue to appear at seven weeks and at 13 weeks for their first blood sample to be taken. We cannot really apply the same rules at seven weeks as we can at 13 weeks.

Cuckle: If they do appear at seven weeks, and very few do, then you can ask them to return a couple of weeks later. If they appear at 13 weeks, you can give them a second trimester triple test.

Wald: This is difficult. Current estimates on free β-hCG and PAPP-A at 10–12 weeks – a point estimate from a couple of studies was about 62% for a 5% false positive rate. You can in the second trimester, with the kind of refinements that are being alluded to, using a scan to determine gestation rate, achieve over 70% for five. Are we going to say that around 62% as a point estimate is similar to 70%, or a little more than 70%? It is an extra 8 or 10 percentage points.
My view is that those percentage points are rather important. You are picking up about a quarter of those that are left to be detected, which would otherwise be missed. It is good enough not to rule out for someone who might want it early on, but it is not good enough to say that it should replace what we have at present. In general, advances in medicine ought to show that what is new is more effective and safer than that which it is intended to replace. At the moment, although it is close, it does not quite meet that target.
I do accept substantially what Professor Cuckle is saying about the lack of evidence, and I am sorry if I am confusing the nuchal translucency and the serum

markers – there is not much evidence of differential effects on miscarriage. The evidence is not overwhelming, however, as Professor Cuckle indicated. Since so much can happen between 10 and 15 weeks, I would probably like some stronger evidence that that was not a problem. That is a secondary point, however. The first point is that however similar it is, the point estimates are still less than the second trimester performance.

Grudzinskas: The point was raised yesterday, and you may choose to develop it today or tomorrow, that it is clear that termination of pregnancy is a safer procedure in the first trimester, or earlier in pregnancy rather than later. That is certainly the case in the US, and I am sure that others have similar data on this side of the Atlantic.

Alberman: I would like to say something about terminology and term, but you may want to leave that until we have worked through this particular question.

Brambati: We have to accept the correction by Professor Wald of the inform-ation that Howard Cuckle gave. We have to accept, at the moment, double marker testing in the first trimester, and a triple test could be a little later. It could be lower. The issue of whether to proceed in the first trimester or in the second trimester will be resolved if we accept the choice of the patient – then it does not matter. We have to underline that at the moment there are some differences in results between different tests but we also have to conclude that, on the basis of current experience, there is sufficient evidence that the detection rate with the first trimester is not less than 60%.

Grudzinskas: I would like to add a statement in here, and those of you who contributed to the report will remember it. The conclusion is: 'The performance of screening, using maternal age, serum free β-hCG, and PAPP-A at ten weeks was better than the double test and similar to the triple test at 15 to 22 weeks.' This report was published on behalf of the International Pre-Natal Screening Research Group in the *British Journal of Obstetrics and Gynaecology* in June. The question of which gestation is better or not (there may be a changing arena, but it has only changed in the last few months) is an important point. There are other aspects which Professor Wald raised here and which will be raised again later, concerning safety and effectiveness. We will come back to those points.

Nørgaard-Pedersen: A few months ago I would have agreed with Professor Wald that intervention studies should not be started yet, but now, with the robustness of the assay systems, we are prepared to do them. Furthermore, I have to correct myself: the detection rate was not in the first – it was in the second trimester, based on the relationship between samples. I should also say that those controlled samples we are using in the study are all samples which gave birth to normal infants.

Marteau: You may perhaps have this comment later, but I wanted to endorse what Professor Wald has mentioned several times – the importance of evaluating first trimester screening in terms of safety and efficacy. We should say what we mean about safety. I would like to have a broader view of what we mean by safety to encompass the psychological consequences of first versus second trimester screening.

We will not come across this at any other point in the programme because tomorrow we shall be talking purely and simply about giving risk information. There is an understandable assumption that earlier detection, if it is as good as or even better than second trimester detection, is better than later detection. That, however, is for those for whom there is a child with Down syndrome. We should recall that the majority of women will be given low risk or negative results, and a proportion will be given false positive results. We know that two of the adverse consequences of any kind of screening test are the anxieties that are raised by false positive results and the false reassurance that some people gain from receiving a negative test result.

By introducing the screening programme into the first trimester, we have the potential to prolong the period of time during which women who are being made anxious will be anxious. So, rather than just being anxious for 24 weeks, in those who have had a false positive result at 16 weeks, we may be giving them 30 weeks of anxiety, and it is the same for false reassurance. For some women, we may be introducing at a very early stage of pregnancy an idea that there is nothing wrong with the pregnancy, leading to a longer period of rehearsal which may make it more difficult for the few who do go on to give birth to a child with Down syndrome to adjust.

Thus, not only might we be introducing longer exposure to adverse psychological effects but also we are introducing them at an earlier stage in pregnancy. That might make it more difficult for women subsequently to adjust to their pregnancy and the birth of their children. These are points which remain to some extent speculative, but in any evaluation where we are looking at first trimester screening, we need to build them into our evaluations, to put them into an equation when trying to work out the pros and cons of first versus second trimester screening.

Simpson: I would have thought it was the opposite. They will be anxious until the results arrive, and you will relieve their anxiety from ten weeks as opposed to having relieved it from 19 weeks. I do not agree.

Marteau: Perhaps I have not explained myself very well. Although there will be some women for whom the anxiety will be allayed, in population based screening programmes women are not presenting with anxiety and so there is not that relief. For the women who are older who have come to a screening programme with that anxiety, you may well be doing that, but for some of those we know from surveys that have been done that around 50% of women going through these screening programmes and falsely believe that there is no risk to their pregnancy of having a child with Down syndrome, or indeed any other problem. Therefore, one has increased the time during which women have false information. For the majority you can discard that, because they will go on to have a child with nothing wrong with it, but for some, where there is a problem, you have given women a greater period of time to have false information. In the majority of cases you will be OK, but there will be more people who have false information for longer. It is similar for those receiving false positive results.

Simpson: If the screening programme and the counselling is telling them for the first time that there are 2–3% of the population with birth defects, I agree. I would submit, however, that there is a different way of handling that, which is obviously a matter of education rather than altering the time in gestation at which one screens.

Brambati: I understand from Professor Marteau that knowledge is equivalent to anxiety. That applies in many situations in life. With regard to fetal abnormalities, the woman should know as early as possible so that she is in a better position to face the problem. In terms of anxiety, which is a psychological term, we have to face this problem if we want to expand prevention in pregnancy as much as possible.

Whittle: There is something else which we should perhaps consider about first trimester screening itself. The consequences of finding a positive result from a screening programme will usually result in an invasive test, probably most frequently CVS. My understanding is that this is a more expensive laboratory test than an amniocentesis – in other words, it costs more to process CVS material than it does amniotic fluid. I am looking for confirmation or otherwise about that, but that also has to be put into the formula when we are looking at first trimester screening. There may be a cost implication downstream from the screening programme itself.

Alberman: I am returning to the point Dr Macintosh made when she talked about term. I find the term 'term' extremely difficult. It is a problem we have all the time. What we are talking about here is a birth, rather than a miscarriage. Even the term 'birth' has changed in this country over the past two and a half years because we have lowered the legal age of a stillbirth from 28 weeks to 24 weeks. The whole question of whether we include stillbirths amongst births is also difficult. I would just make the plea that in whatever recommendations we make, we make it quite clear what we mean by the terms 'birth' or 'term'.

Davies: Just to reiterate something I said yesterday, Professor Wald mentioned a point estimate of detection rate. I think it was a four-marker test of 75%, and he said that the first trimester data we have seen so far is lower than that. I would make the point that the estimated 95% confidence interval on that 75% is about plus or minus 14%. Thus there is no statistical evidence to suggest that they are different.

Cuckle: I would like to know whether people feel that the statement I made is substantially wrong. I know that Nick is the only person who has really addressed that, and seems to be saying, 'it is substantially right, but . . . ' – because of point estimates and relative amounts of data, it may well be that the first trimester double has a slightly lower detection rate. It is certainly lower than the optimal second trimester, which is based on four or five markers.

Practically speaking, at the end of all of this we really need to know whether it is wrong to discourage, not whether we should be encouraging. Are we finishing up where we want to say that we should not be discouraging people from starting first trimester screening in anger – actually doing it, and screening and terminating pregnancies as a result. Should we be discouraging them?

Macri: I am not sure whether you are purposely considering biochemistry in a vacuum in this context, or not. If that is the case, then you are proceeding very well. However, if you are going to decide to move forward with first trimester screening then you must add in the other parameters which are so valuable to you that they will elevate detection to beyond anything that we can conceive of in the second trimester. The procedure here is foreign to me and perhaps I am missing something.

Grudzinskas: No, you are not missing anything. We have tried not to pre-empt what will be said later, and we will weave that together. I would like to bring this part to a close now. I am sure we will come back to this, because we shall be discussing biophysical as well as biochemical tests later.

I sense that there is no dissension this year, as opposed to last year or the year before, that we do actually have phenomena that are identifiable by biochemical tests in the first trimester which are considered by some or many of us here to be worthy of clinical usage or exploitation. The issues we shall attend to later are just how we may consider doing that before we get to our recommendations.

References

Canick, J.A., Kellner, L.H., Saller, D.N. *et al.* (1996) A second level evaluation of urinary gonadotropin peptide as a marker for second trimester Down syndrome screening. *Early Hum Dev* (in press)

Cuckle, H.S., Canick, J.A., Kellner, L.H. *et al.* (1996) Urinary β-core hCG screening in the first trimester. *Prenat Diagn* **16,** 1057–9

Muller, F., Cuckle, H.S., Teisner, B. and Grudzinskas, J.G. (1993) Serum PAPP-A levels are depressed in women with fetal Down syndrome in early pregnancy. *Prenat Diagn* **13,** 633–6

Wald, N.J., Stone, R., Cuckle, H.S. *et al.* (1992) First trimester concentrations of pregnancy associated plasma protein A and placental protein 14 in Down's syndrome. *BMJ* **305,** 28

Wald, N.J., George, L., Smith, D., Densem, J.W. and Petterson, K. (1996) Serum screening for Down's syndrome between 8 and 14 weeks of pregnancy. International Prenatal Screening Research Group. *Br J Obstet Gynaecol* **103,** 407–12

SECTION 5

ULTRASOUND IN SCREENING FOR DOWN SYNDROME IN THE FIRST TRIMESTER

Chapter 18

Ultrasonographic markers of aneuploidy in early pregnancy

Eric Jauniaux

Introduction

Recent years have seen an expansion in the availability of prenatal diagnosis. In particular, during the last decade great advances have been made in ultrasound imaging enabling the investigation of the pregnancy from 5 weeks after the last menstruation of the mother to be. As the availability of new and improved prenatal diagnosis techniques increases, so does the relevance of screening for markers of aneuploidy in early pregnancy. Within this context, three parameters are of pivotal importance: the resolution of the ultrasound equipment used, the dynamics of normal embryological development and the spontaneous evolution of the different types of aneuploidy. This chapter combines a review of the literature on the early ultrasound diagnosis of fetal abnormalities with a discussion on the possibilities and limits of using some of these features as early markers of fetal aneuploidy.

Aneuploidy and early pregnancy loss in humans

Subclinical miscarriages

Retrospective investigations have evaluated that about 60% of all fertilised ova are lost before the end of the first trimester is reached (Miller *et al.* 1980; Edmonds *et al.* 1982). Most of them are lost during the first month after the last menstrual period and are often ignored as conceptions by the patient (Table 18.1). A recent prospective study of 200 presumably fertile couples desiring to achieve pregnancy over 12 menstrual cycles has shown that 82% conceived during that period and that the maximal fertility rate was 30% per cycle in the first two cycles (Zinaman *et al.* 1996). Pregnancy wastage during the first three cycles accounted for 31% of the pregnancies detected and 40% of these losses were seen only by urine human chorionic gonadotrophin (hCG) testing.

The only well-established epidemiological fact about spontaneous abortion is that at least half of them are associated with a chromosomal defect of the conceptus and that the frequency of abnormal chromosomal complement increases over 70% when the embryonic demise occurs earlier in gestation (Edwards 1986; Simpson and Bombard 1987). The other causes of very early pregnancy loss include, endocrine diseases, anatomical abnormalities of the female genital tract, infections, immune factors, chemical agents, hereditary disorders, trauma, maternal diseases and psychological factors (Stephenson 1996). None of these aetiologies can quantitatively be shown to cause more than a small percentage of pregnancy losses in general.

Clinical miscarriages

The rate of pregnancy loss is known to decrease with gestational age. The precise incidence of pregnancy failure at different periods of gestation has been more clearly defined with the routine use of transvaginal ultrasound. In a prospective study of 232 women with positive urinary pregnancy tests and no antecedent history of vaginal bleeding, Goldstein (1994) has demonstrated that pregnancy loss is virtually complete by the end of the embryonic period (70 days after the onset of the last menstrual period). Once a gestational sac has been documented on scan, there is still an 11.5% subsequent loss of viability in the embryonic period. If an embryo has developed up to 5 mm, subsequent loss of viability occurs in 7.2%, with loss rates dropping rapidly after that to 3.3% for embryos of 6–10 mm and to 0.5% for embryos over 10 mm. No pregnancies were lost between 8.5 and 14 menstrual weeks. The fetal loss rate after 14 weeks is about 2% (Table 18.1). The ultrasound screening of a larger group of women with pregnancies between 10 and 13 weeks' gestation has confirmed that the prevalence of pregnancy failure at the end of first trimester is around 2–3% (Pandya *et al.* 1996).

The rate of clinical miscarriage increases with maternal age, a 40-year-old woman carrying twice the risk of a 20-year-old woman and a significant past

Table 18.1. Incidence of early pregnancy failure in humans

Variable	%
Total loss of conception	50–70
Total clinical miscarriages	15–25
Before 6 weeks' gestation	18
Between 6 and 9 weeks' gestation	4
After 9 weeks' gestation	3
EPL in primigravidae	6–10
Risk of EPL after 3 miscarriages	25–30
Risk of EPL of 40-year-old women	30–40

obstetric history (Simpson and Bombard 1987). Among primigravidae, the rate of pregnancy loss is 6% whereas for three or more losses it increases to 25–30% (Simpson *et al.* 1994). Chromosomal abnormalities represent at least 50% of clinically recognised early pregnancy losses (Bouie *et al.* 1976; Simpson and Bombard 1987). Autosomal trisomies are the most common with an incidence of 30–35% followed by triploidies and monosomies X (Jauniaux *et al.* 1996a). All possible autosomal trisomies have been described in cytogenetically abnormal abortions except trisomy 1 which has only been reported, in an 8-cell embryo (Watt *et al.* 1987). Triploidy and tetraploidy are frequent but extremely lethal chromosomal abnormalities and are therefore rarely found in late miscarriages.

The frequency of most trisomies is influenced by maternal age at any gestation suggesting that autosomal trisomies are predictably more likely to arise cytologically in maternal meiosis (90%) than in paternal meiosis (Zaragoza *et al.* 1994). This is true for trisomy 21 and for all the acrocentric chromosomes. Chromosomal complements of successive abortuses in a given family are more likely to be either recurrently normal or recurrently abnormal. If the complement of the first miscarriage is abnormal, the chromosomal complement of the subsequent miscarriage will be abnormal in up to 80% of the cases and the recurrent abnormality is usually a trisomy (Warburton *et al.* 1987). This is supported by the observation that the risk of liveborn trisomy 21 following an aneuploid abortus is about 1–2% (Alberman 1981), compared with 1 in 800 in the general population. However, these chromosomal anomalies are so frequently found in cases of early pregnancy failure that observed adverse outcomes may only be coincidental and their impact on subsequent pregnancies should not be overestimated, particularly, in women with a history of only one chromosomally abnormal miscarriage.

Ultrasonographic findings in miscarriages associated with a chromosomal abnormality

The gestational sac size has been studied as a possible marker of first trimester aneuploidy but its significance has not been extensively documented and is often anecdotal. A small gestational or chorionic sac in the first trimester is a well established factor of poor pregnancy outcome (Table 18.2), even in the presence

Table 18.2. Qualitative evaluation of the predictive value of routine ultrasound/ Doppler measurements in detecting aneuploidies in early pregnancy

Variable	Decreased	Increased	PV
Gestational sac size	EPF T16/Triploid	Multiple gestation Partial mole	+++/+++
Yolk sac size	EPF	EPF	+/+
CRL	EPF T18/Triploid	Early conception	+++/+++
Fetal heart rate	EPF T18/13/16	T21	+++/++
Umbilical artery PI	N/A	T18/Triploid	/++

EPF, early pregnancy failure; N/A, not applicable; +, weak (<50%); ++, average (50–70%); +++, good (>70%).

of embryonic cardiac activity and is associated with an 80–90% incidence of miscarriage (Bromley *et al.* 1991). A small sac, with measurements below the 50th centile is also present in all anembryonic pregnancies and in 62% of all missed abortions (Dickey *et al.* 1994). In this study, the correlation of ultrasound gestational sac measurements with karyotype results has shown that triploidy, trisomy 16 and the presence of satellite bodies on chromosome 22 are significantly associated with a small chorionic sac diameter. A previous retrospective study, not including karyotype analysis, has shown that on scan, partial moles are often associated with an anterior to transverse diameters ratio >1.5 (Fine *et al.* 1989).

Secondary yolk sac measurements are in general of little predictive value in early pregnancy (Jauniaux *et al.* 1991). Although a yolk sac diameter above average for gestation has been reported in a single case of triploidy (Zalel *et al.* 1994), abnormal yolk sac size is a non-specific finding of failed pregnancies and does not correlate to karyotypic status (Goldstein *et al.* 1996).

The value of histological examination

Cell cultures and karyotyping are expensive and time-consuming and cannot, therefore, be routinely offered to all women presenting with a first trimester miscarriage. In 1976, Bouié *et al.* reported the results of pathological and cytogenetic correlation in 1500 spontaneous abortions and described placental histological features of chromosomal anomalies of the conceptus. Although some criteria have been met, the accuracy of histology in these cases is still a matter of controversy. The sensitivity and specificity of microscopic examination in these cases can be improved by adding features of the materno-embryonic interface to classical villous histological criteria (Jauniaux and Hustin 1992). The best correlation has been found in cases of triploidy. This is of importance in the perinatal management of miscarriage associated with this chromosomal anomaly since it is also the most common cause of partial mole which can lead to persisting trophoblastic disease in 1–10% of cases (Goldstein and Berkowitz 1994).

The diagnosis of partial mole is initially based on the ultrasound appearance of the placenta *in utero* or gross examination of the placenta at delivery during the second or third trimester of pregnancy (Jauniaux *et al.* 1996a). If there is no further microscopic examination showing some form of trophoblastic hyperplasia the patient will not be entered in the follow-up registry. In most European countries, miscarriage products are not routinely investigated for partial mole and/or triploidy and it is mainly second- or third-trimester partial mole which have been registered for follow-up. As triploidies are much more common in the first trimester, a large group of women at risk of trophoblastic disease theoretically escape detection and if treatment is required it would only be started at a later stage of the disease. In this context, those women who develop a persistent gestational trophoblastic disease may experience several subsequent episodes of uterine bleeding before the diagnosis is eventually made. Triploidy is less often associated with molar changes in the first trimester of pregnancy than in the second or third trimester (Jauniaux *et al.* 1996a, 1997). The majority of triploid spontaneous abortions, therefore, escape detection on the base of ultrasound or macroscopic examination. The use of standardised criteria detection by microscopic examination is both accurate and reproducible and should play a pivotal role in screening for women at risk of persistent gestational trophoblastic disease.

First trimester markers of aneuploidy

Early fetal biometry

Case reports describing smaller than expected embryos or early fetuses in association with triploidy or trisomy 18 were published in the international literature from the end of the 1980s (Benacerraf 1988; Lynch and Berkowitz 1989). Initial series did not demonstrate a relationship between a small CRL measurement and a chromosomally abnormal fetus (Leelapatana *et al.* 1992). However, the study of larger groups of first-trimester fetuses has subsequently shown that a CRL smaller than dates is associated with a higher risk of chromosomal anomalies than expected for maternal age (Drugan *et al.* 1992; Khun *et al.* 1995). The risk is more than twice in patients with a viable fetus in which the gestational age derived from the CRL was smaller than the menstrual gestational age by at least seven days compared with patients with an ultrasonographically derived gestational age ≤6 days of menstrual age (Drugan *et al.* 1992). The larger the discrepancy, the higher the possibility that the aneuploidy affecting the fetus is of the severe (trisomy 18 or 13) or lethal type (triploidy). By contrast, in early pregnancy, the growth of most fetuses affected by trisomy 21 or sex chromosome abnormalities does not differ from that of euploid fetuses (Khun *et al.* 1995). There has so far been no investigation of the value of other fetal biometric measurements such as femur length in the early screening of aneuploidy. Nuchal fold thickening has been evaluated prospectively in large populations of women with pregnancies before 14 weeks' gestation and may enable the early detection of fetuses with chromosomal abnormalities (see Chapter 19).

Anatomical markers

Theoretically, most ultrasound markers of aneuploidy, classically described around mid-gestation, could be used to screen for chromosomal abnormalities at the end of the first trimester. To date, existing data on the ultrasound diagnosis and significance of most of these anomalies in early pregnancy are derived from case reports or small retrospective series and few have been evaluated prospectively in large populations. The following abnormalities have been diagnosed from the end of the first trimester within the context of aneuploidy ultrasound dectection (Table 18.3).

Abnormalities of the skin and neck

Hydrops fetalis has been defined as a pathological increase of interstitial and total fetal body water that usually appears primarily in serous cavities (pleural, pericardial or intraperitoneal effusion) or as oedema of soft fetal tissue. Trisomy 21 and monosomy X are the most frequently identified chromosomal disorders related to non-immune hydrops fetalis (Jauniaux *et al.* 1990). Trisomy 18, trisomy 13 and trisomy 16 are also commonly found in association with fetal hydrops. Fetal ascites, pericardial effusion or pleural effusion have only been occasionally reported before 15 weeks of gestation whereas generalised skin oedema can be diagnosed from 10 weeks and account probably for an important proportion of fetuses presenting with nuchal fold thickness of more than 3 mm. Increased nuchal translucency thickness is found in more than 80% of the trisomic fetuses between 10 and 14 weeks' gestation (Snijders *et al.* 1996). Chromosomally normal fetuses with large (>4 mm) nuchal fold are at higher risk of abnormalities of the heart and great arteries (Hyett *et al.* 1995) which are the second most common cause of fetal hydrops (Jauniaux *et al.* 1990).

The ultrasound definition of cystic hygroma is often ambiguous and many authors do not differentiate between simple nuchal oedema and nuchal cavitation resulting from an abnormality in development of the lymphatic system. Recent studies have shown that septated or cystic nuchal hygromata diagnosed between 9 and 14 weeks of gestation is associated with up to a 60% risk of aneuploidy with 45,X the most common abnormality (Shulman *et al.* 1994; Trauffer *et al.* 1994). In the presence of a normal karyotype, these fetuses have a normal outcome in about 80% of cases. However, chromosomally normal fetuses presenting with first-trimester cystic hygromata may have other dysmorphic sequelae such as Noonan or Roberts syndrome which diagnosis is based solely on clinical parameters (Trauffer *et al.* 1994). In these cases, the cystic hygroma is usually large and resolves lately in pregnancy or does not resolve until delivery whereas fetuses with

Table 18.3. Early sonographic markers of aneuploidy evaluated by organ systems and in relation to gestational age

Sonographic markers	Gestational age (weeks)	Aneuploidy
Skin and neck		
Generalised oedema	≥10	T21, T18, XO
Cystic hygroma	≥9	XO
Brain		
Dandy-Walker	≥11	Tri
Holoprosencephaly	≥11	T13, Tri
Choroid plexus cyst	≥12	T18[a]
Hydrocephaly	≥15	T21, Tri
Heart		
Atrio-ventricular septal defects	≥13	T21, T18, T13, Tri, XO
Abdomen		
Duodenal atresia	≥14	T21
Exomphalos	≥12	T18, T13, Tri
Hydronephrosis	≥12	T21[a]
Limbs		
Polydactyly	≥13	T13
Syndactyly	≥13	T18, T13, Tri
Placenta and cord		
Partial mole	≥8	Tri
Cord pseudocyst	≥9	T18, T13

[a] Minor anomalies.

small hygroma and early resolution have remarkably few sequelae from their first trimester abnormality.

Brain abnormalities

Dandy-Walker and holoprosencephaly are strong markers of severe aneuploidy such as triploidy and trisomy 13 which can be diagnosed from the end of the first trimester (Blass and Eik-Nes 1996; Weissman and Achiron 1996). A definite diagnosis can often not be reached before 15 weeks of gestation in hydrocephaly resulting mainly from the obstruction of the ventricle drainage with progressive accumulation of cerebrospinal fluid. Furthermore, between 12 and 16 weeks measurements of the lateral ventricle to hemispheric ratio have a large standard deviation and are therefore less accurate in the follow-up of early hydrocephaly.

Heart defects

Atrial and ventricular septal defects are associated with a 16–18% of chromosomal anomalies (Allan *et al.* 1991). In a study of 270 low-risk women and 32 women at high risk, Johnson *et al.* (1992) found that the four-chamber and the great vessels view could only be obtained in less than 75% and 50% of cases, respectively. They conclude that it is unlikely that transvaginal sonography before 16 weeks will replace abdominal scanning at 18 weeks for the screening of low-risk pregnancies but is a valuable addition to the early examination of these women identified as being at high risk of congenital heart disease. Indeed, Gembruch *et al.* (1993) investigating 114 pregnancies between 11 and 16 weeks of gestation, have demonstrated that the four chamber view and the great vessels anatomy can always be visualised from week 13 onward and that 90% of the cardiac malformations can be diagnosed at the end of the first trimester. Similar results have been reported by other teams with more experience in transvaginal scan (Weissman and Achiron 1996).

After week 18 of gestation, transabdominal echocardiography generally gives better results because in the transvaginal approach, the distance between the transducer and fetus increases and therefore, the quality of the image of the fetal heart decreases (Gembruch *et al.* 1993).

Abdominal wall and intra-abdominal defects

Duodenal atresia and exomphalos are severe congenital abnormalities often requiring extensive surgery after delivery. Both anomalies are associated with an incidence of aneuploidy of about 30% when diagnosed antenatally. Exomphalos is associated with chromosomal defects in 39.4% of the cases diagnosed at 12 weeks of gestation decreasing to 27.5% at 20 weeks and 14.4% at birth (Snijders *et al.* 1995). This decrease is mainly due to fetal wastage of aneuploid fetuses with other major abnormalities. Recanalisation of the duodenum is complete by 10 weeks of gestation and fetal swallowing begins only several weeks later. Furthermore, fetal contribution to amniotic fluid is insignificant before 14 weeks and thus, the dilatation of the stomach and the proximal duodenum together with polyhydramnios which are typical of duodenal atresia can only be detected after that period. Similarly, the developmental herniation of midgut through the primitive umbilical ring into the cord during embryogenesis will prevent the diagnosis of exomphalos before 12 weeks of gestation.

Limb defects

Congenital skeletal anomalies or major limb defects such as amelia or phocomelia are not associated with a higher incidence of chromosomal abnormalities. Poly-dactyly and syndactyly are strong markers of aneuploidy but information regard-ing the early diagnosis of these malformations is limited to rare case reports.

Abnormalities of the placenta and cord

More than 90% of partial moles are found in triploid conceptuses. Triploid fetuses almost always present on ultrasound with major malformations and/or with severe asymmetrical growth retardation (Jauniaux et al. 1996b) which are detectable in most cases by ultrasound during the second trimester of pregnancy. Villous hydatidiform appearance is not specific for triploidy and in first trimester spontaneous abortions more that 70% of triploid placentas show no sonographic or macroscopic features suggesting molar transformation (Jauniaux et al. 1996a). Thus, in first trimester pregnancy, when the molar changes may be too small to be seen by ultrasound and the fetal anatomy too difficult to examine in detail, the antenatal screening may rely on other sonographic criteria such as increased fetal nuchal translucency or a discrepancy between CRL and menstrual age and high maternal serum hCG levels (Jauniaux and Nicolaides 1997).

Cord pseudocyst when diagnosed in the second trimester of pregnancy are associated with a high incidence of aneuploidy with trisomy 18 the most common abnormality (Jauniaux et al. 1988; Sepulveda et al. 1994). Vestigial cysts and pseudocysts can sometimes be associated with small abdominal wall defects and a precise early prenatal diagnosis can be more difficult to establish. A large study is required to evaluate the screening value of cord cyst with and without other ultrasound markers of aneuploidy.

Changes in fetal heart rate and umbilical artery flow velocity waveform characteristics

Changes in the fetal heart rate between 11 and 15 weeks of gestation are currently being investigated for the early screening of aneuploidy. Sporadic cases of fetus with Down syndrome presenting with an abnormally low heart rate in the first trimester of pregnancy have been reported. A small series of 25 chromosomally abnormal fetuses, including only five cases of trisomy 21 diagnosed before 15 weeks of gestation, has also indicated a trend towards bradycardia in these cases (Martinez et al. 1996). Van Lith et al. (1992) in a study of 10 chromosomally abnormal fetuses, investigated between 6 and 16 weeks and including five with trisomy 21, found no difference in the fetal heart rate compared to normal fetuses. However, two recent and larger studies have demonstrated a stable and significant increase in the mean fetal heart rate in trisomy 21 pregnancies diagnosed between

10 and 15 weeks of gestation (Hyett *et al.* 1996; Jauniaux *et al.* 1996c). A similar trend has also been observed for fetuses presenting with trisomy 13 and monosomy X whereas the fetal heart rate in trisomy 18 and triploidy is significantly lower than in normal fetuses. Fetuses with Down syndrome are not known to have an increased heart rate in the second half of pregnancy or at delivery, suggesting that the abnormally high fetal heart rate observed earlier in pregnancy may be a temporary phenomenon in those fetuses surviving up to delivery. Furthermore, fetal heart rate measurements obtained before 14 weeks have larger standard deviation than later in pregnancy. Continuous determination of heart rate using computerised analysis over a longer period of time is now mandatory to further explore this phenomenon.

The abnormal development of umbilical artery end diastolic flow (EDF) is an ominous sign of adverse fetal outcome during the second trimester of pregnancy as it is later in pregnancy (Jauniaux and Nicolaides 1996). In chromosomally normal fetuses with an increased nuchal thickness, the development of fetal heart rate and compliance of the umbilicoplacental circulation are within the normal ranges (Jauniaux *et al.* 1996). Some fetuses with trisomy 18 or triploidy may present with an increased resistance to blood flow in the umbilical artery (Fig. 18.1), which is probably due to an abnormal development of the villous vasculature in these cases.

Conclusion

The congenital malformations often encountered on ultrasound during the second half of pregnancy in aneuploidy are less likely to be evidenced in early pregnancy (Tables 18.2 and 18.3). In particular, abnormalities of the digestive tract, hands,

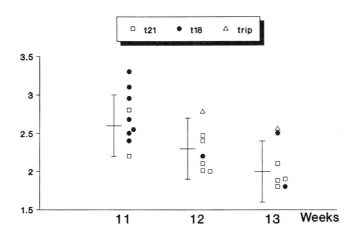

Fig. 18.1. Normal means and ranges (± 1.96SD) by weeks for umbilical artery pulsatility index (PI) and the corresponding individual measurements for the chromosomally abnormal fetuses.

face, amniotic fluid volume and some cardiac defects such as hypoplastic heart syndrome will be difficult to diagnose before the end of the fourth month of pregnancy and may only become apparent in late second trimester (Table 18.3). This is of paramount importance in counselling, about invasive prenatal cyto-genetic testing, mothers with a fetus presenting a 'soft' or minor markers of aneuploidy such as choroid plexus cyst or hydronephrosis which when isolated after 16 weeks does not justify the routine offering of invasive testing (Gross *et al.* 1995; Benacerraf 1996). In most cases, the combined use of transvaginal and transabdominal ultrasound and serial scans may be required before offering the parents a chorionic villus sampling (CVS) or amniocentesis.

References

Alberman, E.D. (1981) 'The abortus as a predictor of future trisomy 21' in F.F. De la Cruz and P.S. Gerald (Eds) *Trisomy 21 (Down Syndrome)*, pp.69–78. Baltimore: University Park Press

Allan, L.D., Sharland, G.K., Chita, S.K., Lockhart, S. and Maxwell, D.J. (1991) Chromosomal anomalies in fetal congenital heart disease. *Ultrasound Obstet Gynecol* **1**, 8–11

Benacerraf, B. (1988) Intrauterine growth retardation in the first trimester associated with triploidy. *J Ultrasound Med* **7**, 153–4

Benacerraf, B. (1996) The second-trimester fetus with Down syndrome: detection using sonographic features. *Ultrasound Obstet Gynecol* **7**, 147–55

Blass, H.G. and Eik-Nes, S.H. (1996) 'Ultrasound assessment of early brain development' in D. Jurkovic and E. Jauniaux (Eds) *Ultrasound and Early Pregnancy*, pp.3–18. Carnforth: Parthenon Publishing

Bouie, J., Philippe, E., Giroud, A. and Boue, A. (1976) Phenotypic expression of lethal anomalies in human abortuses. *Teratology* **14**, 3–20

Bromley, B., Harlow, B.L., Laboda, L.A. and Benacerrraf, B.R. (1991) Small sac size in the first trimester: a predictor of poor fetal outcome. *Radiology* **178**, 375–7

Dickey, R.P., Gasser, R., Olar, T.T. *et al.* (1994) Relationship of initial chorionic sac diameter to abortion and abortus karyotype based on new growth curves for 16th to 49th post-ovulation day. *Hum Reprod* **9**, 559–65

Drugan, A., Johnson, M.P., Isada, N.B. *et al.* (1992) The smaller than expected first-trimester fetus is at increased risk for chromosome anomalies. *Am J Obstet Gynecol* **178**, 1525–8

Edmonds, D.K., Lindsay, K.S., Miller, J.F., Williamson, E. and Wood, P. (1982) Early embryonic mortality in women. *Fertil Steril* **38**, 447–53

Edwards, R.G. (1986) Causes of early embryonic loss in human pregnancy. *Hum Reprod* **1**, 185–98

Fine, C., Bundy, A.L., Berkowitz, R.S., Boswell, S.B., Berezin, A.F. and Doubilet, P.M. (1989) Sonographic diagnosis of partial hydatidiform mole. *Obstet Gynecol* **73**, 414–18

Gembruch, U., Knopfle, G., Bald, R. and Hansmann, M. (1993) Early diagnosis of fetal congenital heart disease by transvaginal echocardiography. *Ultrasound Obstet Gynecol* **3**, 310–17

Goldstein, D.P. and Berkowitz, R.S. (1994) Current management of complete and partial molar pregnancy. *Reprod Med* **39**, 139–46

Goldstein, S.R. (1994) Embryonic death in early pregnancy: a new look at the first trimester. *Obstet Gynecol* **84**, 294–7

Goldstein, S.R., Kerenyi, T., Scher, J. and Papp, C. (1996) Karyotypic ultrasound correlation in patients with failed early pregnancy (Abstract). *Early Preg Med Biol* **2**, 27

Gross, S.J., Shulman, L.P., Tolley, E.A. *et al.* (1995) Isolated fetal choroid plexus cysts and trisomy 18: a review and meta-analysis. *Am J Obstet Gynecol* **172**, 83–7

Hyett, J.A., Moscoso, G. and Nicolaides, K.H. (1995) First-trimester nuchal translucency and cardiac septal defects in fetuses with trisomy 21. *Am J Obstet Gynecol* **172**, 1411–13

Hyett, J.A., Noble, R.J., Snijders, R.J.M., Montenegro, N. and Nicolaides, K.H. (1996) Fetal heart rate in trisomy 21 and other chromosomal abnormalities at 10–14 weeks gestation. *Ultrasound Obstet Gynecol* **7**, 239–44

Jauniaux, E. and Hustin, J. (1992) Histological examination of first trimester spontaneous abortions: the impact of materno-embryonic interface features. *Histopathology* **21**, 409–14

Jauniaux, E. and Nicolaides, K.H. (1996) Placental lakes, absent umbilical artery diastolic flow and poor fetal growth in early pregnancy. *Ultrasound Obstet Gynecol* **7**, 141–4

Jauniaux, E. and Nicolaides, K.H. (1997) Early ultrasound diagnosis and follow-up of molar pregnancies. *Ultrasound Obstet Gynecol* (in press)

Jauniaux, E., Donner, C., Thomas, C., Francotte, J., Rodesch, F. and Avni, E. (1988) Umbilical cord pseudocyst in trisomy 18. *Prenat Diagn* **8**, 557–63

Jauniaux, E., Van Maldergem, L., De Munter, C., Moscoso, G. and Gillerot, Y. (1990) Nonimmune hydrops fetalis associated with genetic abnormalities. *Obstet Gynecol* **75**, 568–72

Jauniaux, E., Jurkovic, D., Henriet, Y., Rodesch, F. and Hustin, J. (1991) Development of the secondary human yolk sac: correlation of sonographic and anatomic features. *Hum Reprod* **6**, 1160–6

Jauniaux, E., Kadri, R. and Hustin, J. (1996a) Partial mole and triploidy: screening in patients with first trimester spontaneous abortion. *Obstet Gynecol* **88**, 616–19

Jauniaux, E., Brown, R., Rodeck, C. and Nicolaides, K.H. (1996b) Prenatal diagnosis of triploidy during the second trimester of pregnancy. *Obstet Gynecol* **88**, 983–9

Jauniaux, E., Gavriil, P., Khun, P., Kurdi, W., Hyett, J. and Nicolaides, K.H. (1996c) Fetal heart rate and umbilicoplacental doppler flow velocity waveforms in early pregnancies with a chromosomal abnormality and/or increased nuchal translucency thickness. *Hum Reprod* **11**, 435–9

Johnson, P., Sharland, G., Maxwell, D. and Allan, L. (1992) The role of transvaginal sonography in the early detection of congenital heart disease. *Ultrasound Obstet Gynecol* **2**, 248–51

Khun, P., Brizot, M.L., Pandya, P.P., Snijders, R.J. and Nicolaides, K.H. (1995) Crown-rump length in chromosomally abnormal fetuses at 10 to 13 weeks' gestation. *Am J Obstet Gynecol* **172**, 32–5

Leelapatana, P., Garrett, W.J. and Warren, P.S. (1992) Early growth retardation in the first trimester: is it characteristic of the chromosomally abnormal fetus? *Aust N Z Obstet Gynaecol* **32**, 95–7

Lynch, L. and Berkowitz, R.L. (1989) First trimester growth delay in trisomy 18. *Am J Perinatol* **6**, 237–9

Martinez, J.M., Comas, C., Ojuel, J., Borrell, A., Puerto, B. and Fortuny, A. (1996) Fetal heart rate patterns in pregnancies with chromosomal disorders or subsequent fetal loss. *Obstet Gynecol* **87**, 118–21

Miller, J.F., Williamson, E., Glue, J., Gordon, Y.B., Grudzinskas, J.G. and Sykes, A. (1980) Fetal loss after implantation. *Lancet* **i**, 554–6

Nicolaides, K.H., Brizot, M.L. and Snijders, R.J. (1994) Fetal nuchal translucency: ultrasound screening for fetal trisomy in the first trimester of pregnancy. *Br J Obstet Gynaecol* **101**, 782–6

Pandya, P., Snijders, R.J.M., Psara, N., Hibert, L. and Nicolaides, K.H. (1996) The prevalence of non-viable pregnancy at 10–13 weeks of gestation. *Ultrasound Obstet Gynaecol* **7**, 170–3

Sepulveda, W., Pryde, P.G., Greb, A.E., Romero, R. and Evans, M.I. (1994) Prenatal diagnosis of umbilical cord pseudocyst. *Ultrasound Obstet Gynecol* **4**, 147–50

Shulman, L.P., Emerson, D.S., Grevengood, C. *et al.* (1994) Clinical course and outcome of fetuses with isolated cystic nuchal lesions and normal karyotypes detected in the first trimester. *Am J Obstet Gynecol* **171**, 1278–81

Simpson, J.L. and Bombard, A.T. (1987) 'Chromosomal abnormalities in spontaneous abortion: frequency, pathology and genetic counselling' in K. Edmonds and M.J. Bennett (Eds) *Spontaneous Abortion*, pp.51–76. Oxford: Blackwell Scientific

Simpson, J.L., Gray, R.H., Queenan, J.T. *et al.* (1994) Risk of recurrent spontaneous abortion for pregnancies discovered in the fifth week of gestation [letter]. *Lancet* **344**, 964

Snijders, R.J.M., Sebire, N.J., Souka, A., Santiago, C. and Nicolaides, K.H. (1995) Fetal exomphalos and chromosomal defects: relationship to maternal age and gestation. *Ultrasound Obstet Gynecol* **6**, 220–5

Snijders, R.J.M., Johnson, S., Sebire, N.J., Noble, P. and Nicolaides, K.H. (1996) First trimester ultrasound screening for chromosomal defects. *Ultrasound Obstet Gynecol* **7**, 216–26

Stephenson, M.D. (1996) Frequency of factors associated with habitual abortion in 197 couples. *Fertil Steril* **66**, 24–9

Trauffer, P.M.L., Anderson, C.E., Johnson, A., Heeger, S., Morgan, P. and Wapner, R.J. (1994) The natural history of euploid pregnancies with first-trimester cystic hygromas. *Am J Obstet Gynecol* **170**, 1279–84

Van Lith, J.M.M., Visser, G.H.A., Mantingh, A. and Beekhuis, J.R. (1992) Fetal heart rate in early pregnancy and chromosomal disorders. *Br J Obstet Gynaecol* **99**, 741–4

Warburton, D., Kline, J., Stein, Z., Hutzler, M., Chin, A. and Hassold, T. (1987) Does the karyotype of a spontaneous abortion predict the karyotype of a subsequent abortion? Evidence from 273 women with two karyotyped spontaneous abortions. *Am J Hum Genet* **41**, 465–83

Watt, J.L., Templeton, A.A., Messinis, I., Bell, L., Cunningham, P. and Duncan, R.O. (1987) Trisomy I in an eight cell human pre-embryo. *J Med Genet* **24**, 60–4

Weissman, A. and Achiron, R. (1996) 'Ultrasound assessment of early brain development' in D. Jurkovic and E. Jauniaux (Eds) *Ultrasound and Early Pregnancy*, pp.95–120. Carnforth: Parthenon Publishing

Zalel, Y., Shalev, E., Yanay, N., Schiff, E. and Weiner, E.A. (1994) Large yolk sac: a possible clue to early diagnosis of partial hydatidiform mole. *J Clin Ultrasound* **22**, 519–21

Zaragoza, M.V., Jacobs, P.A. and James, R.S. (1994) Nondisjunction of human acrocentric chromosomes: studies of 432 trisomic fetuses and liveborns. *Hum Genet* **19**, 411–17

Zinaman, M.J., Clegg, E.D., Brown, C.C., O'Connor, J. and Selevan, S.G. (1996) Estimates of human fertility and pregnancy loss. *Fertil Steril* **65**, 503–9

Chapter 19

First trimester ultrasound screening for chromosomal defects

Kypros H. Nicolaides, Rosalinde J.M. Snijders, Penelope L. Noble,
Maria Brizot and Neil J. Sebire

Screening for chromosomal defects by a combination of fetal nuchal translucency thickness and maternal age is essentially based on two observations made more than 100 years ago. The first observation was by Dr Langdon Down who in 1866 reported that the skin of affected individuals appears to be too large for their body (Down 1866) and the second by Fraser and Mitchell in 1876 who noted an association between the condition and advanced maternal age (Fraser and Mitchell 1876). It is now known that the excess skin of individuals with Down syndrome can be visualised by ultrasonography as increased nuchal translucency (Fig. 19.1) in the first three months of intrauterine life (Nicolaides *et al.* 1992a). Furthermore, increased translucency at 10–14 weeks of gestation is a common phenotypic expression of many chromosomal abnormalities, cardiac defects and genetic syndromes.

Chromosomal defects in relation to maternal age and gestation

Snijders *et al.* (1994, 1995) combined data from studies on mid-trimester amniocentesis and first trimester chorion villus sampling to estimate the prevalence of a wide range of chromosomal defects at different gestations in relation to trisomy 21 in live births. Maternal age and gestational age-specific risks were then calculated by multiplying the maternal age-specific prevalences of trisomy 21 in live births with the relative prevalence at a given gestation (Table 19.1; Fig. 19.2).

For each chromosomal defect it is possible to calculate the rate of intrauterine lethality (Table 19.2; Fig. 19.3) from the differences in prevalence at 40 weeks and prevalence at a given gestation. For example, in trisomy 21, if the prevalence at 40 weeks is 1.00, the prevalence at 16 and 12 weeks of gestation is 1.46 and 1.69,

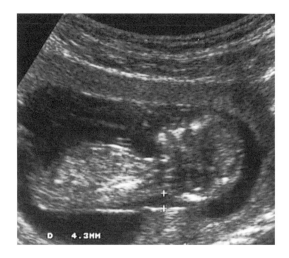

Fig. 19.1. Measurement of fetal nuchal translucency thickness.

Table 19.1. Estimated risk for trisomies 21, 18 and 13 (1/ number given in the table) in relation to maternal age and gestation (Nicolaides *et al.* 1992a)

Maternal age	Trisomy 21			Trisomy 18			Trisomy 13		
	12 wks	20 wks	40 wks	12 wks	20 wks	40 wks	12 wks	20 wks	40 wks
20	898	1175	1527	2484	4897	18013	7826	14656	42423
25	795	1040	1352	2200	4336	15951	6930	12978	37567
30	526	688	895	1456	2869	10554	4585	8587	24856
35	210	274	356	580	1142	4202	1826	3419	9896
40	57	74	97	157	310	1139	495	927	2683

respectively; the rate of intrauterine lethality between 16 weeks and 40 weeks is 32% (1.46−1.00/1.46), and between 12 and 40 weeks is 41% (1.69−1.00/1.69) (Snijders *et al.* 1994, 1995).

Assessment of nuchal translucency thickness

During the second and third trimesters of pregnancy, abnormal accumulation of fluid behind the fetal neck can be classified as nuchal cystic hygromas, which are associated with Turner's syndrome (Azar *et al.* 1991) and nuchal oedema, which has a diverse aetiology including trisomies, cardiovascular and pulmonary defects, skeletal dysplasias, congenital infection and metabolic and haematological disorders (Nicolaides *et al.* 1992b). Furthermore, chromosomally normal fetuses with nuchal oedema have a poor prognosis because in many cases there is an underlying skeletal dysplasia, genetic syndrome or cardiac defect (Nicolaides *et al.*

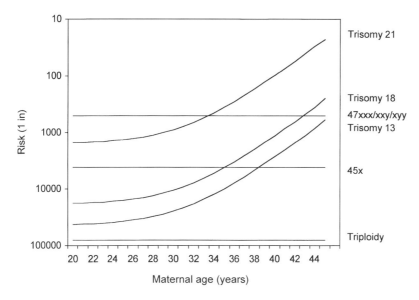

Fig. 19.2. Estimated risks for various chromosomal abnormalities with maternal age.

Table 19.2. Estimates for the rate of spontaneous loss in fetuses with various chromosomal defects (Nicolaides *et al.* 1992a)

Chromosomal defect	Estimated loss rate (%)	
	From 12 to 40 weeks	From 16 to 40 weeks
Trisomy 21	41	32
Trisomy 18	86	74
Trisomy 13	82	71
Turner syndrome	75	52
47,XXX	~5	~3
47,XXY	~5	~3
47,XYY	~5	~3
Triploidy	>99	>99

1992b). In the first trimester the term translucency is used, because this is the ultrasonographic feature that is observed; during the second trimester the translucency usually resolves and in a few cases it evolves into either nuchal oedema or cystic hygromas with or without generalised hydrops.

Measurement

Nuchal translucency can be measured successfully by transabdominal ultrasound examination in about 95% of cases; in the others it is necessary to perform vaginal sonography. The equipment must be of good quality (about £30,000–£40,000) and the average time allocated for each fetal scan should be at least ten minutes. All sonographers performing fetal scans should be capable of measuring reliably the crown–rump length and obtaining a proper sagittal view of the fetal spine. For such sonographers it is easy to acquire, within a few hours, the skill to measure nuchal translucency thickness. Furthermore, it is essential that the same criteria are used to achieve uniformity of results from different operators:

- A good sagittal section of the fetus, as for measurement of fetal crown–rump length, should be obtained.
- The magnification should be such that the fetus occupies at least three-quarters of the image.
- Care must be taken to distinguish between fetal skin and amnion because at this gestation both structures appear as thin membrane. This is achieved by waiting for spontaneous fetal movement away from the amniotic membrane; alternatively the fetus is bounced off the amnion by asking the mother to cough and/or by tapping the maternal abdomen.
- The maximum thickness of the subcutaneous translucency between the skin and the soft tissue overlying the cervical spine should be measured by placing the callipers on the lines as shown in Fig. 19.1. During the scan more than one measurement must be taken and the maximum one should be recorded.

Repeatability

A potential criticism of screening by ultrasound is that scanning requires not only highly skilled operators but it is also prone to operator variability. This issue was addressed by a prospective study at 10–14 weeks of gestation in which the

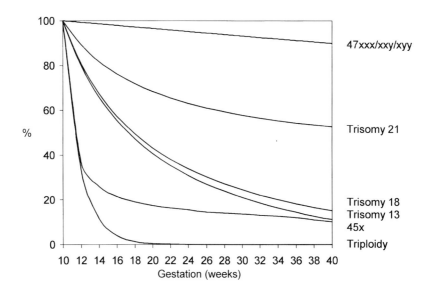

Fig. 19.3. Estimated rates of intrauterine lethality for various chromosomal abnormalities.

translucency was measured by two of four operators in 200 pregnant women (Pandya *et al.* 1995a). This study demonstrated that after an initial measurement, the second one made by the same (intra-) observer or another (inter-) observer varies from the first by less than 0.54 mm and 0.62 mm, respectively, in 95% of the cases. Additionally, the study demonstrated that the caliper placement repeatability was similar to the intra-observer and inter-observer repeatability, suggesting that a large part of the variation in measurements can be accounted for by the placement of the calipers rather than the generation of the image. Digital image processing and automation of caliper placement should reduce the differences in measurement. In the meantime, it is best to take the mean of two good measurements rather than one.

Increase with gestational age

Fetal nuchal translucency thickness increases with crown–rump length (Pandya *et al.* 1995b) and therefore in determining whether a given nuchal translucency thickness is increased it is essential to take gestation into account.

Nuchal translucency and chromosomal defects

In the early 1990s several reports of small series in high-risk pregnancies demonstrated a possible association between increased nuchal translucency and chromosomal defects in the first trimester of pregnancy (Cullen *et al.* 1990; Szabo and Gellen 1990; Nicolaides *et al.* 1992a; Schulte-Vallentin and Schindler 1992; Shulman *et al.* 1992; Suchet *et al.* 1992; Van Zalen-Sprock *et al.* 1992; Ville *et al.* 1992; Wilson *et al.* 1992; Hewitt 1993; Johnson *et al.* 1993; Nadel *et al.* 1993; Savoldelli *et al.* 1993; Pandya *et al.* 1994, 1995c; Trauffer *et al.* 1994; Brambati *et al.* 1995; Comas *et al.* 1995; Szabo *et al.* 1995). Although the mean prevalence of chromosomal defects in 20 series involving a total of 1698 patients was 29%, there were large differences between the studies with the prevalence ranging from 19% to 88%. This variation in results presumably reflects differences in the maternal age distributions of the populations examined and differences in the definition of minimum thickness of the abnormal translucency, ranging from 2 mm to 10 mm.

Subsequently a series of screening studies in high-risk pregnancies were carried out; these involved measurement of nuchal translucency thickness immediately before fetal karyotyping, mainly for advanced maternal age. These studies, involving a total of 1273 pregnancies, reported that the nuchal translucency thickness was above the 95th centile of the normal range in about 80% of trisomy 21 fetuses (Nicolaides *et al.* 1992a, 1994). Similar findings were obtained in an additional four studies of pregnancies undergoing first trimester fetal karyotyping (Schulte-Vallentin and Schindler 1992; Savoldelli *et al.* 1993; Comas *et al.* 1995; Szabo *et al.* 1995). However, in another study involving 1819 pregnancies, nuchal translucency thickness of >3 mm identified only 30% of the chromosomally abnormal fetuses (no data were provided specifically for trisomy 21) and the false positive rate was 3.2% (Brambati *et al.* 1995).

An additional finding of the screening studies in high-risk pregnancies was that the prevalence of chromosomal defects is dependent on both the fetal nuchal translucency thickness and maternal age (Nicolaides *et al.* 1994; Pandya *et al.* 1994, 1995c). For example, in a study of 1015 pregnancies with increased fetal nuchal translucency thickness at 10–14 weeks of gestation the observed number of trisomies 21, 18 and 13 in fetuses with translucencies of 3 mm, 4 mm, 5 mm, and >6 mm was approximately three-times, 18-times, 28-times and 36-times higher than the respective number expected on the basis of maternal age; the incidence of Turner's syndrome and triploidy was nine-times and eight-times higher but the incidence of other sex chromosome aneuploidies was similar to that expected (Pandya *et al.* 1995c).

Screening in unselected populations

The Frimley Park and St Peter's study

Frimley Park Hospital and St Peter's Hospital, Chertsey are general hospitals within the NHS offering routine antenatal care and their combined annual number of deliveries is approximately 6000. Prior to the introduction of nuchal translucency scanning, the policy of these hospitals was to offer amniocentesis to women aged 35 years or older. During 1993 there were 11 fetuses with Down syndrome and only two of these were detected prenatally (Pandya *et al.* 1995d). Subsequently, nuchal translucency screening at 10–14 weeks of gestation was introduced and the implementation of this policy was achieved without the need for increasing the number of staff or the equipment. Women with fetal translucency of 2.5 mm or more were offered fetal karyotyping. In addition women aged 35 years or older were offered amniocentesis at 16 weeks' gestation. The data of the first five months after the introduction of the new policy were analysed following completion of the pregnancies (Pandya *et al.* 1995d). During this period 74% of women delivering in the two hospitals attended for first trimester scanning and the nuchal translucency was successfully measured in all pregnancies. The translucency was raised in 3.6% of cases and the total percentage of invasive procedures was 5.1%. All four cases of Down syndrome that occurred in this period were diagnosed prenatally.

The University College study

In a screening study of 1704 women with singleton pregnancies attending University College Hospital, London, for routine antenatal care at 8–14 weeks of gestation, transabdominal ultrasound examination was performed (Bewley *et al.* 1995). In 20% of cases, the sonographers forgot to measure the fetal nuchal translucency thickness. In a further 18% of those women where a measurement was attempted, this was unsuccessful. In 28% of the 1127 cases where measurements were made, the scans were carried out before ten weeks of gestation. The translucency thickness was ≥3 mm in 6% of the cases. The population contained three fetuses with trisomy 21, all in women aged ≥39 years, and increased translucency was found in one.

The Austrian study

In a screening study of 1972 women with singleton pregnancies attending an NHS hospital in Vienna for routine antenatal care at 10–13 weeks of gestation, transabdominal ultrasound examination was performed and the fetal nuchal translucency thickness was successfully measured in all cases (Hafner *et al.* 1995). The nuchal translucency thickness was ≥2.5 mm in 1.3% of the cases and this group included 73% of those with chromosomal abnormalities.

The multicentre screening study

In a multicentre study, at the Harris Birthright Centre and four District General Hospitals (St Peter's, Chertsey; Frimley Park, Camberley; Queen Mary's, Sidcup; Heatherwood, Ascot), nuchal translucency screening at 10–14 weeks of gestation has been carried out in 20,804 pregnancies, including 164 cases of chromosomal abnormalities (Pandya *et al.* 1995b). This study demonstrated that:

1. in normal pregnancies nuchal translucency thickness increases with gestation,
2. in chromosomally abnormal pregnancies nuchal translucency thickness is increased,
3. the risk for trisomies can be derived by multiplying the background maternal age and gestation-related risk by a likelihood ratio, which depends on the degree of deviation in nuchal translucency from the normal median for crown–rump length,
4. in about 5% of pregnancies the estimated risk for trisomy 21 was at least one in 100 and this group included 80% of fetuses with trisomy 21 and 77% of those with other chromosomal abnormalities. Because the maternal age of the screened population was higher than in Britain as a whole it was estimated that the cut-off risk to include 5% of the British population is 1/300; using this cut-off the sensitivity of the test for trisomy 21 was estimated to be about 80%.

The Fetal Medicine Foundation

The findings of the RADIUS study (Ewigman *et al.* 1993) have demonstrated that inappropriate introduction of new services by inadequately trained personnel and without the provision of audit, can lead to the erroneous conclusion that the new service/technology is not beneficial. In addition, such bad medical practices are inevitably detrimental to the health of patients.

It is for this reason that the Fetal Medicine Foundation, a registered charity, was set up. One of the aims is to provide comprehensive training, support and audit for the proper implementation of the 10–14 week scan. The Foundation is offering, free of charge, training courses on many aspects of first trimester scanning, and has introduced a certificate of competence that can be obtained after passing the appropriate theoretical and practical examinations. The Foundation provides the necessary computer program for calculation of risks only to those sonographers that receive the appropriate certificate of competence and participate in continuing audit of results.

There are now 25 countries with approved centres for carrying out nuchal translucency screening and in Britain alone there are 28 such centres. By 1 July 1996, in 21 centres in Britain a total of 83,327 singleton pregnancies with live fetuses at 10–14 weeks of gestation were examined. The first 61,972 completed pregnancies included 208 with trisomy 21 and 205 with other chromosomal defects (Fig. 19.4); using a cut-off risk of 1 in 300, estimated from the maternal age and fetal nuchal translucency thickness the sensitivity for trisomy 21 was 84% (Tables 19.3 and 19.4).

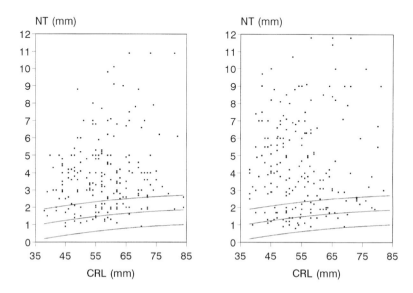

Fig. 19.4. Fetal nuchal translucency thickness with crown–rump length (CRL) in fetuses with trisomy 21 (left) and in fetuses with other chromosome defects (right).

Table 19.3. Results of the Fetal Medicine Foundation multicentre screening project using the combination of maternal age and fetal nuchal translucency thickness at 10–14 weeks of gestation for assessment of the risk for trisomy 21. Data from 61,972 completed singleton pregnancies include 25,295 cases where the woman requested a scan at the Harris Birthright Research Centre and 36,677 cases where women had screening as part of routine antenatal care in their local hospital (DGH)

	HBC		20 DGH		Total	
	All cases	Tr 21	All cases	Tr 21	All Cases	Tr 21
Total number of pregnancies	25,295	123	36,677	85	61,972	208
Maternal age > 37 years	6177	83	2417	33	8591	116
	(24%)	(68%)	(7%)	(39%)	(14%)	(56%)
Estimated risk > 1/300 all cases	4041	107	1861	68	5604	175
	(16%)	(87%)	(5%)	(80%)	(9%)	(84%)
Estimated risk > 1/100 all cases	1215	96	719	55	1934	151
	(5%)	(78%)	(2%)	(65%)	(3%)	(73%)

Table 19.4. Results of the screening study for trisomy 21 based on the combination of maternal age and fetal nuchal translucency thickness at 10–14 weeks of gestation from 61,972 completed singleton pregnancies examined in 21 British centres under the auspices of the Fetal Medicine Foundation

Karyotype	Total	NT >95th centile	Risk >1/300
Trisomy 21	208	153 (74%)	175 (84%)
Trisomy 18	80	59 (74%)	65 (81%)
Trisomy 13	28	22 (79%)	25 (89%)
Other trisomy	13	9 (69%)	11 (85%)
Turner's syndrome	33	29 (88%)	30 (91%)
Sex aneuploidies	20	8 (40%)	13 (65%)
Triploidy	18	11 (61%)	11 (61%)
Other	13	7 (54%)	7 (54%)

Table 19.5. Accuracy of estimated risk for trisomy 21 by a combination of maternal age and fetal nuchal translucency thickness

Estimated risk	n	Trisomy 21	Observed prevalence
<1 in 10	493	105	1 in 5
1 in 10 – 1 in 25	340	28	1 in 12
1 in 25 – 1 in 49	377	7	1 in 53
1 in 50 – 1 in 99	715	10	1 in 72
1 in 100 – 1 in 200	1873	15	1 in 125
1 in 200 – 1 in 500	5629	16	1 in 352
1 in 500 – 1 in 1000	8279	11	1 in 753
1 in 1000 – 1 in 2000	12534	8	1 in 1566
1 in 2000 – 1 in 4000	19099	6	1 in 3183
>1 in 4000	12633	1	–

The 61,972 pregnancies included 25,295 that were examined at the Harris Birthright Research Centre for Fetal Medicine and 36,677 that were screened in 20 other British Centres (Table 19.3). The Harris Birthright Centre recruited self-referred patients and 24% were aged 37 years or more and therefore the prevalence of trisomy 21 was high (approximately one in 200). Consequently, the estimated risk based on maternal age and nuchal translucency thickness was more than 1/300 in 16% of the population, including 87% of the trisomy 21 pregnancies. The other 20 centres offered screening as part of routine antenatal care and the screened patients were more representative of the whole British population. In this group only 7% were aged 37 years or more and 5% had an estimated risk of 1/300; the detection rate for trisomy 21 was 80%.

The results from the Harris Birthright Centre demonstrate that in a population where on the basis of maternal age at least 24% would have been classified as high risk, nuchal translucency screening reduced the need for invasive testing to 16% and yet the sensitivity of the test for trisomy 21 was 87%. The results from the other centres prove that provided there is adequate training and audit nuchal translucency screening, as part of routine antenatal care can identify 80% of trisomy 21 fetuses.

Table 19.5 illustrates the observed prevalence of trisomy 21 according to the predicted risk based on maternal age and fetal nuchal translucency thickness. These results demonstrate the high degree of accuracy of the model.

Lethality of trisomy 21 fetuses with increased translucency

Screening for chromosomal defects in the first rather than the second trimester has the advantage of earlier prenatal diagnosis and consequently less traumatic termination of pregnancy for those couples that chose this option. A potential disadvantage is that earlier screening preferentially identifies those chromosomally abnormal pregnancies that are destined to miscarry. Approximately 40% of affected fetuses die between 12 weeks of gestation and term (Snijders *et al.* 1995). This issue of preferential intrauterine lethality of chromosomal defects is of course a potential criticism of all methods of antenatal screening, including second trimester maternal serum biochemistry; the estimated rate of intrauterine lethality between 16 weeks and term is about 30% (Snijders *et al.* 1995). This section examines the interrelation between increased nuchal translucency in trisomy 21 and fetal lethality.

Decision to continue with the pregnancy after the diagnosis of trisomy 21

In a study of 108 fetuses with trisomy 21 diagnosed in the first trimester because of increased nuchal translucency thickness, in five cases the parents chose to continue with the pregnancy whereas in 103 they had termination; trisomy 21 was also diagnosed in one of the fetuses in a twin pregnancy where the parents elected to avoid invasive prenatal diagnosis or selective fetocide (Pandya *et al.* 1995e). In five of the six fetuses the nuchal translucency resolved and at the second trimester scan the nuchal fold thickness was normal (less than 7 mm). All six trisomy 21 babies were born alive. One had a major atrioventricular septal defect and died at the age of six months. Another two of the babies had small ventricular septal defects and these are being managed conservatively awaiting spontaneous closure. These data suggest that increased nuchal translucency does not necessarily identify those trisomic fetuses that are destined to die *in utero*.

Decision to terminate the pregnancy after the diagnosis of trisomy 21

In a study of 70 pregnancies where trisomy 21 was diagnosed at 12 (range 11–14) weeks of gestation and the parents opted for elective termination which was carried out at 14 (12–20) weeks, ultrasound examination to establish viability was carried out at the time of chorion villus sampling (CVS) and just before termination (Hyett *et al.* 1996). Eight fetuses died in the interval between CVS and termination and the rate of lethality increased with translucency thickness from 5.3% for those with translucency of 0–3 mm to 23.5% for translucency of >7 mm.

Even if one assumes that the relative rate of intrauterine lethality of trisomy 21 fetuses according to translucency thickness stays the same throughout pregnancy, it was estimated that a policy of screening by maternal age and fetal nuchal translucency followed by selective termination of affected fetuses would be associated with at least a 70% reduction in the live birth incidence of trisomy 21 (Hyett *et al.* 1996).

Data from the Fetal Medicine Foundation multicentre study

In the 62,017 completed pregnancies that were screened in the multicentre study there were 208 pregnancies where trisomy 21 fetuses was diagnosed prenatally or at birth. In 175 pregnancies the estimated risk was one in 300 or more (screen positive) and in 33 (16%) the risk was less. It was estimated that 150 babies with trisomy 21 would have been live born had there not been any antenatal screening. This estimate was made from the maternal age distribution of the population and the maternal age-related prevalence of trisomy 21 in live births (Hook and Fabia 1978). In reality there were only 26 (13%) live births with trisomy 21 and nine of these were in the screen positive group (risk more than one in 300) but the parents chose not to have prenatal diagnosis or decided to continue with the pregnancy despite the prenatal diagnosis of trisomy 21.

On the extreme assumption that all 16 screen negative pregnancies with trisomy 21 that were diagnosed antenatally would have resulted in live births had the pregnancies not been terminated, then the number of trisomy 21 live births in the screen negative group would have been 33. In this case, screening by a combination of maternal age and fetal nuchal translucency and selective termination of affected fetuses would have reduced the potential live birth prevalence of trisomy 21 by 78% (117 of 150) (Table 19.6).

Nuchal translucency in multiple pregnancies

Since the 1970s, both the average maternal age and the use of assisted reproduction techniques have increased with consequent increase in the number of multiple pregnancies at high risk of chromosomal defects. In multiple pregnancies compared to singletons, prenatal diagnosis is complicated because first, effective

Table 19.6. Estimated reduction in the birth prevalence of trisomy 21 in 61,972 singleton pregnancies undergoing screening by a combination of maternal age and fetal nuchal translucency thickness

Trisomy 21	*n* (%)
Total diagnosed	208
Total number with risk less than 1 in 300	33 (16%)
Expected live births based on age	150
Actual live births	26 (17%)
Total number with risk less than 1 in 300	33 (22%)

methods of screening, such as maternal serum biochemistry, are not applicable, secondly, the techniques of invasive testing may provide uncertain results or may be associated with higher risks of miscarriage, and thirdly, the fetuses may be discordant for an abnormality in which case one of the options for the subsequent management of the pregnancy is selective fetocide.

In singleton pregnancies the method of choice for fetal karyotyping may be CVS because of the advantages of early diagnosis, whereas in twin pregnancies, the method of choice for fetal karyotyping is amniocentesis. However, cytogenetic results from amniocentesis are not usually available until around 18–20 weeks of gestation; if one fetus is chromosomally abnormal and the parents choose selective fetocide the risk of miscarriage is three times higher than with fetocide before 16 weeks (Evans *et al.* 1994). Therefore, there is a need for selection of the appropriate diagnostic technique depending on the likelihood for selective fetocide; if the risk is high (more than one in 50) then CVS should be the technique of choice, otherwise amniocentesis is preferable (Sebire *et al.* 1996a).

Pandya *et al.* (1995f) examined nuchal translucency thickness of each fetus in eight twin pregnancies where karyotyping at 10–14 weeks of gestation demonstrated that at least one of the fetuses was chromosomally abnormal. Eight fetuses had trisomy 21 and two had trisomy 18. The nuchal translucency thickness was more than 2.5 mm in nine (90%) of the trisomic fetuses and in one of the chromosomally normal ones.

In the Harris Birthright Centre screening study at 10–14 weeks there were 20,543 singleton and 392 twin pregnancies (Sebire *et al.* 1996b). This study demonstrated that in twin pregnancies screening for trisomy 21 by measurement of fetal nuchal translucency thickness and maternal age had a similar sensitivity to that found in singletons. However, the false positive rate of the test is higher in

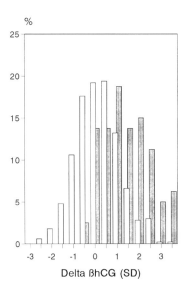 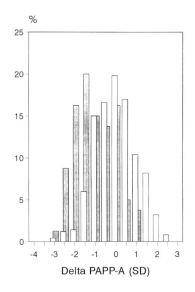

Fig. 19.5. Distribution of maternal serum free β-hCG and PAPP-A measurements in chromosomally normal pregnancies (open bars) and in those with trisomy 21 (closed bars).

twin compared to singleton pregnancies, due to a higher prevalence of increased translucency in chromosomally normal fetuses from monochorionic pregnancies (about 8%, compared to 5% in singletons). The most likely explanation for this high false positive rate is that increased nuchal translucency in one of the fetuses in monochorionic twins is an early manifestation of heart failure due to twin to twin transfusion syndrome.

Nuchal translucency and maternal serum biochemistry

In trisomy 21 during the first trimester of pregnancy the maternal serum concentration of free beta human chorionic gonadotrophin (free β-hCG) is higher and pregnancy associated plasma protein-A (PAPP-A) is lower than in chromosomally normal pregnancies. Pregnancy-specific β-1 glycoprotein (SP-1), alpha fetoprotein and inhibin-A do not provide useful distinction between affected and normal pregnancies(Bersinger *et al.* 1994; Brizot *et al.* 1995a; Noble *et al.* 1997).

Retrospective study

In a study of 80 trisomy 21 pregnancies and 500 matched controls, it was estimated that screening by a combination of maternal age and maternal serum PAPP-A and free β-hCG, the detection rate for trisomy 21 for a false positive rate of 5% would be about 60% (Fig. 19.5). Furthermore, maternal age and fetal nuchal translucency can be combined in calculating risks for fetal trisomies (Brizot *et al.* 1994, 1995a; Noble *et al.* 1996) and it was estimated that the detection rate of about 80% based on maternal age and fetal nuchal translucency can be improved to more than 90% if maternal serum free β-hCG and PAPP-A are included.

Table 19.7. Comparison of detection rates for trisomy 21, for a false positive rate of 5%, by maternal age, maternal serum free β-hCG, fetal nuchal translucency and by a combination of parameters, in a prospective study involving 5434 pregnancies

	Detection rate
Maternal age	11 (31%)
Maternal serum free β-hCG	10 (28%)
Fetal nuchal translucency	28 (78%)
Maternal serum free β-hCG and age	15 (42%)
Fetal nuchal translucency and age	28 (78%)
Maternal serum free β-hCG, age and fetal nuchal translucency	32 (86%)

Prospective study

At the Harris Birthright Centre maternal free β-hCG is now measured prospectively and the data are combined with maternal age and fetal nuchal translucency in the calculation of risk for trisomy 21. In the 5434 pregnancies that were examined by January 1996, the mean maternal age was 33 years and there were 36 trisomy 21 pregnancies. The efficacy of the individual parameters was assessed by comparing detection rates for a 5% false positive rate (Table 19.7). The findings illustrate that with the combination of fetal nuchal translucency and maternal age and serum free β-hCG the detection rate for trisomy 21 was 86%.

Conclusion

Screening for trisomy 21 by a combination of maternal age and fetal nuchal translucency thickness at 10–14 weeks can identify about 80% of affected fetuses for a 5% false positive rate; the detection rate can increase to more than 90% by including data on maternal serum free β-hCG and PAPP-A. In addition, increased nuchal translucency is likely to be a useful marker for a wide variety of fetal abnormalities and genetic syndromes. However, as with the introduction of any new technology into routine clinical practice it is essential that those undertaking the 10–14 week scan are adequately trained and their results are subjected to rigorous audit.

References

Azar, G., Snijders, R.J.M., Gosden, C.M. and Nicolaides, K.H. (1991) Fetal nuchal cystic hygromata: associated malformations and chromosomal defects. *Fetal Diagn Ther* **6**, 46–57

Bersinger, N.A., Brizot, M.L., Johnson, A. *et al.* (1994) First trimester maternal serum pregnancy-associated plasma protein A and pregnancy-specific β1-glycoprotein in fetal trisomies. *Br J Obstet Gynaecol* **101**, 970–4

Bewley, S., Roberts, L.J., Mackinson, M. and Rodeck, C. (1995) First trimester fetal nuchal translucency: problems with screening the general population II. *Br J Obstet Gynaecol* **102**, 386–8

Brambati, B., Cislaghi, C., Tului, L. *et al.* (1995) First-trimester Down's syndrome screening using nuchal translucency: a prospective study. *Ultrasound Obstet Gynecol* **5**, 9–14

Brizot, M.L., Snijders, R.J.M., Bersinger, N.A., Kuhn, P. and Nicolaides, K.H. (1994) Maternal serum pregnancy associated placental protein A and fetal nuchal translucency thickness for the prediction of fetal trisomies in early pregnancy. *Obstet Gynecol* **84**, 918–22

Brizot, M.L., Kuhn P., Bersinger N.A., Snijders R.J.M. and Nicolaides K.H. (1995a) First trimester maternal serum alpha-fetoprotein in fetal trisomies. *Br J Obstet Gynaecol* **102**, 31–4

Brizot, M.L., Snijders, R.J.M., Butler, J., Bersinger, N.A. and Nicolaides, K.H. (1995b) Maternal serum hCG and fetal nuchal translucency thickness for the prediction of fetal trisomies in the first trimester of pregnancy. *Br J Obstet Gynaecol* **102**, 127–32

Comas, C., Martinez, J.M., Ojuel, J. *et al.* (1995) First-trimester nuchal edema as a marker of aneuploidy. *Ultrasound Obstet Gynecol* **5**, 26–9

Cullen, M.T., Gabrielli, S., Green, J.J. *et al.* (1990) Diagnosis and significance of cystic hygroma in the first trimester. *Prenat Diagn* **10**, 643–51

Down, J.L.H. (1866) Observations on an ethnic classification of idiots. *Clinical Lecture Reports, London Hospital,* **3**, 259

Evans, M.I., Goldberg, J.D., Dommergues, M. *et al.* (1994) Efficacy of second-trimester selective termination for fetal abnormalities: international collaborative experience among the world's largest centers. *Am J Obstet Gynecol* **171**, 90–4

Ewigman, B.G., Crane, J.P., Frigoletto, F.D. *et al.* (1993). The effect of prenatal ultrasound screening on perinatal outcome. *N Engl J Med* **329**, 821–7

Fraser, J. and Mitchell, A. (1876) Kalmuk idiocy. Report of a case with autopsy. *J Ment Sci* **98**, 169–79

Hafner, E., Schuchter, K. and Philipp, K. (1995) Screening for chromosomal abnormalities in an unselected population by fetal nuchal translucency. *Ultrasound Obstet Gynecol* **6**, 330–3

Hewitt, B. (1993) Nuchal translucency in the first trimester. *Aust NZ J Obstet Gynaecol* **33**, 389–91

Hook, E.B. and Fabia, J.J. (1978) Frequency of Down syndrome in live births by single-year maternal age interval: results of a Massachusetts study. *Teratology* **17**, 223–8

Hyett, J.A., Sebire, N.J., Snijders, R.J.M. and Nicolaides, K.H (1996) Intrauterine lethality of trisomy 21 fetuses with increased nuchal translucency thickness. *Ultrasound Obstet Gynecol* **7**, 101–3

Johnson, M.P., Johnson, A., Holzgreve, W. *et al.* (1993) First-trimester simple hygroma: cause and outcome. *Am J Obstet Gynecol* **168**, 156–61

Nadel, A., Bromley, B. and Benacerraf, B.R. (1993) Nuchal thickening or cystic hygromas in first- and early second-trimester fetuses: prognosis and outcome. *Obstet Gynecol* **82**, 43–8

Nicolaides, K.H., Azar, G., Byrne, D., Mansur, C. and Marks, K. (1992a) Fetal nuchal translucency: ultrasound screening for chromosomal defects in first trimester of pregnancy. *BMJ* **304**, 867–9

Nicolaides, K.H., Azar, G., Snijders, R.J.M. and Gosden, C.M. (1992b) Fetal nuchal oedema: associated malformations and chromosomal defects. *Fetal Diagn Ther* **7**, 123–31

Nicolaides, K.H., Brizot, M.L. and Snijders, R.J.M. (1994) Fetal nuchal translucency thickness: ultrasound screening for fetal trisomy in the first trimester of pregnancy. *Br J Obstet Gynaecol* **101**, 782–6

Noble, P.L., Abraha, H.D., Snijders, R.J.M., Sherwood, R. and Nicolaides, K.H. (1996) Screening for fetal trisomy 21 in the first trimester of pregnancy: maternal serum free β-hCG and fetal nuchal translucency thickness. *Ultrasound Obstet Gynecol* **6**, 390–5

Noble, P.L., Wallace, E.M., Snijders, R.J.M., Groome, N.P. and Nicolaides, K.H. (1997) Maternal serum inhibin-A and free beta hCG concentrations in trisomy 21 pregnancies at 10–14 weeks of gestation. *Br J Obstet Gynaecol* (in press)

Pandya, P.P., Brizot, M.L., Kuhn, P., Snijders, R.J.M. and Nicolaides, K.H. (1994) First trimester fetal nuchal translucency thickness and risk for trisomies. *Obstet Gynecol* **84**, 420–3

Pandya, P.P., Altman, D., Brizot, M.L., Pettersen, H. and Nicolaides, K.H. (1995a) Repeatability of measurement of fetal nuchal translucency thickness. *Ultrasound Obstet Gynecol* **5**, 334–7

Pandya, P.P., Snijders, R.J.M., Johnson, S.J., Brizot, M. and Nicolaides, K.H. (1995b) Screening for fetal trisomies by maternal age and fetal nuchal translucency thickness at 10 to 14 weeks of gestation. *Br J Obstet Gynaecol* **102**, 957–62

Pandya, P.P., Kondylios, A., Hilbert, L., Snijders, R.J.M. and Nicolaides, K.H. (1995c) Chromosomal defects and outcome in 1015 fetuses with increased nuchal translucency. *Ultrasound Obstet Gynecol* **5**, 15–19

Pandya, P.P., Goldberg, H., Walton, B. *et al.* (1995d) The implementation of first trimester scanning at 10–13 weeks' gestation and the measurement of fetal nuchal translucency thickness in two maternity units. *Ultrasound Obstet Gynecol* **5**, 20–5

Pandya, P.P., Snijders, R.J.M., Johnson, S. and Nicolaides, K.H. (1995e) Natural history of trisomy 21 fetuses with fetal nuchal translucency. *Ultrasound Obstet Gynecol* **5**, 381–3

Pandya, P.P., Hilbert, F., Snijders, R.J.M. and Nicolaides, K.H. (1995f) Nuchal translucency thickness and crown-rump length in twin pregnancies with chromosomally abnormal fetuses. *J Ultrasound Med* **14**, 565–8

Savoldelli, G., Binkert, F., Achermann, J. and Schmid, W. (1993) Ultrasound screening for chromosomal anomalies in the first trimester of pregnancy. *Prenat Diagn* **13**, 513–18

Schulte-Vallentin, M. and Schindler, H. (1992) Non-echogenic nuchal oedema as a marker in trisomy 21 screening. *Lancet* **339**, 1053

Sebire, N.J., Noble, P.L., Psarra, A., Papapanagiotou, G. and Nicolaides, K.H. (1996a). Fetal karyotyping in twin pregnancies: selection of technique by measurement of fetal nuchal translucency. *Br J Obstet Gynaecol* **103**, 887–90

Sebire, N.J., Snijders, R.J.M., Hughes, K., Sepulveda, W. and Nicolaides, K.H. (1996b) Screening for trisomy 21 in twin pregnancies by maternal age and fetal nuchal translucency thickness at 10–14 weeks of gestation. *Br J Obstet Gynaecol* **103**, 999–1003

Shulman, L.P., Emerson, D., Felker, R., Phillips, O., Simpson, J. and Elias, S. (1992) High frequency of cytogenetic abnormalities with cystic hygroma diagnosed in the first trimester. *Obstet Gynecol* **80**, 80–2

Snijders, R.J.M., Holzgreve, W., Cuckle, H. and Nicolaides, K.H. (1994) Maternal age-specific risks for trisomies at 9–14 weeks of gestation. *Prenat Diagn* **14**, 543–52

Snijders, R.J.M., Sebire, N.J. and Nicolaides, K.H. (1995) Maternal age and gestational age specific risk for chromosomal defects. *Fetal Diagn Ther* **10**, 356–67

Suchet, I.B., Van der Westhuizen, N.G. and Labatte, M.F. (1992) Fetal cystic hygromas: further insights into their natural history. *Can Assoc Radiol J* **6**, 420–4

Szabo, J. and Gellen, J. (1990) Nuchal fluid accumulation in trisomy-21 detected by vaginal sonography in first trimester. *Lancet* **336**, 1133

Szabo, J., Gellen, J. and Szemere, G. (1995) First-trimester ultrasound screening for fetal aneuploidies in women over 35 and under 35 years of age. *Ultrasound Obstet Gynecol* **5**, 161–3

Trauffer, M.L., Anderson, C.E., Johnson, A., Heeger, S., Morgan, P. and Wapner, R.J. (1994) The natural history of euploid pregnancies with first-trimester cystic hygromas. *Am J Obstet Gynecol* **170**, 1279–84

Van Zalen-Sprock, M.M., Van Vugt, J.M.G. and Van Geijn, H.P. (1992) First-trimester diagnosis of cystic hygroma – course and outcome. *Am J Obstet Gynecol* **167**, 94–8

Ville, Y., Lalondrelle, C., Doumerc, S. *et al.* (1992) First-trimester diagnosis of nuchal anomalies: significance and fetal outcome. *Ultrasound Obstet Gynecol* **2**, 314–16

Wilson, R.D., Venir, N. and Faquharson, D.F. (1992) Fetal nuchal fluid – physiological or pathological? – in pregnancies less than 17 menstrual weeks. *Prenat Diagn* **12**, 755–63

Chapter 20

Serum parameters and nuchal translucency in first trimester screening for fetal chromosomal abnormalities

Roland Zimmermann, Franz Binkert, Josef Achermann,
Guido Savoldelli, Hans Baumann, Jürg Obwegeser,
Luico Bronz, Verena Geissbühler and Hans Conzin

Introduction

First trimester screening for chromosomal abnormalities would be superior to second trimester screening for many reasons. First, it allows karyotyping by chorionic villous sampling (CVS) which means that the result can be available very early when aspiration termination of pregnancy is possible. Furthermore, direct karyotyping is possible so the time between the positive screening test and the final result is short. In addition in the first trimester the emotional bond to the child is still small as fetal movements cannot be felt. Consequently, most women would opt for a first rather then a second trimester test. Thus substantial efforts have been made for many years to develop a first trimester screening strategy.

During recent years several authors have demonstrated, that in high risk patients an increased sonotranslucent space (>2.5 mm) in the neck and back of the embryo is present at the end of the first trimester (Szabo and Gellen 1990; Nicolaides *et al.* 1992; Savoldelli *et al.* 1993). This sonographic sign, called nuchal translucency (NT), is often present in trisomy 21 embryos but also associated with trisomy 13 and 18, Turner's syndrome, 47,XXY and other sex-chromosome anomalies (Pandya *et al.* 1995).

In addition to sonographic markers, several authors have reported an association between maternal biochemical screening parameters and Down syndrome (DS) in the first trimester. Previous investigations have demonstrated that the median value of pregnancy associated plasma protein A (PAPP-A) in the first trimester in DS pregnancies was significantly lower than in the normal population (Chard and Grudzinskas 1991; Wald *et al.* 1992; Brambati *et al.* 1993, 1994a,b).

For a combination of maternal age and decreased serum PAPP-A levels a detection rate for DS of 62% for a false positive rate of 5% has been reported. Observations on different populations in the first trimester studied in three other centres yielded similar results (Hurley *et al.* 1993; Muller *et al.* 1993), regardless of whether DS was diagnosed at CVS or at term. Spencer and his colleagues (1992) reported that the measurement of elevated maternal serum free beta chorionic gonadotropin levels (free β-HCG) may be useful in the detection of pregnancies affected by DS and trisomy 18, respectively, in the first trimester.

Little, however, is known, whether the combination of sonography with biochemical markers can improve the detection rate of chromosomal abnormalities.

The aim of this study was to evaluate the influence of an increased NT on PAPP-A and free β-hCG levels in chromosomally normal embryos and to analyse whether this ultrasound marker together with the biochemical parameters lead to a higher detection rate of aneuploid pregnancies in the first trimester.

We report here our observations on the combined measurement of nuchal translucency and serum PAPP-A and free β-hCG obtained from 1919 consecutive women at 10–13 weeks' gestation prior to CVS for prenatal diagnosis.

Subjects and methods

A total of 1919 women undergoing CVS between 10 and 13 weeks of pregnancy in various centres in Switzerland and Bregenz, Austria, were enrolled in the study. Indications for the CVS included 1203 cases of advanced maternal age (≥ 35 years), 553 women at low risk (< 35 years, CVS done because of maternal anxiety), 84 with a previous chromosomally abnormal pregnancy, 19 with a fetal nuchal translucency ≥ 3 mm and 60 with other indications including abnormal ultrasound and DNA diagnostic procedures. Nuchal translucency was measured by the physician performing the CVS using different 'middle range' ultrasound equipment (cost=US$70,000$\pm$15,000). All sonographers had had several years of experience in diagnostic ultrasound. An increased nuchal translucency was defined as a sonotranslucent pouch in the neck and back ≥ 3 mm (Szabo and Gellen 1990; Nicolaides *et al.* 1992; Szabo *et al.* 1992; Savoldelli *et al.* 1993). This cut-off point was used since some ultrasound machines do not allow measurement to tenths of a millimetre.

After informed consent 10 ml of venous blood was taken prior to CVS, transported to the genetic laboratories within 2–3 h, centrifuged and stored at $-20°C$ to prevent artefactual increase in the free β-hCG (Zimmermann *et al.* 1994).

Subsequently the samples were thawed once at the Department of Obstetrics, University of Zurich, aliquoted into five Eppendorf tubes and stored at $-70°C$ until measurement of the serum parameters.

All karyotypes were analysed either at the Institute of Medical Genetics, University of Zurich, Switzerland or at Genetica, Cytogenetic Laboratory, Zurich, Switzerland.

Free β-hCG was measured in a blinded manner by immuno radio metric assay (IRMA) (Amerlex-M free β-hCG, Johnson and Johnson, UK) and PAPP-A by a not yet commercially available IRMA (Amerlex-M PAPP-A, Johnson and Johnson, UK). All samples were determined in duplicates in one batch. A total of 446 randomly selected samples of contemporaneous pregnancies with a normal embryo acted as controls in relation to all pregnancies with a chromosomal abnormal embryo and the ones with an increased nuchal translucency but normal karyotype.

In the control group the log values were linearly regressed. The distribution of the residuals showed good accordance with a Gaussian model, allowing the calculation of medians for each gestational day. Subsequently all values were expressed as multiples of the regressed median (MoMs).

The mean MoM in the control group and the group with increased NT but normal karyotype was compared using Mann–Whitney-U test. Comparison of the control group with different subgroups of chromosomal abnormalities was done visually since the number in each group was low.

Stepwise logistic regression was then used to determine whether a combination of different markers provide a better prediction of a chromosomally abnormal embryo.

Results

Of 1919 women undergoing a CVS (1:35), 54 had a sampling with an abnormal karyotype. Only 10 out of these 54 had a trisomy 21 or a mosaicism trisomy 21. In contrast there was an over-representation of trisomy 18 with six cases. Other

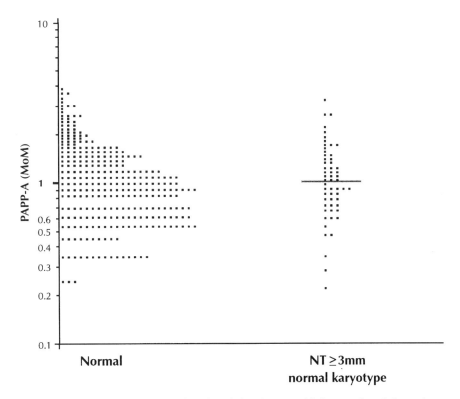

Fig. 20.1. Distribution of the MoMs for PAPP-A in 59 cases with increased nuchal translucency (≥3 mm) and normal karyotype and 446 contemporaneous controls.

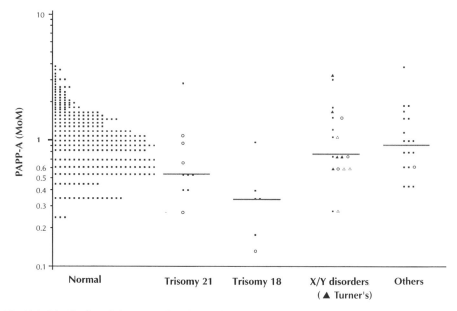

Fig. 20.2. Distribution of the MoMs for PAPP-A in 54 cases with chromosomal abnormalities and 446 contemporaneous controls. The open circles/triangles symbolise cases with an increased nuchal translucency thickness ≥3 mm.

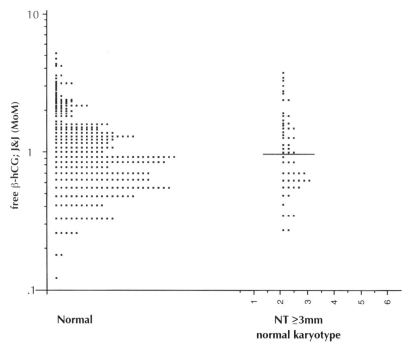

Fig. 20.3. Distribution of the MoMs for free β-hCG in 59 cases with increased nuchal translucency (≥3 mm) and normal karyotype and 446 contemporaneous controls.

chromosomal abnormalities included eight cases with Turner's syndrome, nine with other sex chromosome anomalies, one with trisomy 13 and 20 with other defects.

Of the 72 embryos (3.8%) which had an increased NT, 13 had an abnormal and 59 a normal karyotype. A NT was predominantly present in cases with trisomy 21, trisomy 18, or sex chromosome anomalies but was found only once in other chromosomal abnormalities. A total of 59 additional embryos had an increased nuchal translucency but a normal karyotype. The relative risk for an aneuploidy was 1:5 if an increased NT was present.

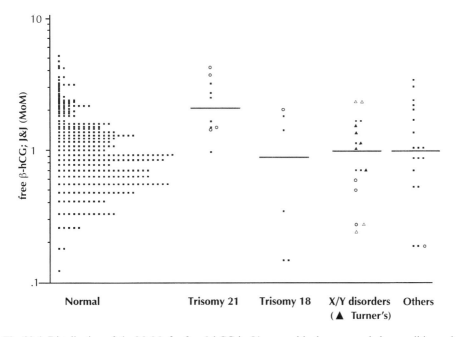

Fig. 20.4. Distribution of the MoMs for free β-hCG in 54 cases with chromosomal abnormalities and 446 contemporaneous controls. The open circles/triangles symbolise cases with an increased nuchal translucency thickness ≥3 mm.

Table 20.1. Mean MoM values for the groups with isolated increased nuchal translucency thickness, trisomy 21, trisomy 18, Turner's syndrome, other X/Y anomalies and other chromosomal abnormalities

MoM	PAPP-A	Free β-hCG	n
Nuchal translucency	1.03	0.96	59
Trisomy 21	0.57	2.07	10
Trisomy 18	0.35	0.90	6
Turner's syndrome	0.76	1.20	8
X/Y disorders	1.10	0.74	9
Others	0.92	1.00	21

Figs. 20.1 and 20.2 give the distribution of MoMs for the control cases and for the cases with increased nuchal translucency but normal karyotype for the parameters PAPP-A and free β-hCG. There was no statistically significant difference seen between the two groups. Figs 20.3 and 20.4 demonstrate the MoM values of the control group compared with the fetuses with trisomy 21, trisomy 18, X/Y-disorders and the cases with other chromosomal abnormalities. The medians for the different groups are listed in Table 20.1.

Logistic regression showed that detection rate for any chromosomal abnormality can be improved if a combination of an increased nuchal translucency in combination with PAPP-A and free β-hCG was used ($p=0.01$).

Discussion

The present study expands the information available on the combination of maternal serum markers and ultrasound as screening tools for Down syndrome in the first trimester in a high risk population.

In this study the most powerful tool, an increased nuchal translucency, was only seen in trisomies and X/Y-disorders but did not contribute to the detection of other chromosomal abnormalities. With a detection rate of 13 out of 54 (24%) the effectiveness of an NT was much lower than reported by others (Nicolaides *et al.* 1994; Szabo *et al.* 1995) but in accord with Brambati *et al.* (1995). The distribution of the present cases with aneuploidy included only 10 pregnancies with trisomy 21, indicating the likely presence of a negative cluster of this disorder. This could in part explain the low overall detection rate. In addition the number of aneuploidies is too small to allow calculation of precise detection rates.

Nevertheless with a positive predictive value of 1 out of 5, an increased nuchal translucency thickness was the single best parameter in this study.

PAPP-A, the single best *biochemical* parameter in first trimester reported to date, shows MoM values in Down fetuses ranging between 0.23 and 0.44 MoM in 63 cases (Chard and Grudzinskas 1991; Wald *et al.* 1992; Brambati *et al.* 1993; Hurley *et al.* 1993; Macintosh *et al.* 1993; Muller *et al.* 1993). These findings could be confirmed in our studies with a calculated median in the Down group of 0.53. In addition PAPP-A was a good parameter to detect cases with trisomy 18 with a MoM of 0.35 with single values ranging from 0.11 to 0.99. In trisomy 21 and 18 PAPP-A levels were low, regardless of whether an increased nuchal translucency was present or not, suggesting PAPP-A to be an independent marker. This is further supported by the observation that the 59 fetuses with an increased nuchal translucency but normal karyotype showed normal levels of PAPP-A. These results are in concordance with the findings of Brizot *et al.* (1994).

Serum free β-hCG MoMs are reported to be elevated in trisomy 21 pregnancies (Spencer *et al.* 1992; Aitken *et al.* 1993; Macintosh *et al.* 1993; Macri *et al.* 1993). The median ranged from 1.85 (Spencer *et al.* 1992) to 2.2 (Macri *et al.* 1993) in a total of 90 cases. Our study with a median of 2.07 confirmed these previous findings for free β-hCG to have good discriminative power. In the cases with trisomy 18 the median did not differ from controls which is in contrast to the data of Spencer who reported a MoM of 0.17 in five cases (Spencer *et al.* 1992). Free β-hCG was not useful in the detection of chromosomal anomalies other than trisomies. Again, in cases with an isolated NT the free β-hCG levels did not differ from controls which confirms results by Brizot *et al.* (1995). Fetuses with Down syndrome and an increased NT did group on both side of the median suggesting no correlation between these to markers.

A logistic regression model, which allows combination of continuous values (MoMs) with dichotomous parameters (increased NT 'yes–no'), showed that the detection rate for any chromosomal abnormality can be significantly improved using a combination of an increased nuchal translucency thickness together with PAPP-A and free β-hCG. Since free β-hCG is high in trisomy 21 and low (or unchanged as in our study) in trisomy 18, risk evaluation should be done separately for these disorders if this parameter is included.

We conclude that the combination of ultrasound and biochemical markers is able to detect a substantial proportion of aneuploidies especially trisomies and X/Y-disorders but will miss most other chromosomal anomalies. Nevertheless this could allow a first trimester multiparameter approach similar to the one already established in second trimester. However, it remains uncertain whether these parameters will identify the abnormal cases which will continue to term or spontaneously miscarry. The report of Pandya *et al.* (1995) on six DS fetuses with increased NT all resulting in live births, however, is encouraging in this respect.

An increased nuchal translucency itself does not seem to be associated with altered levels of the biochemical parameters.

Acknowledgement. This work was partly supported by a grant from Johnson and Johnson Clinical Diagnostics, Cardiff, Wales.

References

Aitken, D.A., McCaw, G., Crossley, J.A. *et al.* (1993) First-trimester biochemical screening for fetal chromosome abnormalities and neural tube defects. *Prenat Diagn* **13**, 681–9

Brambati, B., Macintosh, M.C.M., Teisner, B. *et al.* (1993) Low maternal serum levels of pregnancy associated plasma protein A (PAPP-A) in the first trimester in association with abnormal fetal karyotype. *Br J Obstet Gynaecol* **100**, 324–6

Brambati, B., Tului, L., Bonacchi, I. *et al.* (1994a) Serum PAPP-A and free β-hCG are first-trimester screening markers for Down syndrome. *Prenat Diagn* **14**, 1043–7

Brambati, B., Tului, L., Bonacchi, I. *et al.* (1994b) 'Biochemical screening for Down's syndrome in the first trimester' in J. G. Grudzinskas, T. Chard, M. Chapman and H. Cuckle (Eds) *Screening for Down's Syndrome*, pp.285–94. Cambridge: Cambridge University Press

Brambati, B., Cislaghi, C., Tului, L. *et al.* (1995) First-trimester Down's syndrome screening using nuchal translucency: a prospective study in patients undergoing chorionic villus sampling. *Ultrasound Obstet Gynecol* **5**, 9–14

Brizot, M.L., Snijders, R.J., Bersinger, N.A., Kuhn, P. and Nicolaides, K.H. (1994) Maternal serum pregnancy-associated plasma protein A and fetal nuchal translucency thickness for the prediction of fetal trisomies in early pregnancy. *Obstet Gynecol* **84**, 918–22

Brizot, M.L., Snijders, R.J., Butler, J., Bersinger, N.A. and Nicolaides, K.H. (1995) Maternal serum hCG and fetal nuchal translucency thickness for the prediction of fetal trisomies in the first trimester of pregnancy. *Br J Obstet Gynaecol* **102**, 127–32

Chard, T. and Grudzinskas, J.G. (1991) 'The endocrinology of the fetoplacental unit in the second trimester of pregnancy' in M. Chapman, J.G. Grudzinskas and T. Chard (Eds) *The Embryo: Normal and Abnormal Development and Growth*, pp.181–94. London: Springer Verlag

Hurley, P.A., Ward, R.H.T., Teisner, B. *et al.* (1993) Serum PAPP-A measurements in first-trimester screening for Down syndrome. *Prenat Diagn* **13**, 903–8

Macintosh, M.C.M., Brambati, B., Chard, T. and Grudzinskas, J.G. (1993) First-trimester maternal serum Schwangerschaftsprotein 1 in pregnancies associated with chromosomal anomalies. *Prenat Diagn* **13**, 563–8

Macri, J.N., Spencer, K., Aitken, D. *et al.* (1993) First-trimester free beta (hCG) screening for Down syndrome. *Prenat Diagn* **13**, 557–62

Muller, F., Cuckle, H., Teisner, B. and Grudzinskas, J.G. (1993) Serum PAPP-A levels are depressed in women with fetal Down syndrome in early pregnancy. *Prenat Diagn* **13**, 633–6

Nicolaides, K.H., Azar, G., Byrne, D., Mansur, C. and Marks, K. (1992) Fetal nuchal translucency: ultrasound screening for chromosomal defects in first trimester of pregnancy. *BMJ* **304**, 867–9

Nicolaides, K.H., Brizot, M.L. and Snijders, R.J. (1994) Fetal nuchal translucency: ultrasound screening for fetal trisomy in the first trimester of pregnancy. *Br J Obstet Gynaecol* **101**, 782–6

Pandya, P.P., Kondylios, A., Hilbert, L., Snijders, R.J. and Nicolaides, K.H. (1995) Chromosomal defects and outcome in 1015 fetuses with increased nuchal translucency. *Ultrasound Obstet Gynecol* **5**, 15–19

Savoldelli, G., Binkert, F., Achermann, J. and Schmid, W. (1993) Ultrasound screening for chromosomal anomalies in the 1st trimester of pregnancy. *Prenat Diagn* **13**, 513–18

Spencer, K., Macri, J.N., Aitken, D.A. and Connor, J.M. (1992) Free beta-hCG as first-trimester marker for fetal trisomy. *Lancet* **339**, 1480

Szabò, J. and Gellén, J. (1990) Nuchal fluid accumulation in trisomy-21 detected by vaginosonography in first trimester. *Lancet* **336**, 1133

Szabò, J., Gellén, J. and Szemere, G. (1992) First trimester aneuploid fetuses. Screening by vaginosonography. *Prenat Diagn* **12**, 153s

Szabò, J., Gellén, J. and Szemere, G. (1995) First-trimester ultrasound screening for fetal aneuploidies in women over 35 and under 35 years of age. *Ultrasound Obstet Gynecol* **5**, 161–3

Wald, N., Stone, R., Cuckle, H. S. *et al.* (1992) First trimester concentrations of pregnancy associated plasma protein A and placental protein 14 in Down's syndrome. *BMJ* **305**, 28

Zimmermann, R., Keller, P. J. and Huch, A. (1994) Increased maternal serum free β-human chorionic gonadotrophin concentrations in Down's pregnancies: an artefactual finding? *Br J Obstet Gynaecol* **101**, 257–8

Chapter 21

Screening for Down syndrome with serum and ultrasound markers

Françoise Muller

Introduction

Trisomy 21 screening is based on serial techniques, including first-trimester ultrasonography, second-trimester maternal serum screening and second- and third-trimester ultrasonography. Based on our experience of maternal serum screening in 76 442 pregnancies and 239 trisomy 21 cases, we will examine the relative contribution of these screening techniques to detection of Down syndrome.

Patients and methods

Between 1989 and 1993, first-trimester ultrasound was only performed before 10 weeks in order to date the pregnancy and therefore did not contribute to Down syndrome screening. Detection of trisomy 21 was based on maternal serum screening at 15–17 weeks and on second- and third-trimester ultrasonography.

In 1994, first-trimester ultrasonography at 10–14 weeks was added to the screening programme. However, only 44% of the 29 635 patients included in the study during this period underwent ultrasonography at 10–14 weeks.

Patients were referred to our laboratory by 136 obstetric centres including 16 teaching hospitals, 27 public hospitals, 12 private clinics and 81 private practices. Fifteen centres contributed 50% of the study population.

A questionnaire was completed by the obstetrician in charge of the patient when a maternal blood sample was collected. For each case, gestational age at first-trimester ultrasound was recorded. When known, nuchal appearance was classified as normal or abnormal by the referring obstetrician. No guidelines were provided for sonographers concerning the technique of nuchal measurement, but there was a consensus to consider measurements >3 mm at 10–14 weeks as abnormal. When the nuchal measurement was above 3 mm, patients were offered amniocentesis and were not included in the hCG screening programme.

In France, amniocentesis is offered to patients aged 38 years and over and is free of charge. These patients can request maternal serum screening before amniocentesis. For patients under 38 years, maternal serum screening and consecutive amniocentesis are not free of charge.

Maternal serum screening was based on hCG measurement and on risk calculation as previously described by Muller *et al.* (1993). Our cut-off risk for amniocentesis was 1/100.

Second-trimester ultrasound screening was performed at 20–24 weeks in all pregnancies. When the patient was screened in a high-risk group for trisomy 21 by maternal serum markers, ultrasonography was performed at the time of amniocentesis.

Third-trimester ultrasonography was performed in all continuing pregnancies at 30–33 weeks.

Each pregnancy was followed to delivery, thereby allowing calculation of the overall prevalence of Down syndrome in the study population.

In French law, termination of pregnancy is not limited by gestational age.

Results

The overall incidence of trisomy 21 was 239 out of 76 442. In three cases the trisomy 21 resulted from translocation (translocation and duplication in one case [45, XX,-21t(5; 21; 21) (p15; q11; q11)]. In five cases of trisomy 21 mosaicism was present (mosaicism 45X in one case). All other 281 trisomy 21 cases were free of mosaicism and of translocation.

Maternal age for the 239 trisomy 21 cases was over 38 years in 57 cases (24%), 35–37 in 84 cases, and under 35 in 98 cases (41%).

First-trimester ultrasound screening was performed before 10 weeks for pregnancy dating in most cases. First-trimester ultrasonography at 10–14 weeks for nuchal translucency measurement was introduced in 1994 and concerned only

Table 21.1. Ultrasound signs observed in 48 trisomy 21 cases with abnormal maternal serum screening

Nuchal aspect (isolated)	14
Nuchal aspect + other signs	9
Atrioventricular canal/atrial septal defect	6
Short femur	5
Renal pyelectasia	4
Amniotic fluid volume	3
Facial and extremities anomalies	3
Ventriculomegaly	2
Hydrops	2

13 141 (44%) of the 29 635 patients of this period. A total of 22 cases of trisomy 21 were observed in the group of patients who underwent first-trimester nuchal translucency analysis. None of these 22 cases had abnormal nuchal translucency. The expected prevalence of Down syndrome at birth calculated from maternal age-related risk (Hecht and Hook 1994) was 16/13,141. This value is not significantly different from the observed values of 22 cases. The probability that first-trimester ultrasonography would have picked up more than 25% of Down syndrome cases can be estimated to be lower than 1% based on a Poisson law distribution of trisomy 21 cases (mean 2.5), assuming that (1) all abnormal nuchal translucency cases would have been karyotyped and therefore excluded from our study, (2) nuchal translucency has a 5% false-positive rate and (3) the prevalence of trisomy 21 is 1/600.

Maternal serum hCG screening detected 179/239 cases of trisomy 21 (75%) and 60/98 (61%) for patients under 35 years of age. For patients included in the group at risk for trisomy 21, amniocentesis was proposed and ultrasonography was performed at the time of sampling. For other patients, second-trimester ultrasound screening was performed at 20–24 weeks.

Two miscarriages occurred at 20 weeks before second-trimester ultrasonography (karyotyping performed *post abortum* on fetal tissue).

Of the 179 trisomy 21 cases with abnormal maternal hCG screening, second-trimester ultrasound screening was normal in 131 trisomy 21 cases (73%) and abnormal in 48 (27%). The ultrasound signs are presented in Table 21.1. Abnormal nuchal appearance was seen in 48% of cases.

Of the 60 trisomy 21 cases with normal maternal hCG screening, second-trimester ultrasound screening was normal in 39 (65%). The anomalies observed by ultrasonography in 21 trisomy 21 cases are presented in Table 21.2. Abnormal nuchal appearance was seen in 29% of cases. Two cases of heart malformations were observed at 33 weeks.

At second-trimester ultrasonography, two signs (nuchal appearance and heart malformations) represented 41/69 (59%) of signs allowing the detection of trisomy 21. No differences were observed between trisomy 21 with normal and with abnormal maternal hCG.

Based on a series of 76 441 patients, we observed that 171 of 239 trisomy 21 cases were terminated before 20 weeks due to abnormal maternal serum screening, 17 were terminated at 22–25 weeks due to abnormal second trimester ultrasound

Table 21.2. Ultrasound signs observed in 21 trisomy 21 cases with normal maternal serum screening

Nuchal aspect (isolated)	5
Nuchal aspect + AVC	1
Atrioventricular canal/atrial septal defect	7
Short femur	1
Renal pyelectasia + facial anomalies	1
Hydramnios	1
IUGR	1
Ventriculomegaly	1
Unique umbilical artery	3

signs, and two at 33 weeks due to third-trimester ultrasound signs. Two deaths occurred *in utero* at 16 weeks. A total of 40 infants were born with trisomy 21, 32 of whom had given normal findings in maternal serum screening and second- and third-trimester ultrasonography. In six cases, amniocentesis was refused by the mother (one 36 years of age, and five over 40 years of age). In two cases, amniocentesis was not performed despite observation of abnormal ultrasound signs (hydramnios and cyst of the umbilical cord).

In summary, the combination of maternal hCG screening and second-trimester ultrasonography revealed 85% of trisomy 21 cases, 75% by maternal serum screening and 10% by ultrasonography. At present, in France, first-trimester ultrasound is not effective but is being developed.

References

Hecht, C.A. and Hook E.B. (1994) The imprecision in rates of Down syndrome by one-year maternal age intervals: a critical analysis of rates used in biochemical screening. *Prenat Diagn* **14**, 729–38

Muller, F., Aegerter, P. and Boue, A. (1993) Prospective maternal serum human chorionic gonadotropin screening for the risk of fetal chromosome anomalies and of subsequent fetal and neonatal deaths. *Prenat Diagn* **13**, 29–43

Chapter 22

Ultrasound in screening for Down syndrome in the first trimester

Discussion

Whittle: Professor Brambati has some data he would like to put to us as part of the discussion.

Brambati: Before presenting these new data, I have a question for Professor Nicolaides. When you teach the pupils to use the new methodology for measuring with the calipers, that is putting the marker on-to-on, you said. If you go back to your first paper in 1992, when you described the methodology you said you put the marker just 'in-to-in'. The image you reported – perhaps I am wrong – but in the picture reported in the paper it was clear that the marker was in-to-in and later on you did a report, some multiplication or comment.

I must ask you – because perhaps now you feel that you started to put the markers on-to-on, but it was not clearly reported. In case you started by 'in-to-in', have you done trials to demonstrate that on-to-on is better?

Nicolaides: No. On the first day I started measuring it, I put them on-to-on. In the very first paper I said that we measured the maximum black space. The maximum black space means on-to-on.

Brambati: If you use the grey scale – if you amplify your image, you can extend the grey scale by so much, and then on-to-on becomes in-to-in – it depends on the technique used. Anyway, we all followed your original instructions but it was a pity that it was not clear to us that the calipers should have been on-to-on. But when we set up our prospective study, we published observations on 2000 cases. Currently we have data on 500 new cases and we are continuing with this methodology. The team members are all the same. Perhaps we have spent too much time investigating and not following the exact methodology as you reported it, namely that the fetus should move, the cervical region should be clear, you should be able to distinguish the nuchal fold from the amniotic membrane, and so on, because we do this all the time and our results remain the same; we are unable to improve our detection rate due to some sort of unidentified bias, I think. We have honestly tried to be objective, but certainly we do sound biased.

There is another problem as all these patients, obviously, wish to terminate their pregnancy if we detect abnormalities. For a long time we tried to obtain control data from patients at the time of elective termination, using the trans-abdominal or transvaginal ultrasound. In some cases, for example, in the last stages as here with diploidy, more than ten days after the first ultrasound control, the situation was still the same. In this case, for example, what was 2 mm, became positive because it became 3 mm and so on. I just wish to emphasise the problem of the window of opportunity when the translucency is better evaluated in terms of efficiency. Perhaps we should delay our investigation until ten weeks. In several cases we did a nuchal translucency determination and translucency was not present. This was a problem because of the efficiency of the investigation.

We were also unable to find a high percentage of malformations which tested positive for nuchal translucency. I do not know whether our population is different – I think it may be, because I believe what you say. In more than 80 malformations, only four had a nuchal translucency of more than 3 mm. In our data, the rate of cardiac malformations is not as high in the population that has a nuchal translucency of less than 6 mm.

Finally, we did a trial by abdominal ultrasound, to find out how many cases could be detected. A successful nuchal translucency evaluation was obtained in 87% and in the other cases I used a transvaginal ultrasound. At about the time of our study, I evaluated our population in this trial in comparison with the data of Kornman from Holland in *Prenatal Diagnosis,* which reported that 58% of cases of nuchal translucency were successfully measured within ten minutes (Kornman *et al.* 1996).

It seems that they used a calculation of nuchal translucency from more than five minutes of observation. In our population, if you use five minutes of obser-vation, in 15% nuchal translucency would not be observed.

On reviewing the international experience, it may be that we shall have to learn the details of the techniques in your centre to understand exactly what is relevant to permit achieving the results your groups have been able to report.

Nicolaides: There was a study in 1993 in the *New England Journal of Medicine*, called the RADIUS Study, which showed exactly the same point (Ewigman *et al.* 1993). If people are not trained to the same standard, and they do not use the same terminology, then what they may demonstrate is that ultrasound is completely useless. It is for this reason, and because I recognise the variations in the measurements of nuchal translucency, and the skill necessary to achieve it, that I made an urgent plea to the Royal College of Obstetricians and Gynaecologists along the lines that sooner or later, whether we like it or not, first trimester ultrasound scanning will be introduced.

There is a very large number of publications demonstrating that if there is increased nuchal translucency, then there is a high risk of a chromosomal abnormality. Therefore, that will almost certainly become part of routine practice. In order to avoid a series of potential mistakes when this process, by default or by desire, is introduced, it is important to have a unification of standards. That has not happened, and that is the reason for the recommendation.

It is a reality that there are 20 hospitals doing this, and the hospital staff are ultrasonographers, they are being audited, and there are names and hospital numbers and addresses and their partners' addresses of 62,000 women that have been scanned. Those data are available for anybody to examine. The fact that there are different values reported by different centres goes further in re-iterating the need to have proper and regular audit.

Cuckle: There are two technical differences between studies. One is a straight-forward ultrasound technology, as Professor Nicolaides has described, having the fetus in the right position, and the size of the image and the position of the callipers. It is obviously difficult to compare studies without that.

There is another distinction, which is studies such as Professor Brambati has just presented and we have just heard from Switzerland, where they have used a straight 3mm cut-off. It seems that you just cannot compare those studies with the data that Professor Nicolaides has presented, where they have used a sliding cut-off according to gestational age or serum analytes and taken the maternal age into account. They are just not comparable.

I would like to ask Professor Nicolaides whether, apart from his own series, there are one or two others who are using that sliding cut-off method. Does Szabo use a straight cut-off?

Nicolaides: The problem with many aspects of ultrasound that I wanted to avoid is that, in 1996, after 20 years of ultrasound scanning, up and down the country, there is variation in the interpretation of results; in half of the hospitals, if you diagnose mild hydronephrosis or choroid plexus cysts, you tell the women that they have a one in 200 risk of having a chromosomal abnormality. They have an amniocentesis. And yet, if you were to make a survey tomorrow, and found out from different departments what they mean by pyelectasia – do they have a definition, do they have a gestation, do they have a measurement, do they have a policy? – there are no policies. They want to avoid them.

In the beginning of a series, when you have a small number of cases, you group them, as we learn to do in ultrasound, into normal and abnormal. The cut-off of 3 mm was something that unified the criteria. That was in a paper in 1992, but by 1993 it was already obvious, as the numbers became bigger, that there was a change in NT with gestation, and therefore all our publications refer to values above the 95th centile. That is the first point.

The second point is that from 1993 the data from nuchal translucency were combined with maternal age in calculating the risk.

Cuckle: I know it is in yours, because clearly yours is an enormous series and I am totally convinced by your data, but I was wondering about the rest of the literature. A sceptic would say that, even though there are 20 different hospitals involved in Professor Nicolaides' series, perhaps it does not work in the 21st hospital somewhere else, and they can prove it because there is a series from the 21st hospital. I just wanted to know whether in any of the other published papers outside of yours, has anyone else used a sliding cut-off in risk and so on?

Nicolaides: No, beyond the twenty centres in England, there are now 75 centres in 33 countries. In the audit, whose results I have not presented, in the first country that has 3500 cases which is Greece – because many of the doctors were research fellows of King's before they went back home – their results are exactly the same.

The second country is Brazil, because the second country we have research fellows from is Brazil, and they have found exactly the same in 2500 cases so far. Therefore, the difference is that, for me, it is the mere presence for a few days or a few hours in a centre that does things. Last year, when we had a meeting at this College, I asked and begged that a research fellow or Professor Brambati should come with me to talk about it. He did not – he left unfortunately, because his plane was leaving.

Macintosh: I think Professor Nicolaides' figures are very convincing, for your method in the 19 district general hospitals. We can have no further convincing on that point.

When comparing the studies evaluating nuchal translucency screening for detecting chromosomal abnormalities, that of Dr Zimmerman's group reported that DS accounted for 10 out of the 54 chromosomal abnormalities whereas the Harris Birthright group have reported that DS accounts for 50% of chromosomal abnormalities. This suggests a different population possibly due to gestation or other unaccounted factors.

Nicolaides: Which data are those?

Macintosh: I read it in one of your papers recently, but I also have it from Dr Snijder's thesis work. This was back in 1993, when 79 out of 162 chromosomal abnormalities were Down syndrome. I would like to look at what the differences in the studies are and, apart from cut-off, whether you make adjustments. I find it very interesting that you have ten out of 54, and that the huge series from the Harris Birthright – correct me if I am wrong, because you will have to look at it – has the proportion of DS as about half of all the abnormalities that have been picked up.

Nicolaides: The reason is obvious: in the livebirth data, DS is only one third of all chromosomal abnormalities. If you have a centre, in which, like yours, the results were from women who were undergoing amniocentesis for maternal age, the vast majority of chromosomal abnormalities would be the ones most commonly found in older women.

Macintosh: At what gestational age were your abnormalities from?

Zimmermann: We did CVS at 10–13 weeks, most at weeks 10 and 11.

Macintosh: My understanding is that there were 54 abnormalities, ten of which were DS at that stage.

Zimmermann: That is right. It is an under-representation, a sort of negative cluster of DS.

Cuckle: The most interesting piece of information from Professor Nicolaides is Dr Snijder's calculation of observed and expected births with Down syndrome. That is a convincing figure in itself at 78%. What is the false positive rate which goes with that? I believe the women in this series tend to be older.

Nicolaides: It is two groups – the Harris Birthright group and –

Cuckle: The 78%.

Nicolaides: It is 5%. In the district general hospitals (DGHs) it was 5%, and in the Harris Birthright Centre it was 16%.

Cuckle: With regard to the 78%, in that case, if it is 5%, there is a slight inconsistency in your data, because the model predicted figures are 80% and 5% based on *observed* DS. The observed DS rate, as Professor Wald pointed out earlier today, an 80% rate could be a 67% rate if half of them are going to die. He has already explained that. I would have expected the 78%, based on observed births – this is the calculation that Dr Snijders has done – would have a higher false positive, but it was only 5%.

Nicolaides: There are two groups of patients – the Harris Birthright patients, and the district general hospitals. The 5% is for the district general hospitals, and the Harris Birthright is 16%. With the Harris Birthright, 24% of the women were over the age of 37. The combined detection rate of trisomy 21s was 84% and in the DGHs it was 80%. With the combined results, because I need bigger numbers to allow me to make sequential calculations, the 84% drops to 78% – there is a decrease in the observed calculations where you take everybody as the denominator into the observed over expected at birth, by 6% from 84% to 78%. If we extrapolate from that, and you just have the result from the district general hospitals where there was a 5% false positive rate, then the 80% will at most decrease by those 6% as well.

Nørgaard-Pedersen: Do you have any plans for accreditation? You mentioned certification but one step further would be accreditation of all ultrasound scanning laboratories – as they do in clinical chemistry where they have accreditation and inspection and so on.

Nicolaides: In the United States, as a consequence of various studies, two things happened. The first is that various insurance companies started challenging the value, and therefore the need, for ultrasound. Those that were good at ultrasound started to realise that they needed to defend ultrasound, and the American College is now introducing measures to have certification.

In a process such as the nuchal translucency measurement, it is necessary that that process is a continuous round of audit – and, presumably, that is what you mean by accreditation. That is what we tried to establish with the spot checks of the measurements every few months.

Wald: Professor Nicolaides, I am still rather confused. If you go to district general hospitals outside King's College Hospital, is your current estimate that the observed detection rate was 80% for five, which would reduce to 74% if you allowed for selective fetal loss? Would that be about right?

Nicolaides: Something like that, yes.

Wald: Because one would have expected a somewhat bigger reduction from the selective fetal loss. That is Professor Cuckle's point – he has made the point I wanted to make. That is rather surprising.

There is another aspect of your data that suggests that you do have a higher prevalence. For example, your overall prevalence of DS in your population is 3.3 per thousand, which is over double the population rate and so you are clearly picking up on that double, which might fit with half of them being lost. But if half of them are going to be lost, then you should drop to a point estimate somewhat below 74. We are not talking about many percentage points, it is just that the estimate would take it down to about 67. The broad conclusion would be – and we do not quibble on that small percentage point – that you are getting about three quarters for five – perhaps 70–75, in fact I would have estimated slightly below three quarters. That is what you claim – is that right?

Nicolaides: That is what we found from a study of 62 000 patients in 20 hospitals.

Wald: You keep repeating these large numbers, and saying that it is found and it is proven. One has to try to find the best unbiased estimate. I would suspect that from your data it is something like 67% for five term births. Your adjustment with Dr Snijders gets it to more like 75% for five – a discrepancy of seven percentage points. Do you follow the argument on that?

Nicolaides: No, I do not. That is what we found.

Wald: But it is not actually what you found, because what you found – as you have just pointed out – would be counting the numbers you detected, the ones you missed at birth, and that is subject to bias because the denominators are not comparable.

Grudzinskas: Professor Tim Chard is the Clinical Director of Imaging Services at the Homerton Hospital, one of those district general hospitals doing nuchal translucency screening in the Nicolaides project. He is a well-known and eminent biochemist in his own right. It would be entirely appropriate for Profesor Chard, who has been extremely close to this subject, to report to us here today his conclusions on the basis of the 4000 observations he has spoken about. I would also ask if Dr Jauniaux has something to add in a confirmatory or cautionary sense with respect to the data we have heard on ultrasound today.

Chard: We have indeed recently submitted a paper from the Homerton containing approximately 4000 subjects. It is in the hands of the *British Journal of Obstetrics and Gynaecology* and it is almost certainly also in the hands of other people around this table at this time.
    We are one of those 20 sites working with Professor Nicolaides. It was injected into my backyard over my dead body, as most things generally are, as a dyed-in-the-wool biochemist. We had various problems which I do not think are universal, but undoubtedly are there, with the application of our own type of test in that area. Our findings in respect of the application of nuchal translucency have so far been spotless and would fully confirm everything Professor Nicolaides has said. If you said they are small numbers you would of course be right, but there is a great deal of ancillary evidence which goes with that, but unfortunately I do not have the data with me because I did not come here prepared to make that point. They are documented in a manner which means we would be happy to offer a pre-publication copy to anybody – of the enthusiasm of at least one of those units in

a position very similar to those which Professor Nicolaides described of the other 20 units, endorsing the use of nuchal translucency.

When one is talking about psychology, with anecdotes emerging or whatever, my colleagues and I at the Homerton – whether we are talking about the obstetricians or for that matter the imaging people – are highly convinced of this particular process. I could go on at greater length, but I would only be repeating myself and others.

Jauniaux: There is no doubt that efficiency comes with experience. When you compare the data from the Lindsay Allan team with those from the Hansmann team in terms of detecting cardiac malformation – which, as we know, in the second trimester is a strong marker for chromosomal abnormality – it is likely that the team with the long experience in detecting these malformations but no experience of using nuchal translucency ultrasound would fail, and vice versa. Perhaps a combination of all these markers and better experience would increase the accuracy of ultrasound and improve its sensitivity.

Whittle: It is an issue which perhaps we need to return to later. It is a question about whether we could envisage the first trimester scan replacing the second trimester scan. I have my own views about that. From a resource point of view, it is one of the arguments about which we need to exercise ourselves because scanning is time consuming and resources are at best limited. We have to generate a convincing argument to include both a first trimester nuchal translucency scan with a second trimester anomaly scan to the purchasers. That is the reality of the world in which we live.

My first question is whether Professor Nicolaides would feel, at any point, that a detailed first trimester scan could replace a second trimester scan as most departments in the country have at the moment.

Nicolaides: Yes, the objectives of the second trimester scan will change. I actually want to see three ultrasound scans in pregnancy. I would like to see a pregnancy test scan at seven weeks, and then an anomaly scan at 12–14 weeks, and then an obstetric assessment of the cervix and uterine Doppler scan at 23–24 weeks. These would have different objectives. The anomaly scan will historically move to 12–14 weeks.

Hicks: I would like to broaden the debate, and comment on a point Professor Nicolaides made earlier. A point was made about standards and people improving with experience. Professor Nicolaides said earlier that a number of DGHs had reasonably well-documented fetal losses associated with amniocentesis at 3–4%. He has also described the process of setting standards and professionally led audit resulting in high standards of ultrasound. What role might this group want to consider the profession has in ensuring those standards, not just in the teaching centres but across DGHs for all aspects of the process of screening for Down syndrome.

Nicolaides: On that same basis, Professor Wald and colleagues published a letter in *The Lancet* at the beginning of 1996 in which he said that we accept that there is such a thing as maternal serum biochemistry screening in this country. What is this maternal serum biochemical screening test? What processes has it been through in terms of proving its efficacy, safety and cost effectiveness? When did Professor Wald's, quadruple test which includes inhibin, go through the process of the development of a model, recruitment to a study with informed consent entry, provision of 1500 cases of DS that Mary Macintosh requires to prove that it is effective, and then become introduced into clinical practice?

Serum biochemistry has been a recent introduction. If we look at the rest of serum biochemistry, what does serum biochemistry really mean in England? What percentage of women have just AFP, AFP and hCG, AFP and free β-hCG – or all the various combinations? What is maternal serum biochemistry in the second trimester? And what actually are the results from different centres? In addition, each one of the centres in Britain has results from maternal serum biochemistry screening – have they published those results? Is there a mechanism for knowing? For example, do we know how effective maternal serum biochemistry screening has been in Birmingham or in Nottingham or in Manchester?

Wald: In certain regions there have been audits of it. In principle, wherever that has been done, it has been pretty much as expected. That is the case not only in this country, but around the world. There have been many demonstration projects and many audits. In North Thames, for example, there is an annual audit and all the cases are identified through registries, through the expected rates using the age distribution. By and large, it holds up.

Whittle: So that is a yes. Professor Cuckle?

Cuckle: In the discussion we are not recognising the controversy that is going on here. The controversy is that Professor Nicolaides has a large series and appears to have really good results. There is a feeling that it is only Professor Nicolaides who can do it, and everybody else who tries to do it fails. I do not think there is any evidence for that, given that there are 20 DGHs doing it.

I would like us as a group to be able to come to some kind of conclusion about that – perhaps not to say that everyone should do it tomorrow, but at least to be able to say that there is strong evidence that, with the right kind of education and quality control that Professor Nicolaides is offering, this can achieve the kinds of detection rates that we are seeing in biochemical screening in the second trimester. Even if the detection rate is as low as two thirds rather than three quarters, it is comparable, and that is all people want to know at the moment. Otherwise, if we do not make that kind of statement, people will interpret that as though we are saying that Professor Nicolaides' data are wrong, despite the tens of thousands of results that he has.

Whittle: Thank you very much. That concludes this session. I would like to thank the speakers. I have an uneasy feeling that we have some unfinished business here, and this is an area in which we need to make some careful recommendations about the role of ultrasound screening for Down syndrome and where it fits in with the serum screening.

References

Ewigman, B.G., Crane, J.P., Frigoletto, F.D. *et al.* (1993) Effect of prenatal ultrasound screening on perinatal outcome. *N Engl J Med* **329,** 821–7

Kornman, L.H., Morssink, L.P., Beekhuis, J.R., De Wolf, B.T.H.M., Heringa, M.P. and Mantingh, A. (1996) Nuchal translucency cannot be used as a screening test for chromosomal abnormalities in the first trimester of pregnancy in routine ultrasound practice. *Prenat Diagn* **16,** 797–805

Wald, N.J., Huttly, W., Wald, K. and Kennard, A. (1996) Down's syndrome screening in UK [letter]. *Lancet* **347,** 330

SECTION 6

FETAL CELLS: ALTERNATIVES TO
BIOCHEMICAL SCREENING?

Chapter 23

Detecting aneuploidy by analysis of fetal cells in maternal blood

Joe Leigh Simpson, Dorothy E. Lewis, Farideh Z. Bischoff and Sherman Elias

Introduction

Prenatal genetic diagnosis is clearly possible by analysis of fetal cells in maternal blood (Simpson and Elias 1994a). Fetal sex and Mendelian disorders have been determined from maternal blood by polymerase chain reaction (PCR), and diagnosis of fetal trisomies accomplished by fluorescent *in situ* hybridisation (FISH) with chromosome-specific probes. Attention is now directed toward the choice of specific cell type for enrichment, selection of optimal method(s) of fetal cell enrichment, and determination of sensitivity and specificity indicating aneuploids. We shall review all these issues, updating our previous reports on this topic (Elias and Simpson 1994; Elias *et al.* 1996a; Simpson and Elias 1993, 1994a,b, 1995).

Historical considerations

In 1969, Walknowska *et al.* reported unbanded XY metaphases in maternal blood of pregnant women carrying male fetuses. deGrouchy and Trubuchet (1971) soon detected XY metaphases as well, as did others (Schindler *et al.* 1972; Takahara *et al.* 1972; Whang-Peng *et al.* 1973). However, not all individuals carrying male fetuses showed XY metaphases, and XY metaphases were present in some women carrying female fetuses. Consensus gradually arose that the XY metaphases observed in these studies might have represented cytogenetic misinterpretations.

A different methodology was applied a decade later by Herzenberg and colleagues, who utilised flow cytometry to enrich for fetal cells present in maternal blood (Herzenberg *et al.* 1979; Iverson *et al.* 1981). The strategy was to study HLA-A2-negative women who became pregnant by an HLA-A2-positive male; A2-positive cells recovered from maternal blood should have been fetal in origin because HLA-A2 positive cells in maternal blood could have been present only on fetal cells containing that allele inherited from the father. Y-chromatin was detected in pregnancies in which the fetus was male. Work of the Herzenberg group was widely accepted, but proved difficult to replicate.

Existence of fetal cells in maternal blood was definitively confirmed for the broader scientific community in the late 1980s, using molecular techniques that had only recently become available. Lo *et al.* (1989, 1990) used nested primer PCR to amplify for Y sequences, which usually proved present in maternal blood of women carrying male fetuses. These initial PCR-based studies were performed on unsorted nucleated cells; we and others confirmed these results after various separation schemes (Bianchi *et al.* 1990; Mueller *et al.* 1990; Wachtel *et al.* 1991; Kao *et al.* 1992).

Frequency of fetal cells in maternal blood

In maternal blood there are relatively few nucleated fetal cells compared to nucleated maternal cells. Using an avidin–biotin-based immunoaffinity system, Hall and Williams (1992) estimated that the ratio of fetal nucleated cells to maternal nucleated cells was $1:4.75\times10^6$ to 1.6×10^7. Performing FISH with chromosome-specific probes on unsorted maternal blood and using a DNA probe specific for the repetitive Y DNA sequence DYZI, Hamada *et al.* (1993) estimated the frequencies in the three trimesters to be 0.27, 3.52 and 8.56×10^{-5}, respectively. Wachtel *et al.* (1996) estimate the frequency of fetal cells to be even higher. Using a charge-flow separation system, 2000 fetal nucleated red blood cells were reported recoverable per 20 ml of maternal blood sample. In our experience 0–20 fetal cells can be recovered from a 20 ml blood sample in euploid fetuses. Even acknowledging fetal cells are lost in processing, our estimate and that of most other workers is closer to $1:1\times10^7$ or $1:1\times10^8$ (Price *et al.* 1991).

Irrespective of exact frequency, fetal cells in unsorted samples are so rare that detecting fetal aneuploidy is likely to require enrichment. To accomplish this, one must utilise density gradients or charge flow separation techniques, followed by flow cytometry or magnetic activated cell sorting (MACS). Flow cytometry has proved most useful in our hands, but this technology is more expensive than MACS. Using 'quantitative' PCR and a model system utilising fetal liver cells, Bianchi (1994; Bianchi *et al.* 1996a) concluded that the best enrichment was obtained with fluorescence-activated cell sorting (FACS). Aneuploid cells could be more frequent in maternal blood than euploid cells, presumably reflecting increased leakage or faulty placentation. Indeed, both our group Simpson and Elias (1993) and others Ganshirt-Ahlert *et al.* (1993) found trisomic fetal cells more often than XY cells. Naturally, this would be salutary for prenatal cytogenetic diagnosis.

Persistence of fetal cells after pregnancy

A potential concern is that fetal cells from a prior pregnancy could persist in the maternal circulation and, hence, interfere with diagnosis. Aneuploid cells persisting after a chromosomally abnormal live born offspring or a chromosomally abnormal spontaneous abortion could be especially troublesome.

Hsieh *et al.* (1993) followed 28 women delivered of a male fetus. One week post partum, 26 of the 28 women delivered of males still showed ZFY and SRY sequences in their blood. By four months, 11 of the 28 showed Y-specific sequences; by eight months, two of 23 showed Y-sequences. Our group similarly found prior male pregnancies not to present diagnostic difficulties. No Y-positive cells were observed in eight women delivered of male babies months to years earlier (Elias *et al.* 1996b).

Bianchi *et al.* (1996b) helped clarify the confusion by showing that fetal cells persisting from prior pregnancies could be selected by $CD34^+$ $CD38^+$, a selection criteria different from that used to isolate fetal erythroblasts for diagnostic purposes. Thus, status of prior pregnancies should not interfere with diagnostic accuracy.

Candidate fetal cell types

Diagnosis of fetal sex and Mendelian disorders is possible solely through PCR-based technologies. Fetal cells are present early in pregnancy and consistently detected (Thomas *et al.* 1994). However, detection of fetal chromosomal abnormalities requires enrichment since the search for the rare fetal cells would be tedious and labour intensive by FISH analysis. Prior to addressing the feasibility of achieving prenatal cytogenetic diagnosis, one must consider the various fetal cell types present and the potential methods of this enrichment.

Nucleated fetal red cells (erythroblasts)

The nucleated red cell (erythroblast) is currently receiving the greatest attention as the most promising fetal cell. Attractiveness is based on these cells comprising about 10% of red cells in the 11-week fetus and about 0.5% in the 19-week fetus. Moreover, nucleated red blood cells are rare in peripheral adult blood and are believed to persist no longer than perhaps five days in the adult; thus, fetal cells of this type would not be expected to persist from previous pregnancies (see previous section).

Bianchi *et al.* (1990) were the first to focus on these cells, initially flow-sorting on the basis of transferrin receptor (CD71) positivity. Sorted cells were subjected to PCR for Y sequences. Of eight samples showing a Y sequence, six were derived from pregnancies in which women were carrying male fetuses. Initially failing to confirm this work, we were later successful when sorting not only for CD71 but also for cell size, cell granularity, and glycophorin-A positivity (Wachtel *et al.* 1991; Price *et al.* 1991; Simpson and Elias 1993; Elias and Simpson 1994).

Our search still continues for the optimal selection system. Initially we were pleased with results of positive selection for gylcophorin-A, a major sialoglyco-protein of the erythroid cell membrane (MN blood group). This sialoglycoprotein arises later in the erythroid lineage than CD71, and thus should less likely be present on monocytes and lymphocytes. Using nested PCR primers for a Y sequence, we correctly identified male fetuses in 12 of 12 flow-sorted samples and female fetuses in five of six samples (Wachtel *et al.* 1991). However, in subsequent studies we began to observe clumping with the glycophorin-A antibodies, and have now abandoned this method (Lewis *et al.* 1996). Enrichment strategies have also combined negative selection followed by sorting for CD71 positive cells. For example, removal of lymphocytes on the basis of CD45 expression has been employed. Our recent experience of assessing positive and negative selection criteria is described in detail by Lewis *et al.* (1996).

Trophoblasts

Trophoblasts are attractive candidate cells, given their intimate relationship with the uterus. Syncytiotrophoblasts and cytotrophoblasts are present in relatively high numbers in the maternal circulation early in pregnancy. These cells could represent those being detected early in pregnancy by PCR-based technology (Thomas *et al.* 1994). However, trophoblasts are thought to become sequestered in the lung (Benirschke 1994). This would be consistent with data showing that trophoblasts can be recovered readily from the inferior vena cava and uterine veins of eclamptic women, but fail to be present in peripheral blood (Douglas *et al.* 1959; Holzgreve *et al.* 1992).

A major difficulty encountered in enriching for trophoblasts is lack of monoclonal antibodies specific for placental antigens. Many prospective anti-bodies have been generated but few have proved useful (Covone *et al.* 1984, 1988). Mueller *et al.* (1990) generated 6000 monoclonal antibodies from placental tissue; five were believed specific for fetal tissue. After exposing maternal blood from pregnant women to two of the five monoclonal antibodies, the mixture (including presumptively isolated fetal cells) was subjected to PCR to detect the presence or absence of Y-DNA sequences. Fetal sex was correctly predicted in seven of seven males and in six of seven females. Hawes *et al.* (1994) later applied immuno-histochemical techniques specific for these placental monoclonal antibodies to identify trophoblast fragments in maternal peripheral blood. Further evidence that trophoblasts were indeed being isolated from maternal blood by these antibodies came from molecular analysis of a pregnancy at risk for β-thalassaemia. After enrichment with a 'cocktail' containing three different mono-clonal autobodies, PCR detected a paternally-transmitted haemoglobinopathy. Recently, this same group has discovered that one of their most placental antibodies was in fact directed against human placental lactogen (hPL) (Latham *et al.* 1996).

Sbracia *et al.* (1994) used another approach to recover trophoblasts, enriching through antibodies against HLA-G. Fetal nucleated cells in maternal blood were separated using Ficoll–HistoPaque density gradient, labelled with anti HLA-G monoclonal antibody conjugated to fluorescein isothiocyanate (FITC), sorted by flow cytometry, and collected directly into Eppendorf tubes containing Ham's media. Standard cytogenetic culture techniques were then used. In cultured blood obtained from women with a male fetus, 46,XY cells were recovered in six of ten cases. The ability of Sbracia *et al.* (1994) to obtain a fetal karyotype contrasts markedly with our own failure to obtain fetal metaphases from flow-sorted cells (Tharapel *et al.* 1989, 1993).

A final approach is that of Durrant *et al.* (1994, 1996). Their approach is based on enrichment for cells displaying anti-tumour antibodies.

Pivotal to detecting cytogenetic abnormalities in fetal trophoblasts is the ability to recover mononucleated trophoblasts. Recovering only multinucleated or anucleated cells would make diagnosis by FISH with chromosome-specific probes difficult or impossible, respectively.

One final note concerns the very large number of alleged fetal cells reported recoverable by the charge-flow separation of Wachtel *et al.* (1996). If 2000 fetal cells are indeed present in a 20 ml blood sample as these investigators claim, almost the only plausible cell type would seem to be trophoblasts. Otherwise, the volume of fetal cells in maternal blood could greatly exceed total fetal blood volume. The potential ability to culture such cells using conventional cytogenetic methods devised for lymphocytes would further be a surprise, but consistent with the report of Sbracia *et al.* (1994).

Lymphocytes

Herzenberg and colleagues (1979; Iverson *et al.* 1981) were generally considered to have been sorting for fetal lymphocytes. As noted, this group flow sorted for HLA-A2 positive cells in HLA-A2 negative women whose husbands were A-2 positive. Among 12 pregnancies with male infants, five showed Y-chromatin cells (range 0.3% to 1.6% sorted cells); in seven other women delivered of infants whose lymphocytes failed to react with HLA-A2 antiserum no Y-chromatin cells were found.

Our group was unsuccessful with this technique, at least as assessed by the end point of fetal karyotypes (Tharapel *et al.* 1989, 1993). However, Sargent *et al.* (1994) replicated the work of Herzenberg *et al.* (1979), in at least one case, using Y-specific DNA sequences to determine fetal cells. Obtaining maternal blood at 28 and 32 weeks' gestation and extracting DNA extracted without sorting, paternal HLA-DR sequences were detected (Yeoh *et al.* 1991; Sargent *et al.* 1994).

Even if fetal lymphocytes are present in maternal blood, these cells remain poor candidate cells for enrichment. Specific paternal alleles must be sought in any given family. Any fetal cells persisting from previous pregnancies are also relatively more likely to be lymphocytes.

Granulocytes

Using Ficoll–Paque density gradient centrifugation followed by FISH for a Y-specific DNA probe, Wessman *et al.* (1992) claimed recovery of granulocytes. Y-specific cells were recovered from eight women, seven of whom gave birth to male infants. The sole discrepancy was said to have involved lymphocyte-like cells; thus, the authors claimed total accuracy 'in each case where granulocytes with a Y-specific signal were detected'.

It is also possible that granulocytes are being recovered by some of the protocols we and others are utilising.

Detecting fetal chromosome abnormalities

Sensitivity

Fetal trisomy has now been detected by several groups, principally after enrichment for erythroblasts. We continue to analyse for this cell type. Using glycophorin-A and CD71, we were the first to detect fetal aneuploidy from analysis of maternal blood, initially detecting trisomy 18 (Price *et al.* 1991) and later trisomy 21 (Elias *et al.* 1992). Other groups soon detected trisomies as well (Bianchi and Klinger 1993;Ganshirt-Ahlert *et al.* 1993). Wachtel *et al.* (1996) reported FISH detection of fetal trisomy 18 and trisomy 21 after maternal blood was subjected to their charge flow separation technique.

The sensitivity of detecting fetal trisomic cells is yet to be determined, but we estimate 50–75% as judged by finding a cell or cells with three signals for a chromosome-specific probe (fetal trisomy). Pivotal to this estimate is that in our laboratories cells with three signals are almost never observed in euploid pregnancies. We suspect that fetal trisomic cells may be detectable more readily from maternal blood samples obtained in the late first trimester or at least before 14–15 weeks. We further suspect sensitivity is lower at 16–20 weeks than earlier in pregnancy.

Post-enrichment identification of fetal cells

Even after enrichment fetal cells are vastly outnumbered by maternal cells. Thus, we score up to 3000 cells to analyse the 1–15 fetal cells present. An independent marker to identify fetal cells prior to such laborious analysis would be useful. This would not only greatly decrease microscopy time, but allow fetal XX and maternal XX cells to be distinguished.

Three general approaches seem feasible. First, one could stain enriched cells for fetal haemoglobin (the gene product of γ-globin), identifying the few fetal haemoglobin F-positive cells from among the more common maternal cells. This approach was first used by Zheng *et al.* (1993) and Ferguson-Smith *et al.* (1994), and confirmed by our group (Park *et al.* 1994).

Second, isolation of single cells by micromanipulation is possible. Takabayashi *et al.* (1994) stained with Pappenheim stain to identify unsorted nucleated red blood cells in maternal blood. Cells were then removed with a laser micromanipulator, and subjected to PCR for Y DNA sequences. Nucleated fetal red cells were found in 33 of 60 women between 8 and 23 weeks; 33 of the 39 (85%) showed fetal cells. PCR for Y sequences was performed in 11 cases. No signal was shown in the five pregnancies with female fetuses; however, five of six with male fetuses showed a signal.

Third, Bischoff *et al.* (1995) developed an *in situ* method to detect fetal cells transcribing γ-globin mRNA. An oligonucleotide antisense primer specific to γ-globin cDNA was designed, and added to a mixture containing Taq polymerase, unlabelled dNTPs and dUTP directly labelled with rhodamine. One step annealing and extension occurs, those (fetal) cells abundantly producing HbF showing red fluorescence as a result of labelled dUTP–rhodamine incorporation. β-globin can serve as a marker to indicate adult erythroblasts, whereas γ-globin can serve as a marker for fetal erythroblasts. Although a few adult cells produce HbF (0–1.0%), these cells also produces HbA and, hence, can be identified concurrently through staining prior to sorting with a β-globin–FITC-labelled antibody (greenish fluorescence). FISH analysis with chromosome-specific probes is then performed only on the cells showing red fluorescence. In subsequent work, Bischoff *et al.* (1996a) developed a post-enrichment strategy based on differential expression of beta globin (β-globin) and gamma globin (γ-globin) mRNA. After early embryogenesis, haemoglobin F (HbF, $\alpha_2\gamma_2$) constitutes 90–100% of the total haemoglobin in the fetus. By birth, adult haemoglobin (HbA, $\alpha_2\beta_2$) predominates.

Eight cases studied between 11 and 18 weeks' gestation yielded results consistent with predictions. In three of five male pregnancies, 0.34% of cells (range 1–3 cells/per 30 ml maternal blood sample) showed a signal for a Y-specific DNA probe: none of these cells expressed β-globin but all showed γ-globin mRNA. In the remaining two male pregnancies, no cells were positive (red fluorescence) for γ-globin mRNA and, consistently, none showed a signal for the Y-probe. Presumably no fetal cells were recovered in these two samples. In the three female pregnancies, 0.42% of cells were positive for γ-globin mRNA, a frequency similar to that observed in the first three male pregnancies described above.

US NICHD clinical evaluation

A formal evaluation to determine the sensitivity and specificity of detecting fetal chromosomal abnormalities is underway in the United States. The NICHD has funded several collaborating centres: Baylor College of Medicine/University of Tennessee, Memphis; Jefferson Medical College; Tufts University/New England Medical Center and Wayne State University/University of Basel.

Socioeconomic and demographic information are being gathered on all cases, and collated by a single data management team. Data on cell separation techniques, positive and negative selection criteria, and FISH analysis are recorded. Among questions to be addressed are the time in gestation when fetal cells first appear, frequency of fetal cells at various stages of gestation, potential confounding effect of Rh- or ABO- incompatibilities, and efficacy of the different cell separation techniques. Five colour FISH (X,Y,13,18,21) is recommended; our group uses directly labelled (Vysis, Inc.) probes (Bischoff *et al.* 1996b).

Determining sensitivity and specificity will require analysis of at least 3000 women with the end point detectability for trisomic cells. Enrolled patients are informed both verbally and by written informed consent that the results of analysis will not be made available to them or their physicians. By 1997 data relevant to the propriety of introducing this technology into clinical practice should be available. Until then, traditional invasive CVS or amniocentesis should continue to be offered (de la Cruz *et al.* 1995).

Culturing fetal cells in maternal blood

Conceptionally the simple approach for analysing fetal cells in maternal blood is to culture the fetal cells. No enrichment would be necessary. Indeed, this was the approach taken by Walknowska *et al.* (1969), who were the first to claim recovery of XY metaphases from maternal blood.

There are more recent examples of ostensibly successfully culturing fetal cells, as noted already in this chapter. Sbracia *et al.* (1994) demonstrated 46, XY cells after enrichment for trophoblasts and conventional cytogenetic cultures. Lo *et al.* (1994) cultured maternal blood (11–20 gestational weeks) in erythropoietin-enriched medium. In five women carrying male fetuses, Y cells were detected (per 1/400 to 1/9500 female cells). Wachtel *et al.* (1996) also reported culturing fetal cells.

A culture technique would not only offer the possibility of detecting fetal cells with no prior separation or sorting, but also of obtaining full metaphases by karyotyping. Our group is now working with collaborators (Alter 1994; Kim *et al.* 1996).

Acknowledgement. The authors acknowledge the support of the National Institute of Child Health and Human Development (Contract NO1HD43203), March of Dimes and United States Agency for International Development.

References

Alter, B.P. (1994) 'Biology of erythropoiesis' in J.L. Simpson and S. Elias (Eds) *Fetal Cells in Maternal Blood: Prospects for Noninvasive Prenatal Diagnosis,* pp.36–47. New York: New York Academy of Science

Benirschke, K. (1994) 'Anatomical relationship between fetus and mother' in J.L. Simpson and S. Elias (Eds) *Fetal Cells in Maternal Blood: Prospects for Noninvasive Prenatal Diagnosis,* pp.9–20. New York: New York Academy of Science

Bianchi, D.W. (1994) 'Clinical trials and experience: Boston' in J.L.Simpson, and S. Elias (Eds) *Fetal Cells in Maternal Blood: Prospects for Noninvasive Prenatal Diagnosis,* pp.1–10. New York: New York Academy of Science

Bianchi, D.W. and Klinger, K.W. (1993) ' Prenatal diagnosis through the analysis of fetal cells in the maternal circulation' in A. Milunsky (Ed.) *Genetic Disorders and the Fetus,* 3rd edn, pp.759–70. Baltimore: Johns Hopkins University Press

Bianchi, D.W., Flint, A.F., Pizzimenti, M.F., Knoll, J.H.M. and Latt, S.A. (1990) Isolation of fetal DNA from nucleated erythrocytes in maternal blood. *Proc Natl Acad Sci USA* **87**, 3279–83

Bianchi, D.W., Klinger, K.W., Vadnais, T.J. *et al.* (1996a) Development of a model system to compare cell separation methods for the isolation of fetal cells from maternal blood. *Prenat Diagn* **16**, 289–98

Bianchi, D.W., Zickwolf, G.K., Weil, G.J., Sylvester, S. and DeMaria, M.A. (1996b) Male fetal progenitor cells persist in maternal blood for as long as 27 years postpartum. *Proc Natl Acad Sci USA* **93**, 705–8

Bischoff, F.Z., Lewis, D.E., Nguyen, D. *et al.* (1995) Fetal cells in maternal blood: more efficacious FISH analysis by using gamma globin mRNA to identify fetal cells after flow-sorting. *Am J Hum Genet* **59**, A33

Bischoff, F.Z., Lewis, D.E., Nguyen, D.D. *et al.* (1996a) Greatly increased efficiency of analysis of fetal cells from maternal blood: identification of fetal cells based on CD71 expression, lack of beta globin expression and use of gamma globin mRNA to distinguish fetal (XX) from maternal (XX) cells. *J Soc Gynecol Invest* Abstract 608, p.361A

Bischoff, F.Z., Nguyen, D.D., Murrell, S. *et al.* (1996b) Five-color combinatorial FISH for simultaneous detection of X,Y,13,18 and 21 in fetal cells isolated from maternal blood. *Am J Hum Genet* Abstract 45, p.A11

Covone, A.E., Johnson, P.M., Hutton, D. and Adinolfi, M. (1984) Trophoblast cells in peripheral blood from pregnant women. *Lancet* **ii**, 841–3

Covone, A.E., Kozma, R., Johnson, P.M., Latt, S.A. and Adinolfi, M. (1988) Analysis of peripheral maternal blood samples for the presence of placental-derived cells using Y-specific probes and McAb H315. *Prenat Diagn* **8**, 591–607

de la Cruz, F., Shifrin, H., Elias, S. *et al.* (1995) Prenatal diagnosis by use of fetal cells isolated from maternal blood. *Am J Obstet Gynecol* **173**, 1354–5

deGrouchy, J. and Trubuchet, C. (1971) Transfusion foeto-maternelle de lymphoctyes sanguins et detection du sexe du foetus. *Ann Genet* **14**, 133–7

Douglas, G.W., Thomas, L., Carr, M., Cullen, N.M. and Morris, R. (1959) Trophoblast in the circulating blood during pregnancy. *Am J Obstet Gynecol* **78**, 960–73

Durrant, L.G., McDowell, K.M., Holmes, R.A. and Liu, D.T.Y. (1994) Screening of monoclonal antibodies recognizing oncofetal antigens for isolation of trophoblasts from maternal blood for prenatal diagnosis. *Prenat Diagn* **14**, 131–40

Durrant, L.G., McDowell, K., Holmes, R. and Liu, D. (1996) Non-invasive prenatal diagnosis by isolation of both trophoblasts and fetal nucleated red blood cells from the peripheral blood of pregnant women. *Br J Obstet Gynaecol* **103**, 219–22

Elias, S., Price, J., Dockter, M., Wachtel, S., Tharapel, A. and Simpson, J.L. (1992) First trimester prenatal diagnosis of trisomy 21 in fetal cells from maternal blood. *Lancet* **340**, 1033

Elias, S. and Simpson, J.L. (1994) 'Prenatal diagnosis of aneuploidy using fetal cells isolated from maternal blood: University of Tennessee, Memphis experience' in J.L. Simpson and S. Elias (Eds) *Fetal Cells in Maternal Blood: Prospects for Noninvasive Prenatal Diagnosis*, pp. 80–91. New York: New York Academy of Science

Elias, S., Lewis, D.E., Bischoff, F.Z. and Simpson, J.L. (1996a) Isolation and genetic analysis of fetal nucleated red blood cells from maternal blood: the Baylor College of Medicine experience. *Early Hum Dev* **47** (Suppl.) 585–8

Elias, S., Lewis, D.E., Simpson, J.L. *et al.*. (1996b) Isolation of fetal nucleated red blood cells from maternal blood: persistence of cells from prior pregnancy is unlikely to lead to false positive results. *J Soc Gynecol Invest* **3**, 359A

Ferguson-Smith, M.A., Zheng, Y.L. and Carter, N.P. (1994) 'Simultaneous immunophenotyping and FISH on fetal cells from maternal blood' in J.L. Simpson, S. Elias (Eds) *Fetal Cells in Maternal Blood: Prospects of Noninvasive Prenatal Diagnosis*, pp.73–9. New York: New York Academy of Sciences

Ganshirt-Ahlert, D., Borjesson-Stoll, R., Burschyk, M. *et al.*. (1993) Detection of fetal trisomies 21 and 18 from maternal blood using triple gradient and magnetic cell sorting, *Am J Reprod Immunol* **30**,194–201

Hall, J.M. and Williams, S.J. (1992) Isolation and purification of CD34++ fetal cells from maternal blood. *Am J Hum Genet* **51**, A257

Hamada, H., Arinami, T., Kubo, T., Hamaguchi, H. and Iwasaki, H. (1993) Fetal nucleated cells in maternal peripheral blood: frequency and relationship to gestational age. *Hum Genet* **91**, 427–32

Hawes, C.S., Suskin, H.A., Kalionis, B. *et al.*. (1994) 'Detection of paternally inherited Mutations for β-thalassemia in trophoblast isolated from peripheral maternal blood' in J.L. Simpson and S. Elias (Eds) *Fetal Cells in Maternal Blood: Prospects of Noninvasive Prenatal Diagnosis*, pp.181–5. New York: New York Academy of Sciences

Herzenberg, L.A., Bianchi, D.W., Schroder, J., Cann, H.M. and Iverson, G.M. (1979) Fetal cells in the blood of pregnant women: detection and enrichment by fluorescence-activated cell sorting. *Proc Natl Acad Sci USA* **76**, 1453–5

Holzgreve, W., Garritsen, H.S.P. and Ganshirt-Ahlert, D. (1992) Fetal cells in the maternal circulation. *J Reprod Med* **37**, 410–18

Hsieh, T.T., Pao, C.C., Hor, J.J. and Kao, S.M. (1993) Presence of fetal cells in maternal circulation after delivery. *Hum Genet* **92**, 204–5

Iverson, G.M., Bianchi, D.W., Cann, H.M. and Herzenberg, L.A. (1981) Detection and isolation of fetal cells from maternal blood using the fluorescence-activated cell sorter (FACS). *Prenat Diagn* **1**, 61–73

Kao, S.M., Tang, G.C., Hsieh, T.T., Young, K.C., Wang, H.C. and Pao, C.C. (1992) Analysis of peripheral blood of pregnant women for the presence of fetal Y chromosome-specific ZFY gene deoxyribonucleic acid sequences. *Am J Obstet Gynecol* **166**, 1013–19

Kim, J.I., Bischoff, F.Z., Alter, B.P. *et al.* (1996) Culturing fetal cells in maternal blood: multi-color FISH is necessary for reliable detection and analysis. *Am J Hum Genet* Abstract 1886, p.A324

Latham, S.E., Suskin, H.A., Petropoulos, A., Hawes, C.S., Jones, W.R. and Kalionis, B. (1996) A monoclonal antibody to human placental lactogen hormone facilitates isolation of fetal cells from maternal blood in a model system. *Prenat Diagn* **16**, 813–21

Lewis, D.E., Schober, W., Murrell, S. *et al.* (1996) Rare event selection of fetal nucleated erythrocytes in maternal blood by flow cytometry. *Cytometry* **23**, 218–27

Lo, Y.-M.D., Wainscot, J.S., Gilmer, M.D.G., Patel, P., Sampietro, M. and Fleming, K.A. (1989) Prenatal sex determination by DNA amplification from maternal peripheral blood. *Lancet* **ii**, 1363–5

Lo, Y.-M.D., Patel, P., Sampietro, M., Gillmer, M.D.G., Fleming, K.A. and Wainscoat, J.D. (1990) Detection of single-copy fetal DNA sequence from maternal blood. *Lancet* **335**, 1463–4

Lo, Y.-M.D., Morey, A.L., Wainscoat, J.S. and Fleming, K.A. (1994) Culture of fetal erythroid cells from maternal peripheral blood. *Lancet* **344**, 264–5

Mueller, U.W., Hawes, C.D., Wright, A.E. *et al.* (1990) Isolation of fetal trophoblast cells from peripheral blood in pregnant women. *Lancet* **336**, 197–200

Park, V.M., Bravo, R.R., Price, J.O., Simpson, J.L. and Elias, S. (1994) 'A model system using fetal hemoglobin to distinguish fetal cells enriched from maternal blood' in J.L. Simpson and S. Elias (Eds) *Fetal Cells in Maternal Blood: Prospects for Noninvasive Prenatal Diagnosis,* pp.133–5. New York: New York Academy of Science

Price, J., Elias, S., Wachtel, S.S. *et al.* (1991) Prenatal diagnosis using fetal cells isolated from maternal blood by multiparameter flow cytometry. *Am J Obstet Gynecol* **165**, 1731–7

Sargent, I.L., Choo, Y.S. and Redman, C.W.G. (1994) 'Isolating and analysing fetal leukocytes in maternal blood' in J.L. Simpson and S. Elias (Eds) *Fetal Cells in Maternal Blood: Prospects for Noninvasive Prenatal Diagnosis,* pp.147–53. New York: New York Academy of Science

Sbracia, M., Scapellini, F., Lalwani, S., Grasso, J.A. and Scarpellini, L. (1994) 'Possible use of an unusual HLA antigen to select trophoblast cells from the maternal circulation to perform early prenatal diagnosis' in J.L. Simpson and S. Elias (Eds) *Fetal Cells in Maternal Blood: Prospective for Noninvasive Prenatal Diagnosis,* pp.170–4. New York: New York Academy of Science

Schindler, A.M., Graf, E. and Martin-Du-Pan, R. (1972) Prenatal diagnosis of fetal lymphocytes in the maternal blood. *Obstet Gynecol* **40**, 340–6

Simpson, J.L. and Elias, S. (1993) Isolating fetal cells from maternal blood: advances in prenatal diagnosis through molecular technology. *JAMA* **270**, 2357–61

Simpson, J.L. and Elias, S. (1994a) 'Fetal cells in maternal blood: overview and historical perspective' in J.L. Simpson and S. Elias (Eds) *Fetal Cells in Maternal Blood: Prospects for Noninvasive Prenatal Diagnosis,* p.108. New York: New York Academy of Science

Simpson, J.L. and Elias, S. (1994b) Isolating fetal cells in maternal circulation for prenatal diagnosis. *Prenat Diagn* **14**, 1229–42

Simpson, J.L. and Elias, S. (1995) Isolating fetal cells in the maternal circulation. *Hum Reprod* **1**, 409–18

Takabayashi, H., Kuwabara, S., Ukita, T. and Igarashi, T. (1994) 'Fetal nucleated erythrocyte retrieval from maternal blood' in H. Zakut (Ed.) *7th International Conference on Early Prenatal Diagnosis,* pp.45–52. Bologna: Monduzzi Editore

Takahara, H., Kadotani, I., Kusumi, I. and Makino, S. (1972) Some critical aspects of prenatal diagnosis of sex in leukocyte cultures from pregnant women. *Proc Jpn Acad* **48**, 603–7

Tharapel, A.T., Jaswaney, V., Dockter, M. *et al.*(1989) Can fetal cells in maternal blood be selected through cytogenetic means? *Am J Hum Genet* **45**(S), 271

Tharapel, A.T., Jaswaney, V.L., Dockter, M.E. *et al.* (1993) Failure to detect fetal metaphases in lymphocytes flow sorted by maternal-fetal HLA differences. *Fetal Diagn Ther* **8**, 95–101

Thomas, M.R., Williamson, R., Craft, I., Yazhani, N. and Rodeck, C.H. (1994) Y chromosome sequence DNA amplified from peripheral blood in women in early pregnancy. *Lancet* **343**, 413–14

Wachtel, S.S., Sammons, D., Manley, M. *et al.* (1996) Fetal cells in maternal blood: recovery by change flow separation. *Hum Genet* **98**, 162–6

Wachtel, S.S., Elias, S., Price, J. *et al.* (1991) Fetal cells in the maternal circulation: isolation by multiparameter flow cytometry and confirmation by PCR. *Hum Reprod* **6**, 1466–9

Walknowska, J., Conte, F.A. and Grumback, M.M. (1969) Practical and theoretical implications of fetal/maternal lymphocyte transfer. *Lancet* **i**, 1119–22

Wessman, M., Ylinen, K. and Knutila, S. (1992) Fetal granulocyte in maternal venous blood detected in in situ hybridization. *Prenat Diagn* **12**, 993–1000

Whang-Peng, J., Lettin, J.S., Harris, C., Lee, E. and Stites, J. (1973). The transplacental passage of fetal leukocytes into the maternal blood. *Proc Soc Exp Biol Med* **142**, 50–3

Yeoh, S.C., Sargent, I.L., Redman, C.W.G., Wordsworth, B.P. and Thein, S.L. (1991) Detection of fetal cells in maternal blood. *Prenat Diagn* **11**, 117–23

Zheng, Y-L, Carter, M.P., Price, C.M. *et al.* (1993) Prenatal diagnosis from maternal blood: simultaneous immunophenotyping and FISH of fetal nucleated erythrocytes isolated by negative magnetic cell sorting. *J Med Genet* **30**, 1051–6

Chapter 24

Prenatal detection of fetal aneuploidies and single gene defects using transcervical cell samples

Matteo Adinolfi, Jon Sherlock and Charles Rodeck

Introduction

Recent investigations have shown that trophoblastic cells can be detected in transcervical samples retrieved from pregnant women between seven and 17 weeks of gestation (Adinolfi *et al.* 1995a; Adinolfi 1996). Molecular analysis of transcervical cell (TCC) samples obtained by lavage of the endocervical canal have documented the presence of fetal cells as judged by the detection of Y-derived DNA sequences using polymerase chain reaction (PCR) (Griffith-Jones *et al.* 1992; Adinolfi *et al.* 1995a) or fluorescent *in situ* hybridisation (FISH) assays (Adinolfi *et al.* 1993). Using PCR procedures Rh(D) DNA sequences have also been detected in TCC samples obtained from Rh(D) negative mothers with Rh(D)-positive fetuses (Adinolfi *et al.* 1995b).

In the course of investigations aimed at comparing two methods – lavage and aspiration – for the collection of transcervical samples, several cases of fetal chromosome disorders have been detected (Sherlock *et al.* 1997). In two cases, clumps of cells were isolated from the whole transcervical samples by micromanipulation under an inverted microscope (Tutschek *et al.* 1995) and the diagnosis of triploidy and sex chromosome aneuploidy (XYY) confirmed using FISH and PCR.

The isolation of clumps of fetal cells free of maternal contaminants also offers the opportunity of performing prenatal diagnoses of fetal single gene disorders as well as chromosome aneuploidies as shown in a study targeted at performing prenatal diagnosis of haemoglobinopathies (Adinolfi *et al.* 1997).

Materials and methods

TCC and maternal peripheral blood samples were collected from pregnant women between seven and 13 weeks' gestation prior to termination of pregnancy (TOP).

A sample of placenta was retrieved after the TOP procedure. Standard FISH protocols were performed using probes specific for chromosomes X and Y using dual colour FISH, the centromere of chromosome 18; the centromere of chromosome 1, two cosmid contigs specific to chromosome 21.

Using micromanipulation clumps of cells with the morphology of trophoblasts were removed from the fresh TCC sample. They were tested by FISH and/or to quantitative fluorescent duplex PCR with primers specific for a polymorphic short tandem repeat (STR) on chromosome 21, D21S11 (Mansfield 1993; Pertl *et al.* 1995, 1996) and the amelogenin region of the sex chromosomes (Nakahori *et al.* 1991). Prenatal diagnosis was also performed on six pairs of parents known to be carriers of haemoglobin (Hb) mutations by testing TCC samples, retrieved prior to chorionic villus sampling, (CVS), by aspiration of cervical mucus. The Hb mutations affecting each subject are shown in Table 24.1. Fetal prenatal diagnosis was independently determined on CVS tissue using the Amplification Refractory Mutation System (ARMS). For the detection of the thalassaemia mutation, DNA amplification was performed by nested PCR and the amplification product tested by gel electrophoresis and silver staining (Orita *et al.* 1989; Adinolfi *et al.* 1997). Details of the amplification of the thalassaemia deletions and of the haemoglobin S mutation are reported by Adinolfi *et al.* (1996).

Results

Chromosome anomalies

In a 42-year-old patient intrauterine lavage was carried out eight days after CVS, prior to TOP. FISH tests, performed on the TCC sample with a chromosome 18 specific centromeric probe, documented the presence of 26% of cells with trisomy 18. In a second case, a TCC sample was obtained by intrauterine lavage prior to

Table 24.1. Results of testing clumps of cells from TCC samples for Hb mutations

| Case | Mutations[a] | | | Clumps | | | | | | |
	Mother	Father	CSV	1	2	3	4	5	6	7
1	+/I10	+/I10	+/+	+/+	+/+	+/I10	...	...	...	...
2	+/5	+/C30	+/+	+/5	+/5	+/5	+/5	...	...	...
3	+/HbS	+/5	+/5	HbS/5	HbS/5	HbS/5	...	...	...	...
4	+/I10	+/6	+/6	+/6	+/6	+/6	...	...	...	...
5	+/I10	+/I10	+/I10	+/I10	+/I10	+/I10	+/I10	...	...	...
6	+/del 1	+/del 2	del 1/ del 2	del 1/ del 2	del 1/ del 2	del 1/ del 2	del 1/ del 2	+/ del 1	+/ del 1	+/ del 1

[a] Mutations causing β-thalassaemia in introns 1=5, 6, 110 and exon 1=C30. In mother 3, the HbS mutation was in exon 1. Four bp deletion in mother 6 (del 1); 619 bp deletion in father 6 (see text).
In cases 1 and 4 the correct diagnosis of thalassaemia on some clumps (case 1=normal fetus; case 2=fetus carrying the paternal mutation) was performed. In cases 5 and 6, although the correct diagnosis was performed, the possibility of maternal cell contamination could not be excluded.

TOP from a woman at risk of carrying a fetus with trisomy 21 due to advanced maternal age. FISH analysis carried out without knowledge of the karyotype of the fetus documented the presence of trisomy 21 cells. Samples of placenta obtained following TOP were subsequently karyotyped, confirming the result of fetal trisomy 21.

In the course of a study aimed at comparing the results of collecting endo-cervical cells by aspiration and lavage, a sample of cervical mucus was retrieved by aspiration before obtaining a further sample by lavage from a 24-year-old primigravida, at seven weeks of gestation. A maternal peripheral blood sample and placental tissue were also collected after TOP.

The results of the FISH tests showed that 6.7% (7 out of 111) nuclei from the aspirated sample and 2.7% (3 out of 111) nuclei from the lavage exhibited two green (XX) and one red (Y) signal thus suggesting that the fetus could have a 47, XXY chromosomal abnormality or could be triploidy. Further FISH tests with

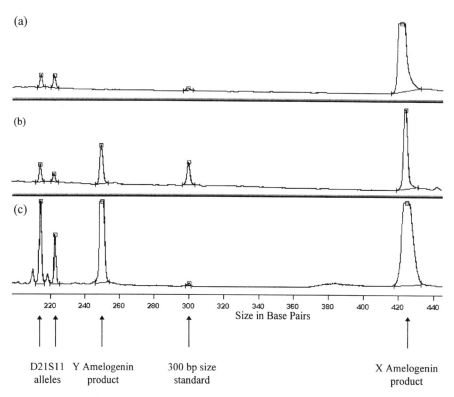

Fig. 24.1. Quantitative multiplex PCR analysis from an XXY triploid pregnancy. DNA was amplified from maternal blood (a), placenta (b) and a clump of cells isolated from the transcervical mucus aspirate (c). Relative abundance of D21S11 alleles and amelogenin PCR products are compared. The two D21S11 alleles (chromosome 21 marker) with a signal intensity ratio of 2:1 in both the placental and isolated cell clump indicate the presence of three copies of chromosome 21. These results combined with both X- and Y-specific PCR products co-amplified at the amelogenin locus, are consistent with the FISH diagnosis of fetal triploidy.

a chromosome 1-derived probe documented the presence of nuclei with three chromosomes 1 in the endocervical samples. The diagnosis of triploidy was then confirmed by FISH analysis of the isolated placental cellular elements.

Using an inverted microscope, small clumps of cells – with the morphological characteristics of syncytio- or cytotrophoblastic cellular elements – were isolated from the endocervical samples retrieved by aspiration or lavage. Nuclei prepared from these cells, as well as cells present in the TCC samples and from dissociated placental cellular elements, were analysed by dual colour FISH using X and Y chromosome specific probes labelled with FITC (green) or rhodamine (red). All nuclei from seven aspiration samples and from four clumps isolated from lavage samples contained two X and one Y signals.

Another isolated cell-clump was tested by quantitative multiplex fluorescent PCR with a polymorphic STR marker on chromosome 21 (D21S11) co-amplified with primers specific for the amelogenin region of the sex chromosomes. This assay displayed the same pattern as tested placental DNA, two STR allele sizes with a quantitative ratio of 2:1 due to the presence of three chromosome 21s, and X and Y-specific PCR products. These results are consistent with the cells being of fetal origin and with the FISH diagnosis of triploidy (Fig. 24.1).

In the fourth case a twin pregnancy with two distinct placentae was detected using ultrasound prior to TOP at 11 weeks' gestation. TCC, placenta and fetal tissue samples were collected together with peripheral maternal blood. Interphase FISH analysis of the TCC samples revealed the presence of two populations of cells: the first with two X and one Y chromosome signals; the second with one X and two Y signals. FISH tests carried out on umbilical cord and placental tissue from both twins, showed that the two cell populations were present in all fetal samples, but with a different ratio (Table 24.2).

All maternal peripheral blood cells tested by interphase FISH showed two chromosome X and one Y signals. Conventional cytogenetic analysis of chromosomes samples revealed the presence of a 15p/Yq translocation and thus a maternal karyotype of 46,XX, t(Y;15) (qh;pter). These findings suggest that both fetuses were chimeras with different ratios of XX+Yqh and XY+Yqh cells, probably as a result of early interchange of embryonic cells.

Finally, in case 5, transcervical CVS performed at 10 weeks of fetal gestation revealed a fetal karyotype of 47, XYY. The TCC sample collected 6 days after CVS, contained 95% of cells 47, XYY and 5% 46 XY. Clumps of cells isolated using an inverted microscope also contained one X and two Y chromosomes when tested by FISH.

Table 24.2. Samples of placenta were taken from two different regions, A and B

Sample	Twin A		Twin B	
	% XXY	% XYY	% XXY	% XYY
Placenta (site A)	93	7	20	80
Placenta (site B)	94	6	16	84
Umbilical cord	95	5	30	70

Detection of Hb mutations

Prenatal diagnosis was performed on six pairs of parents known to be carriers of Hb mutations; TCCs were retrieved, prior to CVS, by the aspiration of cervical mucus from pregnant women from 10–12 weeks of gestation. Fetal prenatal diagnosis of the haemoglobinopathies were independently performed on CVS tissue using ARMS. As shown in Table 24.1, in the first case, two out of three clumps contained cells with normal Hb alleles. It was, therefore, possible to conclude that the fetus was not affected. This was in agreement with the prenatal test performed on CVS. In case 4 all three clumps showed heterozygosity for the paternal mutation and a normal HbS allele, a finding confirmed by the CVS analysis. In the last two cases, even if the diagnosis was correct, it was not possible to exclude the possibility of maternal contamination of the samples.

Discussion

In 1971 Shettles suggested that, during pregnancy, chorionic cellular elements from the degenerating villi were shed into the endocervical canal and could be analysed to assess the sex of the fetus. Recent investigations have confirmed that trophoblastic cells are present in the endocervical canal and that fetal DNA specific sequences can be identified using FISH or the PCR assay (Adinolfi 1996).

The recovery of fetal cells is dependent on the time of gestation and the method employed to retrieve the TCC samples. Trophoblastic cells are shed into the endocervical canal between seven and 13 weeks of gestation. Aspiration of the mucus has been shown to provide samples with fetal cells in about 60% of cases whereas, by lavage with 10 ml of saline, about 90% of TCC samples may contain trophoblastic cellular elements (Adinolfi 1996).

Aspiration of endocervical mucus has also been successfully employed to collect TCC samples from pregnant women prior to CVS without any risk for the mother or the fetus (Adinolfi et al. 1995a).

The present findings confirm the possibility of using TCC samples for the prenatal diagnoses of chromosomal abnormalities in the first trimester of pregnancy. We have also shown that by a simple micromanipulation procedure, it is possible to obtain clumps of cells free from maternal contaminants. This offers the possibility of performing tests for the prenatal diagnosis of single gene disorders using clumps of fetal cells isolated from TCC samples. Work is now in progress to further improve the methods for the collection of TCC samples and to develop new approaches for the isolation of fetal cells.

If the procedures for the collection of the TCC samples and the isolation of the trophoblastic cells can be improved, then, perhaps, this minimally invasive prenatal diagnostic assay could be used selectively on young pregnant women not at risk of having fetuses with chromosomal disorders or on women suspected of having an affected fetus, according to borderline biochemical or ultrasound results

Acknowledgements. We would like to thank the Dunhill Medical Trust and the Birth Defects Foundation for their financial support.

References

Adinolfi, M. (1996) Detection of fetal cells present in transcervical cell samples. *Fetal Maternal Med Rev* **8**, 1–10

Adinolfi, M., Davies, A., Sharif, S., Soothill, P. and Rodeck, C. (1993) Detection of trisomy 18 and Y-derived sequences in fetal nucleated cells obtained by transcervical flushing. *Lancet* **342**, 403–4

Adinolfi, M., Sherlock, J., Tutschek, B., Halder, A., Delhanty, J. and Rodeck C. (1995a) Detection of fetal cells in transcervical samples and prenatal diagnosis of chromosomal abnormalities. *Prenat Diagn* **15**, 943–51

Adinolfi, M., Sherlock, J., Kemp, T. *et al.* (1995b) Prenatal detection of fetal RhD DNA sequences in transcervical samples. *Lancet* **345**, 318–19

Adinolfi, M., El-Hashemite, N., Sherlock, J., Ward, R.H.T., Petrou, M. and Rodeck, C. (1997) Prenatal detection of Hb mutations in transcervical cells. *Prenat Diagn* (in press)

Griffith-Jones, M.D., Miller, D., Lilford, R.J., Scott, J. and Bulmer, J. (1992) Detection of fetal DNA in trans-cervical swabs from the first trimester of pregnancies by gene amplification: a new route to prenatal diagnosis? *Br J Obstet Gynaecol* **99**, 508–11

Mansfield, E.S. (1993) Diagnosis of Down syndrome and other aneuploidies using quantitative polymerase chain reaction and small tandem repeat polymorphisms. *Hum Mol Genet* **2**, 43–50

Nakahori, Y., Takenaka, O. and Nakagome, Y. (1991) A human X-Y homologous region encodes 'amelogenin'. *Genomics* **9**, 264–9

Orita, M., Iwahana, H., Kanazawa, H., Hayashi, K. and Sekiya, T. (1989) Detection of polymorphisms of human DNA by gel electrophoresis as single-strand conformation polymorphisms. *Proc Natl Acad Sci USA* **86**, 2766–70

Pertl, B., Yau, S.C., Sherlock, J., Davies, A.F., Mathew, C.G. and Adinolfi, M. (1995) Rapid molecular method for prenatal detection of Down syndrome. *Lancet* **343**, 1197–8

Pertl, B., Weitgasser, U., Kopp, S., Kroisel, P.M., Sherlock, J. and Adinolfi, M. (1996) Rapid detection of trisomy 21 and 18 and sexing by quantitative fluorescent PCR. *Hum Genet* **98**, 55–9

Sherlock, J., Halder, A., Tutschek, B., Delhanty, J.D.A., Rodeck, C. and Adinolfi, M. (1997) Prenatal detection of fetal aneuploidies using transcervical cell samples. *J Med Genet* (in press)

Shettles, L.B. (1971) Use of the Y chromosome in prenatal sex determination. *Nature* **230**, 52–3

Tutschek, B., Sherlock, J., Halder, A., Delhanty, J., Rodeck, C. and Adinolfi, M. (1995) Isolation of fetal cells from transcervical samples by micromanipulation: diagnosis of fetal aneuploidy and molecular confirmation of fetal origin. *Prenat Diagn* **15**, 951–61

Chapter 25

Fetal cells: alternatives to biochemical screening?

Discussion

Chard: If the likely success of this topic were to be judged by the quality of the basic science that we have just heard, then my predictions would prove to be very pessimistic. No one could fail to be impressed. Let us throw it open to the rest of the group for comments or questions.

Davies: The expectation of fetal cells is that this is a diagnostic test. That may be the wrong expectation. The first question is, how many women do you see where you are unable to isolate any fetal cells? Following that, the second point is that that limits the detection rate to the limit of the number you can find.

Simpson: This is a question for which we do not have the definitive answer at present, for several reasons. First, the biggest set of data we have relates to the issue of male cells that are detected in pregnant women carrying male fetuses. That is definitely not the question to ask. The question is what is the frequency of trisomic cells. It has recently become clear that there will probably be more trisomic cells than euploid cells, and therefore we need to generate the trisomic numbers in order to answer Dr Davies' question.

The answer with respect to male cells is that probably we are missing a good 40% at present – that is male, euploid cells, and it is a very soft number which I probably will not be willing to defend for too much later than this.

It is clear that we are missing many cells in a given pregnancy, and that is why I was cautious to point out that we would not recommend a single selection criterion. We continue to run through a series of different selection criteria and we continue to look at such things as how we fix the cells and how they are collected from the flow sorting system to ensure that we have not lost cells.

There are two problems. First, we need data on trisomics, and not on simple gender differences, and second, we need better simple technology in order to prevent additional loss of cells. Until we have that, it is not a fair question to ask. That is why I am not prepared to say that we will be ready in 24 months to put this out commercially.

Cuckle: There are all sorts of other technologies around, apart from those which have just been described. We have the bi-annual meetings of the Fetal Cell Group in Britain which are attended by people from all over the world. You see all sorts of different technologies and from time to time people go over the top about particular technologies – we have seen this with magnetic and self-sorting and so on.

We have one at Leeds which we have patented, which is to do with the panning method. There is a commercial one which does not use any antibodies, but uses the haematological properties of different kinds of cells in a funny tube which is spun and then water and different chemicals are added at different times. They all seem to have the same kind of properties – that you can concentrate by many different methods the ratio of fetal to maternal cells so that they are in the kinds of proportions that you would like to start looking down a microscope at, but at every stage you lose fetal cells. I do not think anyone has yet come up with a technology that both concentrates the cells to a reasonable degree and does not dramatically reduce the number of fetal cells in the sample. That is the problem.

Aitken: I am sure a number of you will remember from the fore-runner meeting to this one, that there was a suggestion from the audience that the fundamental problem here is that there are insufficient fetal cells present to begin with. Is there no legitimate or ethical way in which one could increase the number of fetal cells in the maternal circulation to make the current procedures that much more effective?

Simpson: I do not think it will be necessary. At a practical screening level, it would not be terribly well accepted by the patients. There is at least one study which has attempted to look at the number of fetal cells that are present before and after rolling the patient around and rubbing the uterus, but the problem is that the end point was not FISH with chromosome specific probes, but a morpho-logical criterion for what looked like erythroblasts.

In my opinion, all those studies are neither valid nor useful, because it is impossible to distinguish a maternal erythroblast from a fetal erythroblast. There will be better techniques. All we need is a slightly better antibody to select for or against, and if we improved our recovery only by a small amount we would easily have sufficient cells to work with.

SECTION 7

INVASIVE TESTS IN THE DIAGNOSIS OF DOWN SYNDROME

Chapter 26

A comparison of chorionic villus sampling and amniocentesis for prenatal diagnosis in early pregnancy

Eric Jauniaux

Introduction

Ultrasonography has changed our perception of human development after conception and the fetus is now perceived as an individual, influencing patient attitudes toward the different methods of prenatal diagnosis. The advent of high resolution ultrasound imaging has enabled direct access to the different constituents of the gestational sac from the second half of the first trimester of pregnancy. The diagnosis of fetal abnormalities during the second half of pregnancy brings on a variety of difficult issues for patients and health care professionals alike. The primary advantage of early prenatal diagnosis is that karyotype results can be obtained earlier, before fetal movements have been perceived by the mother or when the pregnancy has become obvious to others. Demand for early prenatal diagnosis is increasing rapidly, especially among women of advanced maternal age with higher education and socioeconomic levels. Several medical, social, ethical and financial implications have been raised by the rapid development of these new invasive procedures. In particular, the post-procedure complication rate and pregnancy outcome after early sampling of the fetal adnexae is the matter of permanent debate. This chapter reviews and discusses the use and advantages of invasive procedures in early pregnancy and their potential risks and complications to the developing fetus.

Early amniocentesis

History

Mid-second trimester amniocentesis was introduced in the 1960s by Steele and Breg (1966) and is still the most commonly used invasive technique for prenatal diagnosis. Its safety, when performed under ultrasound guidance, has rapidly increased its acceptance worldwide. Early amniocentesis (10–14 weeks) has theoretically most of the practical advantages of late amniocentesis (Hanson *et al.* 1987; Evans *et al.* 1989) and, therefore, has the potential as an attractive alternative for fetal karyotyping and DNA analysis. Although, amniotic fluid biochemical analysis could be investigated before 12 weeks for the detection of structural fetal abnormalities including neural tube defects, ventral wall defects or urinary tract obstruction (Crandall and Chua 1995), its routine clinical value is limited because the corresponding fetal organs are not always functionally mature at this stage.

Complications

Gestational age has a direct influence on the procedure related risks of early amniotic fluid sampling. The amniotic space is obviously narrower in the first trimester and the risk of fetal injury during early amniocentesis is higher than with second trimester amniocentesis. The definitive placenta is only formed from 10 weeks of gestation. Before that period, the vascularised villi of the chorion frondosum surround the whole gestational sac making the transplacental entry of the needle in the amniotic cavity almost inevitable, therefore, increasing the risk of intra-amniotic and/or feto-maternal haemorrhage (Jauniaux and Rodeck 1995). During the first three months of pregnancy, the amniotic cavity is separated from the placenta by the exocoelomic cavity (Jauniaux *et al.* 1992) and the chorion frondosum fuses completely with the uterine wall between 11 and 13 weeks of gestation increasing the risk of membrane tenting (Jauniaux and Rodeck 1995). Transvaginal amniocentesis which is technically easier (Jauniaux *et al.* 1991) than the transabdomial procedure and not associated with higher rates of fetal loss than chorionic villus sampling (CVS) when performed after 10 weeks of gestation (Shalev *et al.* 1994) should be evaluated by a large randomised study.

During an early amniocentesis a greater proportion of the amniotic fluid is withdrawn and the damage this may induce for fetal organs such as the developing lungs (Hislop and Fairweather 1982) may be less reversible than later in pregnancy. The risk of pulmonary hypoplasia in fetuses born after early amniocentesis has been recently investigated (Calhoun *et al.* 1994) but the numbers are still too small to allow any conclusion (Sundberg *et al.* 1991). Within this context, amnio-filtration with removal of the cells for culture and reinjection of the fluid at the end of the procedure is a logical approach which may decrease this long-term risk of early amniocentesis.

Pregnancy outcome after early amniocentesis

When early amniocentesis was first reported expectations were that this technique would be as safe and accurate as traditional amniocentesis (Elejade *et al.* 1990; Penso *et al.* 1990; Hackett *et al.* 1991; Kennerknecht *et al.* 1992; Jorgensen *et al.* 1992; Kerber and Held 1993; Lockwood and Neu 1993). If the accuracy of cytogenetic investigation performed on early amniotic fluid samples is similar to that of mid-trimester amniocentesis, the post-procedure complication rates of early amniocentesis are difficult to evaluate from the data presented in these studies because of crucial drawbacks, small sample numbers and unbalanced gestational age distribution with an excess of cases over 12 weeks of gestation. Several authors have found a much higher post-procedure loss rate after early than after late amniocentesis (Penso *et al.* 1990; Stripparo *et al.* 1990). The only, but partially, randomised trial comparing early amniocentesis with CVS performed at the same gestational age period has demonstrated that early amniocentesis is associated with 3% less chance of successful pregnancy outcome than CVS performed at the same gestational age (Nicolaides *et al.* 1994, 1996). A recent retrospective study has also shown that early (11–14 weeks) amniocentesis was associated with a significantly higher risk of post-procedure vaginal bleeding (1.9 versus 0.2%), amniotic fluid leakage (2.9 versus 0.2%) and fetal loss within 30 days (2.2 versus 0.2%) than late (16–19 weeks) amniocentesis (Brumfield *et al.* 1996).

Chorionic villus sampling (CVS)

History

In the early 1980s, Rodeck *et al.* (1983) and Ward *et al.* (1983) showed that chorionic villi can be successfully aspirated with a flexible catheter inserted through the cervical canal under abdominal ultrasound guidance and Simoni *et al.* (1983) showed that karyotyping was possible from these samples. In 1984, Smidt-Jensen and Hahnemann proposed a transabdominal method of sampling which is being used increasingly often by prenatal diagnosis centres through-out the world. With the advent of high-resolution ultrasound, CVS has been performed routinely transabdominaly from six weeks of gestation until the third trimester using the freehand ultrasound-guided single needle aspiration technique described by Brambati *et al.* (1988). Several refinements have been proposed in the last decade including the use of biopsy forceps (Dumez *et al.* 1984), a double needle system (Maxwell *et al.* 1986) or an automatic puncturing apparatus (Popp and Ghirardini 1990).

Transcervical versus transabdominal CVS

There are no medical contraindications to invasive procedure with the transabdominal method whereas an active vaginal infection is a contraindication for a transvaginal or transcervical invasive procedure. In early series, up to 30% of the catheters used for the procedure were reported to be colonised by bacteria and there was some concern about secondary intrauterine infection (Hammarstrom and Marsk 1990; Silverman *et al.* 1994). However, the rate of fetal loss is not directly associated with bacterial colonisation of the cervix and life-threatening infections have not been encountered since the use of a single catheter for repeated insertions has been abandoned. It has also been shown that transabdominal single-needle aspiration causes more placental disruption and feto-maternal haemorrhage than transcervical biopsy forceps (Rodeck *et al.* 1993). Thus, within this context, trauma is a major factor as is gestational age.

Pregnancy outcome after early CVS

Vaginal spotting or bleeding is the most common (1–4%) immediate complications of a CVS procedure and is mainly (up to 20% of the cases) observed after a transcervical sampling (Rhoads *et al.* 1989). Direct vascular injury of small branches of the utero-placental or umbilico-placental circulations may also lead to a retro-placental haematoma and/or a subchorionic haemorrhage and subsequently to a miscarriage. The formation of a haematoma inside the gestational sac often becomes apparent during or within a few minutes after the procedure. Intrauterine infection and chronic amniotic fluid leakage are two possible complications of CVS, occurring within a few days to three weeks after the procedure. Intrauterine infection after CVS is a rare (<0.1%) but serious complication which can lead to maternal septic shock (Barela *et al.* 1986) and, therefore, requires immediate evacuation of the uterine contents (Fisk and Anderson 1987). The oligohydramnios sequence is a less dramatic complication with a good fetal outcome in most cases (Turnpenny *et al.* 1990; Bronshtein and Blumenfeld 1991). No accurate information documents its frequency but it is probably a rare complication of CVS as this technique does imply the puncture of the amniotic sac.

A long-term possible teratogenic effect of CVS has been raised by different groups of investigators (Boyd *et al.* 1990; Firth *et al.* 1991; Gruppo Italiano Diagnosi Emrio-Fetali 1993), resulting in intense debate and contradictory information. The background frequency of limb reduction defect in the general population is low and varies between 0.04 and 0.06% of birth (Castilla *et al.* 1995;

Table 26.1. Incidence of limb reduction defect (LRD) per live birth from three multicentric registries and three series of consecutive CVS cases

Reference Country	Number of cases with follow-up	Gestational age at CVS (weeks)	LRD (%)
GIDEF (1993) Italy 5 centres	2759	6–16	1.49
Hsieh *et al.* (1995) Taiwan 165 centres	78,742	7–12	0.29
Froster and Jackson (1996) WHO 63 centres	138 966	6–20	0.06
Firth *et al.* (1991) UK	289	8–9.5	1.73
Blakemore *et al.* (1993) USA	4105	8–12	0.84
Wapner *et al.* (1996) USA	20 040	6–20	0.03

GIDEF, Gruppo Italiano Diagnosi Emrio-Fetali; WHO, World Health Organisation.
Incidence of limb defects in the surveyed general population:
North America (British Columbia): 0.06%
South America (Castilla *et al.* 1995): 0.05%
Taiwan (Hsieh *et al.* 1995): 0.03%

Froster and Jackson 1996). Several authors have agreed that very early CVS may be associated with an overall ten-fold increase in the incidence of limb reduction defects and oromandibular–limb hypogenesis. This pattern and much higher (2–3 times) incidence in limb reduction deformities before 9 weeks compared with sampling after 9.5 weeks suggest a causal relation (Brambati et al. 1992; Rodeck 1993). Furthermore, about 20% of CVS-exposed infants with limb disruption defects may also present at birth with one or more haemangiomatae (Burton et al. 1995). The incidence of haemangioma is particularly high after transcervical CVS and is not influenced by gestational age at sampling, sample size or the number of sampling attempts. The spectrum of limb defects reported after CVS by Firth and colleagues (1991) seems to be more severe than the limb defects seen in the general population and directly related to the timing of CVS during pregnancy. It must be stressed that, the larger the series, the lower the risk of limb defect (Table 26.1). The World Health Organisation (WHO) has initiated an international registration of post-CVS complications including limb defects. From May 1992 to May 1994, 77 infants or fetuses out of 138,996 pregnancies which had a CVS were reported with defects of the lower or upper limbs to the WHO CVS registry (Froster and Jackson 1996). These figures are in agreement with the distribution of limb defects in several large population-based studies and they suggest that there is no difference from the background population in the overall frequency or pattern distribution of limb deficiencies after CVS. There was also no correlation between gestational age at CVS and severity of defects. The debate should remain open for some time.

Early amniocentesis versus early CVS

Most clinical trials on the safety of invasive procedures during pregnancy have compared the outcome of CVS in the first trimester with second trimester amniocentesis and it is only recently that data on early amniocentesis have been incorporated (Table 26.2). According to the first analyses (MRC 1991; Smidt-Jensen et al. 1991; Lippman et al. 1992), CVS resulted in an 0.5–4% increase of the risk of post-procedure pregnancy loss compared to late amniocentesis. Considerable differences in study design and, in particular, in the number and experience of operators involved, size of the study groups and sampling approaches makes the comparison and interpretation of these data difficult. In most of these studies, the sampling procedure failure rate is at least three times higher for CVS than for amniocentesis which is directly related to the greater experience of operators in performing mid-trimester amniocentesis than CVS. Furthermore, the spontaneous miscarriage rate between the CVS period (9–12 weeks) and the amniocentesis period (15–17 weeks) is at least 3% and should be clearly indicated in the final statistics and correlated with not only gestational but also maternal age. Another major bias is the definition of post-procedure fetal loss which includes complicated cases from three weeks after the procedure to any lethal complications up to 28 weeks of gestation.

Early amniocentesis and CVS after 10 weeks of gestation have theoretically similar success rates in obtaining cell culture and chromosomal analysis and similar harvest time (Byrne et al. 1991). However, before 10 weeks of gestation,

Table 26.2. Comparison of the rate of post-procedure miscarriage (PPM) before the end of the second trimester and total fetal loss (TFL) observed after CVS and amniocentesis in four randomised (R) and four non-randomised (patient or operator choice) studies

	CVS			Amniocentesis		
Reference	No. of cases	GA (weeks)	PPM/TFL (%)	No. of cases	GA (weeks)	PPM/TFL (%)
MRC (1991)(R)	1609	9–12 (TC)	5.3/9.0	1592	15–17 (TA)	1.6/5.8
Smidt-Jensen et al. (1991)(R)	1175 1191	9–11 (TC) 9–11 (TA)	6.8/10.1 2.4/6.2	1041	15–16 (TA)	1.0/6.3
Ammala et al. (1993)(R)	400	9–11 (TC)	3.0/7.8	400	16 (TA)	0.8/8.3
Nicolaides et al. (1994)[a]	250	10–13 (TA)	1.2/1.2	238	10–13 (TA)	4.2/5.9
Shalev et al. (1994)	356	9–12 (TC)	1.7/2.9	356	14–21 (TA) 10–12 (TV)	0.6/0.9 1.7/3.2
Palo et al. (1994)	821	10–15 (TA)	1.9/6.7	771	13–17 (TA)	0.3/4.4
Shulman et al. (1994)	250	9–13 (TA)	1.2/2.0	250	9–15 (TA)	2.4/3.6
Nicolaides et al. (1996)	652	10–13 (TA)	2.1/5.5	840	10–13 (TA)	4.9/7.0

GA, gestational age; TA, transabdominal; TC, transcervical; TV, transvaginal; S, significant difference between the methods.
[a] Only randomised data are presented in the table.
TFL includes preprocedure spontaneous loss, elective abortion and loss from procedure time to end of neonatal period.

amniotic fluid samples contain fewer cells and compared to villus samples, they require longer harvest times (up to 40 days more) and their success rate in culture is only about 50% (Evans et al. 1989; Penso et al. 1990; Hackett et al. 1991; Kennerknecht et al. 1992).

Counselling on an invasive procedure at 10–14 weeks

Post-procedure abortion rates

It is imperative to be able to discuss the possibility of fetal loss or damage with couples contemplating the various techniques of invasive fetal sampling, because in most instances this is the couple's major concern. The earlier the procedure is performed, the higher the risk of subsequent miscarriage. The rate of spontaneous abortion is 'naturally' high before 10 weeks of gestation and is directly influenced by maternal age. In a prospective study of 232 women with positive urinary pregnancy tests and no antecedent history of vaginal bleeding, Goldstein (1994) has demonstrated that once a gestational sac has been documented on scan, subsequent loss of viability in the embryonic period is 11.5%. If an embryo has developed up to 5 mm, subsequent loss of viability will occur in 7.2%. Loss rates drop rapidly after that to 3.3% for embryos of 6–10 mm and to 0.5% for embryos over 10 mm. The fetal loss rate after the end of the first trimester is 2%. The ultrasound screening of a larger group of women with pregnancies of 10–13 weeks' gestation has confirmed that the prevalence of pregnancy loss at the end of the first trimester is around 2–3% (Pandya et al. 1996). These findings, together with the possible small risk of limb reduction defect before 10 weeks, suggest that no invasive procedure should be performed during the first nine weeks of gestation.

Technical considerations

From 10 weeks of gestation, the uterus is more stable and tends to rotate less on attempting to insert the needle through the myometrium. The double needle system produces samples of better quality and is probably less traumatic than single needle or catheter aspiration. Biopsy forceps produce clean atraumatic samples and are being increasingly used. For both amniocentesis and CVS, the transabdominal route is more practical than the transcervical route and is associated with less secondary bleeding. In cases of a posterior placenta or in obese patients, the transcervical or transvaginal approach is probably safer and should be considered for a CVS. Conversely, if an amniocentesis is planned and the placenta is anterior and obstructing, a transabdominal CVS would be more appropriate and probably safer.

There is little doubt that the CVS procedure-related accident is related to the operator experience and in particular to the number of attempts needed to obtain a sufficient villous sample (Rhoads et al. 1989; Silver et al. 1992). Amniocentesis was developed before real-time ultrasound was available and its safety was evaluated before the recent time of randomised controlled studies. The Danish randomised controlled trial (Tabor et al. 1986) which demonstrated that mid-trimester amniocentesis was associated with a 1% risk of fetal loss came from a centre with considerable experience in ultrasound-guided procedures. Within this context, the operator experience and/or the expert use of ultrasound imaging should be audited for each individual centre offering an amniocentesis to determine more precisely the risks associated with this technique.

Laboratory failure and mosaicism

CVS produces larger samples which are convenient when rapid cell culture and DNA analysis are planned. However, short-term culture increases the technicians' workload in the laboratory and may be difficult to offer on a routine basis because of the increased cost. Direct preparations are not always feasible and there is a 5–10% failure rate in most laboratories.

Repeat cytogenetic analyses from initially unsuccessful CVS demonstrate a higher incidence of aneuploidy than initially successful procedures (Donnenfeld et al. 1993). Preliminary results also suggest that failure of amniotic fluid cell growth may also be related to fetal aneuploidy (Persutte and Lenke 1995).

Cytogenetic results following CVS may be obscured by contamination of the sample by mosaicism and pseudomosaicism which occur in 1 and 0.4% of cases, respectively (Smidt-Jensen *et al.* 1993). Overall, amniotic fluid samples are about 10 times less often altered by inherent mosaicism problems than villous samples. The risk of fetal mosaicism when placental mosaicism is diagnosed by CVS is about 10% (Phillips *et al.* 1996). Patients should be counselled about the risk of mosaicism in CVS and be aware of the need in this case of follow-up amniocentesis or fetal blood sampling.

Multiple gestations

CVS is an efficient technique for first-trimester prenatal diagnosis in multiple pregnancies and carries in these cases no greater risk of pregnancy loss than that associated with singleton pregnancies (Pergament *et al.* 1992). The risk of amniocentesis in twin gestations has only been evaluated after 14 weeks.

Epidemiology of missed abortion

CVS in cases of intrauterine embryonic death provides the greatest chances of successfully obtaining a karyotype than other postmortem investigations (Johnson *et al.* 1990). From an epidemiological point of view and in the context of parental anxiety this represents a possible new application for CVS. However, as first trimester clinical miscarriage (which represents about 20% of clinical pregnancies) is associated with chromosomal abnormalities in 60–70% of cases, the value of routine CVS in these cases is questionable and certainly not financially justifiable for patients with only one episode. Indeed, the association between a chromosomally abnormal miscarriage and subsequent pregnancies affected by the same defect or another aneuploidy remains controversial and finding trisomy 21 which has an incidence of 1 in 800 newborns in the general population is probably coincidental.

References

Ammala, P., Hiilesmaa, V.K., Liukkonen, S., Saisto, T., Teramo, K. and Von Koskull, H. (1993) Randomized trial comparing first-trimester transcervical chorionic villus sampling and second-trimester amniocentesis. *Prenat Diagn* **13**, 919–27

Baird, P.A., Yee, I.M.L. and Sadovnick, A.D. (1994) Population-based study of long-term outcomes after amniocentesis. *Lancet* **344**, 1134–6

Barela, A.I., Kleinman, G.E., Golditch, I.M., Menke, D.J., Hogge, W.A. and Golbus, M.S. (1986) Septic shock with renal failure after chorionic villus sampling. *Am J Obstet Gynecol* **154**, 1100–2

Blakemore, K., Filkins, K., Luthy, D.A. *et al.* (1993) Cook obstetrics and gynecology catheter multicenter chorionic villus sampling trial: comparison of birth defects with expected rates. *Am J Obstet Gynecol* **169**, 1022–6

Boyd, P.A., Keeling, J.W., Selinger, M. and Mackenzie, I.Z. (1990) Limb reduction and chorion villus sampling. *Prenat Diagn* **10**, 437–41

Brambati, B. (1993) Genetic disorders: methods of avoiding the birth of an affected child. *Hum Reprod* **8**, 1983–2000

Brambati, B., Tului, L., Simoni, G. and Travi, M. (1988) Prenatal diagnosis at 6 weeks. *Lancet* **ii**, 397

Brambati, B., Simoni, G., Travi, M. *et al.* (1992) Genetic diagnosis by chorionic villus sampling before 8 gestational weeks: efficiency, reliability, and risks on 317 completed pregnancies. *Prenat Diagn* **12**, 789–99

Bronshtein, M. and Blumenfeld, Z. (1991) First- and early second-trimester oligohydramnios: a predictor of poor fetal outcome except in iatrogenic oligohydramnios post chorionic villus sampling. *Ultrasound Obstet Gynecol* **1**, 245–50

Brumfield, C.G., Lin, S., Connor, W., Cosper, P., Davis, R.O. and Owen, J. (1996) Pregnancy outcome following genetic amniocentesis at 11–14 versus 16–19 weeks' gestation. *Obstet Gynecol* **88**, 114–18

Burton, B.K., Schulz, C.J., Angle, B. and Burd, L.I. (1995) An increased incidence of haemangiomas in infants born following chorionic villus sampling (CVS). *Prenat Diagn* **15**, 209–14

Byrne, D., Marks, K., Azar, G. and Nicolaides, K. (1991) Randomized study of early amniocentesis versus chorionic villus sampling: A technical and cytogenetic comparison of 650 patients. *Ultrasound Obstet Gynecol* **1**, 235–40

Calhoun, B.C., Brehm, W. and Bombard, A.T. (1994) Early genetic amniocentesis and its relationship to respiratory difficulties in paediatric patients: a report of findings in patients and matched controls 3-5 years post-procedure. *Prenat Diagn* **14**, 209–12

Castilla, E.E., Cavalcanti, D.P., Dutra, M.G., Loez-Camelo, J.S., Paz, J.E. and Gadow, E.C. (1995) Limb reduction defects in South America. *Br J Obstet Gynaecol* **102**, 393–400

Crandall, B.F. and Chua, C. (1995) Detecting neural tube defects by amniocentesis between 11 and 15 weeks' gestation. *Prenat Diagn* **15**, 339–43

Donnenfeld, A.E., Librizzi, R.J., Weiner, S. and Bolognese, R.J. (1993) Increased risk of aneuploidy in women having unsuccessful chorionic villus sampling. *Br J Obstet Gynaecol* **100**, 826–7

Dumez, Y., Goosens, M., Poenaru, L. and Henrion, R. (1984) La biopsie de villosite choriale a la pince sous controle ultrasonore: technique et resultats. *J Genet Hum* **32**, 335–44

Elejade, B.R., de Elejade, M.M., Acuna, J.M., Thelen, D., Trujillo, C. and Karrmann, M. (1990) Prospective study of amniocentesis performed between weeks 9 and 16 of gestation: its feasibility, risks, complications and use in early prenatal diagnosis. *Am J Med Genet* **35**, 188–96

Evans, M.I., Drugan, A., Koppitch, F.C., Zador, I.E., Sacks, A.J. and Sokol, R.J. (1989) Genetic diagnosis in the first trimester: the norm for the 1990s. *Am J Obstet Gynecol* **160**, 1332–9

Firth, H.V., Boyd, P.A., Chamberlain, P., Mackenzie, I.Z., Lindenbaum, R.H. and Huson, S.M. (1991) Severe limb abnormalities after chorionic villus sampling at 56-66 days' gestation. *Lancet* **337**, 741–6

Firth, H.V., Boyd, P.A., Chamberlain, P., Mackenzie, I.Z., Morriss-Kay, G.M. and Huson, S.M. (1994). Analysis of limb reduction defects in babies exposed to chorionic villus sampling. *Lancet* **343**, 1069–71

Fisk, N.M. and Anderson, J.C. (1987) Avoidance of maternal morbidity in acute intrauterine infection following chorionic villus sampling. *Obstet Gynecol* **69**, 501–3

Froster, U.G. and Jackson, L. (1996) Limb defects and chorionic villus sampling: results from an international registry, 1992-94. *Lancet* **347**, 489–94

Goldstein, S.R. (1994) Embryonic death in early pregnancy: a new look at the first trimester. *Obstet Gynecol* **84**, 294–7

Gruppo Italiano Diagnosi Emrio-Fetali (1993) Transverse limb reduction defects after chorion villus sampling: a retrospective cohort study. *Prenat Diagn* **13**, 1051–6

Hackett, G.A., Smith, J.H., Rebello, M.T. *et al.* (1991) Early amniocentesis at 11–14 weeks' gestation for the diagnosis of fetal chromosomal abnormality: a clinical evaluation. *Prenat Diagn* **11**, 311–15

Hammarstrom, M. and Marsk, L. (1990) First trimester live pregnancy and subsequent loss: the impact of transcervical CVS and colonization of the cervix. *Gynecol Obstet Invest* **30**, 19–22

Hanson, F.W., Zorn, E.M., Tennant, F.R., Marianos, S. and Samuels, S. (1987). Amniocentesis before 15 weeks' gestation: outcome, risks and technical problems. *Am J Obstet Gynecol* **155**, 1524–31

Hislop, A. and Fairweather, I. (1982) Amniocentesis and lung growth: an animal experiment with clinical implications. *Lancet* **ii**, 1340–1

Hsieh, F.J., Shyu, M.K., Sheu, B.C., Lin, S.P., Chen, C.P. and Huang, F.Y. (1995). Limb defects after chorionic villus sampling. *Obstet Gynecol* **85**, 84–8

Jauniaux, E. and Rodeck, C. (1995) Use, risks and complications of amniocentesis and chorion villus sampling for prenatal diagnosis in early pregnancy. *Early Pregn Biol Med* **1**, 245–52

Jauniaux, E., Jurkovic, D., Gulbis, B., Gervy, C., Ooms, H.A. and Campbell, S. (1991) Biochemical composition of exocoelomic fluid in early human pregnancy. *Obstet Gynecol* **78**, 1124–8

Jauniaux, E., Burton, G.J. and Jones, C.P.J. (1992) 'Early human placental morphology' in E.Barnea, J. Hustin and E. Jauniaux (Eds) *The First Twelve Weeks of Gestation*, pp.45-64. Heidelberg: Springer-Verlag

Johnson, M.P., Drugan, A., Koppitch, F.C., Uhlmann, W.R. and Evans, M.I. (1990) Postmortem chorionic villi sampling is a better method for cytogenetic evaluation of early fetal loss than culture of abortus material. *Am J Obstet Gynecol* **163**, 1505–10

Jorgensen, F.S., Bang, J., Lind, A.M., Christensen, B., Lundsteen, C. and Philip, J. (1992) Genetic amniocentesis at 7–14 weeks of gestation. *Prenat Diagn* **12**, 277–83

Kennerknecht, I., Baur-Aubele, S., Grab, D. and Terinde, R. (1992) First trimester amniocentesis between the seventh and 13th weeks: evaluation of the earliest possible genetic diagnosis. *Prenat Diagn* **12**, 595–601

Kerber, S. and Held, K.R. (1993) Early genetic amniocentesis: 4 years' experience. *Prenat Diagn* **13**, 21–7

Lippman, A., Tomkins, D.J., Shime, J. and Hamerton, J.L. (1992) Canadian multicentre randomized clinical trial of chorion villus sampling and amniocentesis: final report. *Prenat Diagn* **12**, 385–476

Lockwood, D.H. and Neu, R.L. (1993) Cytogenetic analysis of 1375 amniotic fluid specimens from pregnancies with gestational age less than 14 weeks. *Prenat Diagn* **13**, 801–5

Maxwell, D., Lilford, R., Czepulkowski, B., Heaton, D. and Coleman, D. (1986) Transabdominal chorionic villus sampling. *Lancet* **i**, 123–6

MRC Working Party on the Evaluation of Chorion Villus Sampling (1991) Medical Research Council European trial of chorion villus sampling. *Lancet* **337**, 1491–9

Nicolaides, K., Brizot, M., Patel, F. and Snijders, R. (1994) Comparison of chorionic villus sampling and amniocentesis for fetal karyotyping at 10-13 weeks' gestation. *Lancet* **344**, 435–9

Nicolaides, K., Brizot, M., Patel, F. and Snijders, R. (1996) Comparison of chorion villus sampling and early amniocentesis for karyotyping in 1,492 singleton pregnancies. *Fetal Diagn Ther* **11**, 9–15

Palo, P., Piiroinen, O., Honkonen, E., Lakkala, T. and Aula, P. (1994) Transabdominal chorionic villus sampling and amniocentesis for prenatal diagnosis: 5 years' experience at a university centre. *Prenat Diagn* **14**, 157–62

Pandya, P.P., Snijders, R.J.M., Psara, N., Hibert, L. and Nicolaides, K.H. (1996) The prevalence of non-viable pregnancy at 10–13 weeks of gestation. *Ultrasound Obstet Gynecol* **7**, 170–3

Penso, C.H., Sandstrom, M.M., Garber, M.F., Ladoulis, M., Stryker, J.M. and Benacerraf, B.B. (1990) Early amniocentesis: report of 407 cases with neonatal follow-up. *Obstet Gynecol* **76**, 1032–6

Pergament, E., Schulman, J.D., Copeland, K. *et al.* (1992) The risk and efficacity of chorion villus sampling in multiple gestations. *Prenat Diagn* **12**, 377–84

Persutte, W.H. and Lenke, R.R. (1995) Failure of amniotic-fluid-cell growth: is it related to fetal aneuploidy. *Lancet* **345**, 96–7

Phillips, O.P., Tharapel, A.T., Lerner, J.L., Park, V.M., Wachtel, S.S. and Shulman, L.P. (1996) Risk of fetal mosaicism when placental mosaicism is diagnosed by chorionic villus sampling. *Am J Obstet Gynecol* **174**, 850–5

Popp, L.W. and Ghirardini, G. (1990) The role of transvaginal sonography in chorion villi sampling. *J Clin Ultrasound* **18**, 315–22

Rhoads, G.G., Jackson, L.G., Schlesselman, S.A. *et al.* (1989) The safety and efficacy of chorionic villus sampling for early prenatal diagnosis of cytogenetic abnormalities. *N Engl J Med* **320**, 609–17

Rodeck, C.H. (1993) Fetal development after chorionic villus sampling. *Lancet* **341**, 468–9

Rodeck, C.H., Morsman, J.M., Nicolaides, K.H., McKenzie, C., Gosden, C.M. and Gosden, J.R. (1983) A single operator technique for first trimester chorion biopsy. *Lancet* **ii**, 1340–1

Rodeck, C.H., Sheldrake, A., Beattie, B. and Whittle, M.J. (1993) Maternal serum alphafetoprotein after placental damage in chorionic villus sampling. *Lancet* **341**, 500

Shalev, E., Weiner, E., Yanai, N., Shneur, Y. and Cohen, H. (1994) Comparison of first-trimester transvaginal amniocentesis with chorionic villus sampling and mid-trimester amniocentesis. *Prenat Diagn* **14**, 279–83

Shulman, L.P., Elias, S., Phillips, O.P., Grevengood, C., Dungan, J.S. and Simpson, J.L. (1994) Amniocentesis performed at 14 weeks' gestation or earlier: comparison with first-trimester transabdominal chorionic villus sampling. *Obstet Gynecol* **83**, 543–8

Silver, R.K., Macgregor, S.N. and Hobart, E.D. (1992) Factors associated with multiple-pass procedures during chorionic villus sampling: a video analysis. *Prenat Diagn* **12**, 183–8

Silverman, N.S., Sullivan, M.W., Jungkind, D.L., Weinblatt, V., Beavis, K. and Wapner, R.J. (1994) Incidence of bacteremia associated with chorionic villus sampling. *Obstet Gynecol* **84**, 1021–4

Simoni, G., Brambati, B., Danesino, C. *et al.* (1983) Efficient direct chromosome analyses and enzyme determination from chorionic villi samples in the first trimester of pregnancy. *Hum Genet* **63**, 349–57

Smidt-Jensen, S. and Hahnemann, N. (1984) Transabdominal fine needle biopsy from chorionic villi in the first trimester. *Prenat Diagn* **4**, 163–9

Smidt-Jensen, S., Permin, M. and Philip, J. (1991) Sampling success and risk by transabdominal chorionic villus sampling, transcervical chorionic sampling and amniocentesis: a randomized study. *Ultrasound Obstet Gynecol* **1**, 86–90

Smidt-Jensen, S., Lind, A.M., Permin, M., Zachary, J.M., Lundsteen, C. and Philip, J. (1993) Cytogenetic analysis of 2928 CVS samples and 1075 amniocentesis from randomized studies. *Prenat Diagn* **13**, 723–40

Steele, M.W. and Breg, W.R. (1966) Chromosome analysis of human amniotic fluid cells. *Lancet* **i**, 383–5

Stripparo, L., Buscaglia, M., Longatti, L. *et al.* (1990) Genetic amniocentesis: 505 cases performed before the sixteenth week of gestation. *Prenat Diagn* **10**, 359–64

Sundberg, K., Smidt-Jensen, S. and Marsal, K. (1991) Amniocentesis with increased cell yield, obtained by filtration and reinjection of the amniotic fluid. *Ultrasound Obstet Gynecol* **1**, 91–5

Tabor, A., Philip, J., Madsen, M., Bang, J., Obel, E.B. and Nørgaard-Pedersen, B. (1986) Randomized controlled trial of genetic amniocentesis in 4606 low-risk women. *Lancet* **i**, 1287–93

Turnpenny, P.D., Hakim, M.M., Thwaites, R.J. *et al.* (1990) Oligohydramnios sequence in a live-born infant following chorionic villus sampling. *Prenat Diagn* **10**, 675–6

Wapner, R., Jackson, L., Evans, M. and Johnson, M.P. (1996) Limb reduction defects (LRD) are not increased following first trimester chorionic villus sampling (CVS). *Am J Obstet Gynecol* **174**, 310

Ward, R.H.T., Modell, B., Petrou, M., Karagozlu, F. and Douratsos, E. (1983) Method of sampling chorionic villi in the first trimester of pregnancy under guidance of real time ultrasound. *BMJ* **286**, 1542–4

Chapter 27

Invasive tests in the diagnosis of Down syndrome

Discussion

***

Simpson: Dr Jauniaux referred to one of the transvaginal papers as 'crazy', and I should perhaps respond. It is actually a very good technique to use in a retroflexed, retroverted uterus and it is probably much safer than some of the lateral transabdominal procedures in which we worry about hitting the maternal bowel. You might want to re-think that.

For historical accuracy, you will find that some of the early amniocentesis that Fritz Fuchs performed were not done intracervically, but were done by pulling the cervix down and going transvaginally into the amniotic cavity from a vaginal route as opposed to an abdominal route. They tried it several ways, but that was the most typical.

We ought to realise one thing about the Smidt-Jensen study which should not go uncorrected (Smidt-Jensen *et al.* 1992). That is that they were the developers of transabdominal CVS, and so the randomised study of amniocentesis versus transcervical and transabdominal routes came many years after they had had extensive experience in the transabdominal procedure. It is probably not fair to put in transcervical at the same time in that group since they have had far more experience in one technique than the other.

Another quick comment is that the group should be aware that there are two other ongoing randomised studies which will bear upon the question of safety in this area. The Canadians are conducting an early amniocentesis versus traditional amniocentesis randomised trial (Johnson *et al.* 1996). This is the only way you can have an early procedure in Canada, since they do not do CVS in Canada – thus, if you want an answer at ten or eleven weeks, this is the only way to obtain it. They are successfully randomising and we will have results from that in the next several years.

Finally, we in the US have just received funding from the NICHD to look at the window of 11–14 weeks' gestation, and there we will randomise early amniocentesis versus late CVS. The reason we chose 11–14 weeks is that we have a strong suspicion that the week by week variation will be tremendously important in terms of the safety of early amniocentesis. My prediction is that 13 and 14 will not be much different from 16 and 17, whereas that may or may not be the case for 11 to 12 weeks.

Barry-Kinsella: We have dismissed early amniocentesis far too easily out of hand. There is a great deal of evidence to suggest that when you include data such as the gauge of the needle, crossing the placenta, and the amount of liquor removed, and when you take those variables into consideration, early amniocentesis may be much safer than we are led to believe.

Jauniaux: This is a recent literature review. I have not found these data relating to the size of the needle and the liquor removed with the outcome of pregnancy in the very small group of patients who have been studied.

I would like to widen the debate to something else, and expand this investigating technique to remove the incidence of complication after amniocentesis at 12 weeks versus 14 weeks or 16 weeks, carried out by experienced operators, or more experienced in one technique than another.

We have to go back to basics because, if we introduce one of these screening programmes, either ultrasound or nuchal translucency or any other programme in a district general hospital, in a community hospital, the doctors there will feel that they have the right then to go on and perform the invasive procedures. Most of the registrars in this country have been to these hospitals, and one of the first questions I ask them when they come to the ante-natal clinic is how they perform amniocentesis? Most of the hospitals do not perform CVS, as has been said.

How do they perform amniocentesis? Most of the time, the registrar is sent during his first week on duty to the labour ward where amniocentesis is being performed. He watches a few, and then after a week he is able to do them himself. If early amniocentesis is not a serious risk – with a risk of 3% or 2.5% – this is not really an issue. This issue is, what is the risk in the general population? We should not focus on these specialised papers – I had to do so because it was the topic of my chapter – but we should really focus on the experience of the operator and set up a decent programme to ensure that the same quality of care is available to all the patients who undergo screening.

Harper: If we are to summarise what we have said in this session and make some recommendations from it, we would probably not be deciding that any one particular technique is better than another but that perhaps we should make some recommendations as you suggest about the training and experience of the operator.

Whittle: Just looking at amniocentesis, there are guidelines coming out from the College about amniocentesis and the need to do it under ultrasound control. Even the fact that there is a need for a guideline indicating that amniocentesis should be carried out under ultrasound control is in itself extraordinary in this day and age. But there is a need for that.

That document also indicates something about the requirements for training, and for the continuance of operator experience. It sometimes happens that doctors can perform only one, two or three a year, and the College has grasped that particular nettle about the need to identify training requirements and also the continuation of experience and skill. Those are important issues which we should underline from this group.

Macintosh: I would like to return to the issue of what the College expects for training requirements, and whether it will be in fetal medicine units in tertiary unit centres, or do they anticipate that the training will be adequate in district general hospitals? With our purchaser/provider situation, people are loathe to refer up to tertiary centres and therefore we must be looking at the training which will go ahead in the district general hospital.

I would also love to know the source of the figures of miscarriage rates of 3% and 4%. Are they attributable to the amniocentesis in the district general hospital? Is this published, and have we seen it? I become concerned when I see figures like that.

I know it is obvious that we should be using ultrasound when we are doing amniocentesis, but the only paper that we all talk about on risks is the randomised controlled trial from Denmark, which showed a 1% risk of miscarriage from amniocentesis in the younger women. Did she actually use ultrasound then? Was it direct ultrasound?

Whittle: [*Yes*]

Brambati: In my opinion, there are no problems in terms of danger to the patient if first trimester screening is to be done. The only invasive, well-established procedure evaluated at this time is CVS, done, as the study demonstrated, between 9 and 12 weeks, and the traditional amniocentesis at 15 or more weeks.

There should be another item included in the list of possibilities of earlier amniocentesis. Personally, I meet a lot of people to justify ethically the study that the Canadians are doing. I asked Dr Wilson, who heads it, how they justified doing it but he could not give me an answer. I would also like to ask my American friends what they will be able to do. I think Professor Simpson is rather sceptical about the possibilities, but basically, I read so-called informed consent that the American people will give the patient, and it is also what is written there – it is impossible following the logic of informed consent to justify the randomised study.

Simpson: You know that I am a big devotee of CVS and I do not need to defend my credentials in that area. I certainly would prefer that we do early CVS, probably followed by late CVS, followed by traditional amniocentesis. The reality is that that is not what is happening in the United States. The reality is that large numbers of individuals in their private offices have traditionally performed traditional amniocentesis. Some of the district hospitals were loathe to refer the patients out because they were losing money or they were being charged for specialist care, and so they are *de facto* performing the procedure, whether we like it or not, at 12 or 13 weeks.

This is really an effort, once and for all, to look to see whether or not our biases are correct, and early amniocentesis particularly at 11–12 weeks, will be as unsafe as you and I have suspected. My guess is that we may have a problem at 11–12 weeks, but I really doubt that we will have a problem at 14 weeks and probably at 13 weeks as well – if the patient is properly selected.

Reynolds: Since I am from a laboratory, it is probably terribly politically incorrect if I make comments about obstetrics. However, in the lab, if we do 50 tests a year, then it is actually better to refer it somewhere else. The anaesthetists in our hospital have the policy that as we do so few emergency paediatric cases there are only two designated anaesthetists.

Is it sensible for the group policy to say that if you do not more than 50 amniocenteses every year, then you should not be allowed to perform any? Is there a minimum limit which the College should advise?

Harper: I think we are recommending that.

Nicolaides: I hoped that early amniocentesis was going to be much better than CVS. I performed a study and showed it was disastrously worse. However, that study was one of the few that spent a great deal of time on the patients and methods. Usually, when we do studies, we do not say what the protocols are and the specific details. So people can now actually examine and find possible reasons for the different results.

There are two factors. One is the size of the needle, and I will always remain convinced that it is completely irrelevant. If you use a 20 gauge needle, you suck out the fluid much faster so that you finish earlier, and if you use a 29 gauge needle, it takes about 20 hours to suck it out so that the damage produced by doing this is much greater. I do not think the size of the needle is important.

What is important, however, and certainly from looking at the results of Dr Dornan in Belfast, is the logic that I had to desperately try to avoid the placenta whereas Jim Dornan got good results by definitely going through the placenta (Dornan, personal communication). I am aware of an extremely good study that will be published very soon from Denmark with Karen Sundberg who compared amniofiltration with CVS at the same gestation. Again, she deliberately went through the placenta (Sundberg, personal communication).

The most obvious cause of the much higher miscarriage rate from amniocentesis is the coelomic cavity – the membranes that are not yet stuck onto the uterus. If you go through the placenta, that is one place where the membranes have stuck, and in this way the results are much better. So there is perhaps a place for a controlled study.

The other factor which was very obvious from my results is that, as the pregnancy advances, the safety of amniocentesis becomes better. So perhaps at 14 or 15 weeks, they will be equally good as with CVS.

Harper: Certainly in a study we are currently performing in Belfast with 285 completed pregnancies, we had eight miscarriages less than four weeks after the procedure and in none of them was the placenta traversed. There may well be something in that. I would comment that we are quite selective in choosing patients for the procedure: we do not perform the procedure on someone who is already bleeding heavily. I think some of Professor Nicolaides' patients were actively bleeding at the time.

Nicolaides: For me, bleeding is an indication, not a contraindication for fetal karyotyping.

Simpson: I would add that in the US study, there is a safety committee, as there has been in our previous studies, which is independent of the investigators. It has access to the data and can stop the study as a whole, at any week of gestation, at any time that the data indicate that there is an early problem. We are certainly cognisant of what the results could be.

Harper: Thank you very much, Dr Jauniaux and all the discussants.

References

Johnson, J.M., Wilson, R.D., Winsor, E.J.T., Singer, J., Dansereau, J. and Kalousek, D.K. (1996) The early amniocentesis study: a randomized clinical trial of early amniocentesis versus midtrimester amniocentesis. *Fetal Diagn Therapy* **11**, 85–93

Smidt-Jensen, S., Permin, M., Philip, J. *et al.* (1992) Randomised comparison of amniocentesis and transabdominal and transcervical chorionic villus sampling. *Lancet* **340**, 1237–44

SECTION 8

COUNSELLING ABOUT RISK ASSESSMENT

Chapter 28

What risks should be given?

Mary C.M. Macintosh

The definition of risk is 'the chance of a bad outcome'. The objective of giving a 'risk' is to provide information to enable an individual to make an informed decision of the future course of the pregnancy and in this case usually the potential of avoiding the birth of a Down syndrome baby.

History of 'quoting risks associated with Down syndrome'

The association of raised maternal age and Down syndrome (DS) was first described by Shuttleworth (1909). The extra G chromosome in DS was discovered in 1959 by both Lejeune *et al.* and Jacobs *et al.* and subsequently identified as chromosome 21. Antenatal diagnosis by amniocentesis was introduced in the early 1970s and in keeping with a new technology was offered to those deemed to be at highest risk. By the early 1980s all health regions in the United Kingdom offered amniocentesis to women with age limits varying between 35 and 40.

The 'serendipitous' discovery of the association of low alpha fetoprotein with chromosomally abnormal pregnancies (Merkatz *et al.* 1984) and subsequently other markers in particular human chorionic gonadotrophin (hCG) and oestriol along with the concept of converting biochemical measurements into a risk value (Baumgarten 1985) enabled statistical models to be developed which predicted that 65% of cases of Down syndrome would be detected for a 5% screen positive rate (Cuckle *et al.* 1987; Palomaki and Haddow 1987). The first prospective studies evaluating these predictions were underway in 1989 and summarised by the RCOG working party in 1993.

Since the early 1990s ultrasound measurement of fetal nuchal translucency thickness has been used to provide an individual risk for Down syndrome and aneuploidies. Controversy has existed over whether this is an effective method of screening (Bewley1996; Mol *et al.* 1996) with some studies not reproducing the results (Roberts *et al.* 1995; Bewley *et al.* 1995; Zimmermann *et al.* 1996) that have been found by others (Szabo *et al.* 1992; Savoldelli *et al.* 1993; Snijders *et al.* 1996). The predominant arguments against this technology centre around poor reproducibility of the measurement and the preponderance of the initial findings based at a tertiary referral centre rather than in an unselected population.

The derivation of a risk factor from measurement of the nuchal translucency like that of biochemistry has been refined over time. Adjustment factors include the crown–rump length and fetal heart rate.

Provision of risk based on biochemical screening

There are no official statistics on the provision of Down syndrome screening policies but surveys recording uptake have been carried out among health authorities and laboratories performing the tests. These show that in 1991 about one-third of pregnant women were undergoing screening (Wald *et al.* 1992) and that by 1994 this proportion had risen to around one-half (Wald *et al.* 1996). Uptake reflects both availability and acceptance by the individual. However, the majority but not all districts provide a prenatal screening service for Down syndrome to younger women (Wald *et al.* 1996).

Biochemical screening in comparison with raised maternal age screening is a more efficient way of detecting Down syndrome from the objective of number of cases detected for a fixed number of invasive tests. However, the choice to provide such screening in the United Kingdom depends on agreements between the purchaser and provider who prioritise the provision of health service. This from one perspective enables the health professional to protect patients from what may appear to be an inappropriate desire for knowledge but also allows health professionals to impose their views of the value of prenatal diagnosis on their patient.

Age restricted policies

The initial statistical concept of screening was based on offering the test to the entire maternity population. Since then some have argued from a cost perspective that it may be advantageous to restrict screening to the 'thirties and over' (Fletcher *et al.* 1995). A survey of laboratories belonging to the National External Quality Assurance Scheme (NEQAS) which is a voluntary scheme to which the majority of laboratories in the United Kingdom subscribe reported that 14% (10/72) had some form of age restricted policy within their hospitals. There was no consistent choice of age restriction which ranged from offering the test to: 'older women' only where the 'older' was 25, 29, 30, 35 and 36 and above; to 'younger women' only where 'younger' was 38 and less; and to defined age ranges such as 27–36 years (Macintosh *et al.* submitted). The commonly quoted '65% detection rate for a 5% screen positive rate' will no longer apply if the screening is applied to an age-restricted population. This is due to the change in the denominator population. For example, assuming a fixed cut-off of around 1 in

250 offering the test to the 'over thirties' will result in approximately 20% of those taking the test being classified as screen positive.

Provision of risk based on ultrasound screening

Analogous to the situation with biochemistry there are no official statistics regarding the provision of nuchal translucency screening within the UK. Most reports originate from the Harris Birthright centre where the risk is computed after measurement of the nuchal translucency, the crown–rump length and fetal heart rate. These values are entered into a software package which calculates the corresponding likelihood ratios and subsequently adjusts the age specific rates. To date this approach has been formally evaluated in 19 district general hospitals (Snijders *et al.* 1996). However, the original publications described likelihood ratios for varying measurements of nuchal fold thickness and this lesser refined application may be used in other units. The effectiveness of the latter approach is debatable.

Precision and accuracy of risk values

Age-specific risks

Initially maternal age risks were cited only for five-year intervals so there was no distinction in risk made between a 35- and a 39-year-old women. The need to provide improved genetic counselling and cost–benefit analysis of prenatal diagnosis programmes acted as the stimuli for estimation of age-specific incidences. These were first presented by Hook and Chambers (1977) and were based on birth certificate data of white babies in New York. Subsequently there have been numerous other live birth studies estimating age-specific risks in Down syndrome and eight of these have been combined to give a more precise estimate (Cuckle *et al.* 1987). Although there was a degree of variation in the risks (for example between 1/272 and 1/491 at the age of 35 years) the numerical risk was stressed less than the maternal age in defining the boundary cut-off.

Current risk estimates of Down syndrome live births may be higher than in earlier studies because of better perinatal care than 20 years ago (Halliday *et al.* 1995).

Biochemical adjusted risks

With the advent of biochemical screening the numerical risk has taken on a greater apparent importance. Prior to this, maternal age tended to define the boundary cut-off for offering invasive testing. The correctness of the categorisation into a screen-positive and screen-negative group depends not only on the methods used for adjustment of the observed biochemical markers but also on the initial maternal age specific rate used for calculation. Neither figure is an absolute but is an estimate of the true value. The precision of a test result refers to the repeatability of the result. Confidence intervals or standard errors are the general method of expressing precision and are applicable to commonly used measurements such as a mean or a proportion of a sample. However, no such equivalent calculation exists for the individual risk value resulting and so the theoretical precision of the risk value is illusory.

Reproducibility within the population

This refers to assessment of the performance of the screening test when applied to an unselected population. To date there have been 17 prospective studies which when combined include 389 cases of DS and 279 000 screened women (Cuckle 1996). The detection rate is 257/389 (66%) for a 4.5% false positive rate. The positive predictive value (the average chance in all those designated as screen positive) is 1 in 48 and negative predictive value (average chance in those designated as screen negative) is 1 in 1900 (Cuckle 1996).

Reproducibility within the individual

Although the theoretical precision of the risk is illusory, the reproducibility of the risk result for an individual may be assessed by sending the same blood sample to different laboratories, a process performed by NEQAS. They have demonstrated wide spreads in reported risk values (coefficient of variation 46%). For example, a sample sent to 19 laboratories using AFP and intact hCG as markers found a range between 1 in 115 and 1 in 550 (Seth and Ellis 1994). Choice of cut-off varies between laboratories and coupled with the variation in calculated risk results in a lack of consensus in the classification into high or low risk (Seth and Ellis 1994).

The accuracy of an individual test refers to how near the correct value the result is. For example, in a group of 250 women given the risk of 1 in 250 an 'accurate' test will result in one affected pregnancy. To determine this requires a database of the outcomes of large numbers of tested pregnancies which involves an enormous administrative effort which is not feasible in the majority of laboratories. Thus the accuracy of the test for an individual risk value remains unproven.

There is little information regarding the repeatability of the risk result in the same individual. Selective repeat testing has not been thought to substantially improve screening efficiency and correlation coefficients between the three markers in 142 paired samples are described (Cuckle *et al.* 1994).

Ultrasound adjusted risks

The same issues also pertain to the risk calculated from nuchal translucency screening.

Reproducibility within populations

Concerns have focused around the issue of the setting of the study in a tertiary referral centre where the higher prevalence of affected pregnancies, sophistication of ultrasound equipment and operator skill may derive optimistic results not able to be extrapolated to other more general settings (Roberts *et al.* 1995; Bewley *et al.* 1995). Studies failing to reproduce the results in unselected populations (Bewley *et al.* 1995; Hafner *et al.* 1995) are based on three and four cases of Down syndrome, respectively. They are too small to either prove or refute the efficiency of nuchal translucency derived risk as a screening test for Down syndrome. The first (the University College Hospital, UCH study) used a cut off of ≥3 mm and three cases of Down syndrome in an unselected population of 1127 women. Only one of the three cases had a nuchal translucency greater than 3 mm (Bewley *et al.* 1995). The second (the Austrian study) was based on a cut off of ≥2.5 mm and four cases of Down syndrome in an unselected population of 1972 women. Two of the four cases were identified (Hafner *et al.* 1995). The largest multicentre study involving 19 district general hospitals with 43 cases of Down syndrome and 22 076 women (Pandya *et al.* 1995; Snijders *et al.* 1996). Using a risk of 1 in 100 or greater, as determined by measurement of the nuchal translucency as a proportion of the crown–rump length, 28 of the 43 cases (68%) were 'screen positive' and overall there was a 2% (518/22,706) screen-positive rate.

Reproducibility within the individual

The contribution of operator variability has been addressed. The intra-observer and inter-observer variation was less than 0.54 mm and 0.62 mm in 95% of the 200 cases, respectively. The caliper placement was described as accounting for most of the variation rather than the image generation (Pandya *et al.* 1995). There is no comment on the effect on risk assessment. The latter was addressed in the University College Hospital study where by repeating the measurements with a different operator, the same operator using a different still image or the same operator using the same still image 18.8%, 17.5% or 12.4% (of 43 fetuses) changed their classification of normal or abnormal where the cut off was 3 mm (Roberts *et al.* 1995).

Quality control of risk values

The National External Quality Assurance Scheme has existed since 1989 and the majority but not necessarily all laboratories providing biochemical screening belong. There is a large variation in workload ranging from under 1000 to over 10 000 tests annually. The existence of this scheme enables estimates of the uptake of screening services, reviews of the variation in practice and identification of quality control issues with respect to the production of the biochemical risk value.

The equivalent to quality control for ultrasound-adjusted risk is the Fetal Medicine Foundation, a registered charity, with the objective of training and audit of the implementation of nuchal translucency screening. Polaroid photos of nuchal measurements are assessed looking at aspects such as calliper placement and magnification of image. It is possibly unfortunate that the provision of the necessary quality control is by the pioneer of the technology as it may be, rightly or wrongly, considered to be non-objective.

Combining ultrasound and biochemical risk

Adjusting second trimester biochemical risks

Ultrasound findings have been used in the second trimester to adjust biochemical risks. However, the accuracy of the adjusting factors remains problematical. Meta-analysis of second trimester ultrasonography findings in Down syndrome pregnancies has been attempted (Vintzileos and Egan 1995). The presence of a normal scan reduced the biochemical risk by a factor of 10. However, the appropriateness of this technique in the light of unexplained heterogeneity of the combined studies should and has been questioned (Palomaki and Haddow 1995). In practice a half (9/18) of Down syndrome cases in 395 women with screen positive biochemistry had normal ultrasonography (Nyberg *et al.* 1995).

Given the variation in biological variability and scanning expertise the ability to accurately adjust the risk value seems unlikely to be introduced. Caution should be applied in the degree of reassurance that a normal second trimester scan has for a women with an increased biochemical risk.

Combining biochemistry with nuchal translucency risk

The most promising first trimester markers for Down syndrome pregnancies are pregnancy-associated plasma protein A (PAPP-A) and free beta human chorionic gonadotropin (free β-hCG). Initial studies have found no significant relationship between fetal nuchal translucency thickness and serum PAPP-A or free β-hCG in either affected or unaffected pregnancies (Brizot *et al.* 1994, 1995; Zimmermann *et al.* 1996), implying that the biochemical and ultrasound risks may be combined.

Serial risks

The relationship between ultrasound findings and biochemistry remain uncertain. There are insufficient data regarding their dependence or independence. Serial testing rather than combining the risks will necessarily increase the screen-positive rate with a limited increase in detection rates. From a population perspective this is inefficient, however from an individual's perspective (especially those wishing to avoid invasive testing) this approach may serve as a pragmatic approach to the decision of whether to proceed or not to further testing.

Risk at different gestations

Initial age-related risks were derived from birth studies and so referred to the likelihood of an affected baby at term. Subsequent amniocentesis and chorionic villus data have enabled age-specific risks for earlier stages of pregnancy to be derived in older women. Meta-analysis of published studies provide the most precise risks (Table 28.1) (Snijders *et al.* 1994; Macintosh *et al.* 1995).

Risks in women aged 20–35 years for early pregnancy are estimated from birth risks adjusted by the miscarriage rates of Down syndrome pregnancies and are based on the assumption that fetal loss rates are independent of age. The latter have been estimated by comparison of the prevalence at 10 weeks, 16 weeks and at term. The loss rates between the time of CVS and amniocentesis have been estimated at approximately 31% and between CVS and term at 53% (Snijders *et al.* 1994; Halliday *et al.* 1995; Macintosh *et al.* 1996). Lesser loss rates (corresponding to 17% and 32%) have been estimated by Halliday and colleagues (1995), using the Perinatal Data Collection Unit in Victoria, Australia. They attribute their lower figures to the better perinatal care resulting in a higher live birth prevalence of Down syndrome than in the original birth studies 20 years ago.

The risk figures at different stages may be useful if women want to know their risks of a Down syndrome fetus being detected by a prenatal diagnostic test. A review of biochemical report forms has demonstrated inconsistency and at times confusion over which gestation the risk is referring to (Macintosh *et al.* 1996). In an already perplexing topic it would seem reasonable to standardise the approach of citing risks and so it would seem most appropriate to cite only term risks since this could be deemed to be ultimately the most relevant figure.

Risks of other aneuploidies

Although the primary purpose of screening was the detection of Down syndrome there is a significant chance that another unexpected chromosome abnormality is detected. Trisomy 21 accounted for 51.1% (613/1200) of all chromosome aberrations in the large European Collaborative study of amniocentesis (Ferguson-Smith and Yates 1984). Trisomy 18 (121/1200; 10.1%) was the next most frequent. Similar trends occur in chorionic villus sampling where 48.8% (79/162) were trisomy 21 and 13.6% (22/162) were trisomy 18 (Snijders 1993). The difficulties in counselling and prediction of the fetal phenotype with the other autosomal and sex chromosome arrangements is as likely to occur as that of a trisomy 21 pregnancy.

Trisomy 18

There is no equivalent to the Down syndrome national cytogenetic register but crude estimates from the Oxford Human Genetic and Chromosome Anomaly Register suggest there are less than 100 cases in England and Wales annually. The six month survival of trisomy 18 is 5% (Goldstein and Nielsen 1988). It appears that a greater proportion of trisomy 18 are detected prenatally than trisomy 21 (Oxford Human Genetic and Chromosome Anomaly Register). This is likely to be due to more obvious ultrasound markers present in this condition. Thus for such an infrequent lethal condition laboratories routinely offering risks for this condition should monitor their screen positive rates and positive predictive value of karyotyping. Assuming a detection rate of 65% of trisomy 18 cases then to keep the number of amniocenteses down to 50 to 1 the screen positive rate has to be less than 0.5%. A recent survey of the 75 laboratories registered with NEQAS in 1995 found that only four laboratories routinely provided a risk for trisomy 18 but that 30 laboratories would notify the clinician if they thought the risk was high (Macintosh et al. 1996). There was a variety of methods used to classify high risk for Edwards' syndrome. From the 25 reporting details 12 calculated a risk and used a cut-off between 1 in 50 and 1 in 600. The remainder look for unexpectedly low results and suggest follow-up if the multiples of the normal median (MoM) of all the analytes are below some defined limit (range 0.2–0.5 MoMs).

Provision of risk in multiple pregnancies

A 'pseudo-risk' may be calculated for twin pregnancies from the biochemical measurements. The level of the analyte in a series of unaffected twin pregnancies was compared with unaffected singleton pregnancies and this factor is used to modify the measured serum values and provide the 'pseudo-risk' (Wald and Densem 1994). If the latter is above the cut-off then the pregnancy is considered to be 'at risk' although an accurate figure is not possible. This publication

Table 28.1. Odds of having a Down syndrome pregnancy at the time of CVS (about 10 weeks' gestation), at amniocentesis (about 16 weeks' gestation) and at term (Macintosh et al. 1995)

Maternal age (completed years)	CVS	Amniocentesis	At term
35	1:208	1:218	1:384
36	1:156	1:177	1:307
37	1:117	1:144	1:242
38	1: 87	1:117	1:189
39	1: 65	1: 95	1:146
40	1: 49	1: 77	1:112
41	1: 36	1: 63	1: 85
42	1: 27	1: 51	1: 65
43	1: 20	1: 41	1: 49
44	1: 15	1: 33	1: 37
45	1: 11	1: 27	1: 28
46	1: 8	1: 22	1: 21
47	1: 6	1: 18	1: 15
48	§	§	1: 11
49	§	1: 11	1: 8

§ risk not estimated as no cases of Down syndrome were observed.

provided estimates of false-positive rates but not of detection rates. No pro-spective experience of this has been reported. Statistical modelling predicts that by using this method an overall detection rate of 53% of all twin pregnancies (73% monozygotic and 43% dizygotic) would be made for a 5% screen-positive rate (Neveux *et al.* 1996).

Ultrasound has the advantage of being able to give risks according to each fetus present. The detection rates for trisomy 21 appear to be similar to that in singleton pregnancies but the specificity is lower because the translucency is also increased in chromosomally normal monochorionic twin pregnancies (Sebire *et al.* 1996). However, prenatal diagnosis and its consequences in a twin pregnancy is a considerably more complex issue than in a singleton.

Other risk information

To enable a balanced decision the risks of the invasive procedure need to be known. Figures based on published studies may be quoted which will not necessarily reflect local practice. Loss rates attributable to amniocentesis range between 0.5 and 1%, whereas those attributable to CVS range between 0.5 and 2%. The accuracy will depend on whether this is based on local audit or not. Other aspects which should be mentioned include the chance of an unexpected chromosome anomaly and problems of interpretation of the karyotype such as mosaicism.

Framing of risk

The screening process offers uncertainty. The most that can be offered is possible outcomes and their probable occurrence. The language of figures is fraught with ambiguity. There is a lack of consensus among practitioners regarding the level of probability of 'high' and 'low' (Parsons and Atkinson 1992). The severity of the disorder can affect the perception of the actual risk figure, and a low risk of a severe disorder may be actually seen as a high risk (Frets *et al.* 1990). The actual figure may be of less concern to the patient than the fact that they are in a state of being 'at risk' (Lippman-Hand and Fraser 1979).

There is increasing evidence that the way in which the numerical results are expressed has a significant influence on: physicians' willingness to prescribe drugs (Naylor *et al.* 1992; Forrow *et al.* 1992; Bobbio *et al.* 1994; Bucher *et al.* 1994); patients' perception of benefit from treatment (Malenka *et al.* 1993) and health purchasing decisions (Fahey *et al.* 1995). Applying these principles to the description of a woman's individual risk it is likely that the nature of the presen-tation influences her decision. For example, a 33-year-old woman has an age-related risk of the birth of a Down syndrome baby of 1:600 and subsequently her biochemistry measurements result in an adjustment of 1:300. The information given to her may be: your risk is 1:300 which is considered to be low risk; your risk is 1:300 which is classified as screen negative; you are twice as likely as a woman your age to have a child with Down syndrome. The latter is describing the relative risk which may magnify the likelihood of the condition especially when the incidence of the event is infrequent.

Future work will involve structuring the information process, identifying areas of inconsistency in its provision and systematically assessing the effects of varying the presentation form.

Conclusions

Although there is ample evidence of the efficacy of biochemical screening, in practice there is wide variation in the quality of the production of the risk. Similar issues pertain to risk derived from nuchal translucency measurements. There is a need to provide and demonstrate a quality control of the technology producing the risk value. Paralleling this is the equally important requirement to develop a quality control system for the information process and its delivery.

References

Baumgarten, A. (1985) AFP screening and Down syndrome. *Lancet* **i**, 751

Bewley, S. (1996) Screening of fetal trisomies by maternal age and fetal nuchal translucency thickness at 10 to 14 weeks of gestation. *Br J Obstet Gynaecol* **103**, 1054

Bewley, S., Roberts, L.J., Mackinson, A.-M. and Rodeck, C.H. (1995) First trimester fetal nuchal translucency: Problems with screening the general population. *Br J Obstet Gynaecol* **102**, 386–8

Bobbio, M., Demichelis, B. and Giustetto, G. (1994) Completeness of reporting trial results: effect on physicians' willingness to prescribe. *Lancet* **343**, 1209–11

Brizot, M.L., Snijders, R.JM., Bersinger, N.A., Kuhn, P. and Nicolaides, K.H. (1994) Maternal serum pregnancy-associated plasma protein A and fetal nuchal translucency thickness for the prediction of fetal trisomies in early pregnancy. *Obstet Gynecol* **84**, 918–22

Brizot, M.L., Snijders, R.J.M., Butler, J., Bersinger, N.A. and Nicolaides, K.H. (1995) Maternal serum hCG and fetal nuchal translucency thickness for the prediction of fetal trisomies in the first trimester of pregnancy. *Br J Obstet Gynaecol* **102**, 31–4

Bucher, H.C., Weinbacher, M. and Gyr, K. (1994) Influence of method of reporting study results on decision of physicians to prescribe drugs to lower cholesterol concentration. *BMJ* **309**, 761–4

Cuckle, H. (1996) Established markers in second trimester maternal serum. *Early Hum Dev* **47**, S27–9

Cuckle, H.S., Wald, N.J. and Thompson, S.G. (1987) Estimating a woman's risk of having a pregnancy associated with Down's syndrome using her age and maternal serum alpha-fetoprotein level. *Br J Obstet Gynaecol* **94**, 387–402

Cuckle, H., Densem, J. and Wald, N. (1994) Repeat maternal serum testing in multiple marker Down's syndrome screening programmes. *Prenat Diagn* **14**, 603–7

Fahey, T., Griffiths, S. and Peters, T.J. (1995) Evidence based purchasing: understanding results of clinical trials and systematic reviews. *BMJ* **311**, 1056–60

Ferguson-Smith, M.A. and Yates, J.R.W. (1984) Maternal age specific rates for chromosome aberrations and factors influencing them. Report of a collaborative European Study on 52,965 amniocentesis. *Prenat Diagn* **45**, 43–8

Fletcher, J., Hicks, N.R., Kay, J.D.S. and Boyd, P.A. (1995) Using decision analysis to compare policies for antenatal screening for Down's syndrome. *BMJ* **311**, 351–6

Forrow, L., Taylor, W. and Arnold, R. (1992) Absolutely relative: how research results are summarised can effect treatment decisions. *Am J Med* **92**, 121–4

Frets, P.G., Duivenvoorden, H.J., Verhage, F. *et al.* (1990) Factors influencing the reproductive decision after genetic counselling. *Am J Med Genet* **35**, 496–502

Goldstein, H. and Nielsen, K. (1988) Rates and survival of individuals with trisomy 13 and 18: data from a 10 year period in Denmark. *Clin Genet* **34**, 366–72

Hafner, E., Schuchter, K. and Phillip, K. (1995) Screening for chromosomal abnormalities in an unselected population by fetal nuchal translucency. *Ultrasound Obstet Gynecol* **6**, 330–3

Halliday, J.L., Watson, L.F., Lumley, J., Danks, D.M. and Sheffield, L.J. (1995) New estimates of Down syndrome risks at chorionic villus sampling, amniocentesis, and livebirth in women of advanced maternal age from a uniquely defined population. *Prenat Diagn* **15**, 455–65

Hook, E.B. and Chambers, G.M. (1977) Estimated rates of Down syndrome in live births by one year maternal age intervals for mothers aged 20–49 in a New York State study – implications of the risk figures for genetic counselling and cost benefit analysis of prenatal diagnosis programs. *Birth Defects: Original Article Series* XIII **34**, 123–41

Jacobs, P., Baikie, A., Court-Brown, W. and Strong, J. (1959) The somatic chromosomes in Mongolism. *Lancet* **i**, 710

Lejeune, J., Gautier, M. and Turpin, R. (1959) Les chromosomes humains en culture de tissus. *CR Acad Sci* **248**, 602

Lippman-Hand, A. and Fraser, F.C. (1979) Genetic counselling – the post counselling period: 1. Parents' perceptions of uncertainty. *Am J Med Genet* **4**, 51–71

Macintosh, M.C.M., Wald, N., Chard, T., *et al.* (1995) The selective miscarriage of Down's syndrome from 10 weeks onwards *Br J Obstet Gynaecol* **102**, 798–801

Macintosh, M.C.M., Wald, N., Chard, T. *et al.* (1996) The selective miscarriage of Down's syndrome from 10 weeks of pregnancy (letter). *Br J Obstet Gynaecol* **103**, 1172–3

Malenka, D.J., Baron, J.A., Johansen, S., Wahrenberger, J.W. and Ross, J.M. (1993) The framing effect of relative and absolute risk. *J Gen Intern Med* **8**, 543–8

Merkatz, I., Nitowsky, H., Macri, J. and Johnson, W. (1984) An association between low maternal serum a-fetoprotein and fetal chromosomal abnormalities. *Am J Obstet Gynecol* **148**, 886–94

Mol, B.W., Pajkrt, E., van Lith, J.J.M. and Bilardo, C.M. (1996) Screening for fetal trisomies by maternal age and fetal nuchal translucency thickness at 10 to 14 weeks of gestation. *Br J Obstet Gynaecol* **103**, 1051–2

Naylor, C.D., Chen, E. and Strauss, B. (1992) Measured enthusiasm: does the method of reporting trial results alter perception of therapeutic effectiveness? *Ann Intern Med* **117**, 916–21

Neveux, L.M., Palomaki, G.E., Knight, G.J. and Haddow, J.E. (1996) Multiple marker screening for Down syndrome in twin pregnancies. *Prenat Diagn* **16**, 29–34

Nyberg, D.A., Luthy, D.A., Cheng, E.Y., Sheley, R.C., Resta, R.G. and Williams, M.A. (1995) Role of prenatal ultrasonography in women with positive screen for Down syndrome on the basis of maternal serum markers. *Am J Obstet Gynecol* **173**, 1030–5

Palomaki, G. and Haddow, J. (1987) Maternal serum α fetoprotein, age and Down syndrome risk. *Am J Obstet Gynecol* **156**, 460–3

Palomaki, G.E. and Haddow, J.E. (1995) Can the risk for Down syndrome be reliably modified by second-trimester ultrasonography? *Am J Obstet Gynecol* **173**, 1639–40

Pandya, P.P., Altman, D., Brizot, M.L., Pettersen, H. and Nicolaides, K.H. (1995) Repeatability of measurement of fetal nuchal translucency thickness. *Ultrasound Obstet Gynecol* **5**, 334–7

Pandya, P.P., Goldberg, H., Walton, B. *et al.* (1995) The implementation of first-trimester scanning at 10–13 weeks' gestation and the measurement of fetal nuchal translucency thickness in two maternity units. *Ultrasound Obstet Gynecol* **5**, 20–5

Parsons, E.P. and Atkinson, P.A. (1992) Lay construction of genetic risk. *Soc Health Illness* **14**, 437–55

Roberts, L.J., Bewley, S., Mackinson, A.M. and Rodeck, C.H. (1995) First trimester fetal nuchal translucency: problems with screening the general population. *Br J Obstet Gynaecol* **102**, 381–5

Royal College of Obstetricians and Gynaecologists (1993) *Report of the RCOG Working Party on Biochemical Markers and the Detection of Down's Syndrome*. London: RCOG Press

Savoldelli, G., Binkert, F., Achermann, J. and Schmid, W. (1993) Ultrasound screening for chromosomal anomalies in the first trimester of pregnancy. *Prenat Diagn* **13**, 513–18

Sebire, N.J., Snijders, R.J.M., Hughes, K., Sepulveda, W. and Nicolaides, K.H. (1996) Screening for trisomy 21 in twin pregnancies by gestational age and fetal nuchal translucency thickness at 10–14 weeks of gestation. *Br J Obstet Gynaecol* **103**, 999–1003

Seth, J. and Ellis, A.R. (1994) 'The United Kingdom National External Quality Assessment Scheme for screening for Down's syndrome' in J.G. Grudzinskas, T. Chard, M. Chapman and H. Cuckle (Eds) *Screening for Down's Syndrome*. Cambridge: Cambridge University Press

Shuttleworth, G.E. (1909) Mongolian imbecility. *BMJ* **2**, 661

Snijders, R.J.M. (1993) Screening by ultrasound for fetal chromosomal abnormalities. Thesis. Elinkwijk BV, Utrecht, The Netherlands

Snijders, R.J.M., Holzgreve, W., Cuckle, H. and Nicolaides, K.H. (1994) Maternal age-specific risks for trisomies at 9–14 weeks' gestation. *Prenat Diagn* **14**, 543–52

Snijders, R.J.M., Johnson, S., Sebire, N.J., Noble, P.L. and Nicolaides, K.H. (1996) First-trimester ultrasound screening for chromosomal defects. *Ultrasound Obstet Gynecol* **7**, 216–26

Szabò, J., Gellén, J. and Szemere, G. (1992) First trimester aneuploid fetuses. Screening by vaginosonography. (Abstract) *Prenat Diagn* **12**, (Suppl) S153

Vintzileos, A.M. and Egan, J.F.X. (1995) Adjusting the risk for trisomy 21 on the basis of second trimester ultrasonography. *Am J Obstet Gynecol* **172**, 837–44

Wald, N.J. and Densem, J.W. (1994) Maternal serum free beta-human chorionic gonadotrophin levels in twin pregnancies: implications for screening for Down's syndrome. *Prenat Diagn* **14**, 19–20

Wald, N.J., Cuckle, H., Hu, T. and George, L. (1991) Maternal serum unconjugated oestriol and human chorionic gonadotropin levels in twin pregnancies: implications for screening for Down's syndrome. *Br J Obstet Gynaecol* **98**, 905–8

Wald, N., Wald, K. and Smith, D. (1992) The extent of Down's syndrome screening in Britain in 1991. *Lancet* **340**, 494

Wald, N.J., Huttly, W., Wald, K. and Kennard, A. (1996) Down's syndrome screening in UK [letter]. *Lancet* **347**, 330

Zimmermann, R., Hucha, A., Savoldelli, G., Binkert, F., Achermann, J. and Grudzinskas, J.G. (1996) Serum parameters and nuchal translucency in first trimester screening for fetal chromosomal abnormalities. *Br J Obstet Gynaecol* **103**, 1009–14

Chapter 29

Communicating risk information: gaps between policy and practice

Theresa M. Marteau

Screening for Down syndrome involves determining the probability that a fetus is affected by the condition. Over the past 20 years this has been done on the basis of maternal age, those older than 35 years of age and hence with higher risk being offered amniocentesis. Developments in biochemistry and ultrasound now provide additional, more precise methods of prediction. One of the key issues surrounding these new tests is how best to inform women about the tests and their results. The aim of this chapter is to address this issue. Following discussion of what comprises risk information and the purpose of providing it to pregnant women, the next section considers how health professionals provide such information and how women respond to it. Given that there are as yet no published data concerning communication of risk information during first trimester screening for Down syndrome, this section draws on research conducted on prenatal screening conducted during the second trimester. The next section considers optimal methods of providing risk information about Down syndrome. The final section considers why, despite evidence of poor communication, these methods are not being incorporated into screening programmes for Down syndrome.

Risk information

Risk entails two key components: uncertainty and a negative event (Brun 1994). Communicating about risks of Down syndrome therefore involves communicating about the chance of Down syndrome occurring in a pregnancy as well as about Down syndrome itself.

Purpose of providing risk information

The great majority of reports on serum screening for Down syndrome and other tests for fetal abnormality in pregnancy emphasise the importance of providing good information to allow women and their partners to make informed decisions about their use of such tests. Extracts from some of these reports are given below.

> Mothers must be made aware in advance of the limitations and implications of screening and their consent sought.
>> Joint Study Group on Fetal Abnormalities (1989)

> Adequate information should be given to women eligible for screening or diagnostic tests for fetal abnormality.
>> Recommendation from the 23rd Study Group of the Royal College of Obstetricians and Gynaecologists (Drife and Donnai 1991)

> Serum screening should only be undertaken with the knowledge and consent of the woman. Whatever her decision it should be respected.
>> Report of the RCOG Working Party on Biochemical Markers and the Detection of Down's Syndrome (1993)

> (Prenatal) screening is only acceptable if it rests on free and informed consent.
>> *Human Genetics: The Science and its Consequences*
>> House of Commons Science and Technology Committee (1995)

Obstetricians and midwives presentations of risk information

There are at least three stages of testing for Down syndrome during which risk information may be given: when presenting the test; when presenting test results; and when presenting the results of any subsequent diagnostic tests.

Presenting tests

The majority of obstetricians when surveyed say that their policy is to provide screening to detect fetal abnormalities not as routine tests, but as tests that women should decide for themselves whether they wish to undergo them (Farrant 1985; Green 1994). In contrast with this, observational studies of obstetricians and midwives presenting prenatal screening and diagnostic tests show that often very little and, occasionally inaccurate information is given. In one study, routine consultations between 102 pregnant women and an obstetrician or midwife were tape-recorded to determine how AFP screening for neural tube defects and Down syndrome were presented (Marteau *et al.* 1992b). Overall, little information was provided about the test. This was particularly so for risk information. The chance that the fetus was affected was never mentioned. Descriptions of the two conditions for which screening was being offered were provided on just four occasions. The extent to which these findings reflect current practice is not known.

There is a large body of evidence showing that many women have a poor understanding of screening for Down syndrome (for review, see Marteau 1995). It has been suggested that understanding among women undergoing tests conducted privately and by post may be even poorer than that of women participating in

NHS clinic-based screening programmes (Boyd 1994). Interviews with genetic counsellors in the US suggest that many women undergoing serum screening for Down syndrome are also poorly informed before undergoing the test (Burke and Kolker 1994).

The consequences of being poorly informed about tests include undergoing tests that, with more information, would not have been undergone (Round and Hamilton 1993; Thornton *et al.* 1995) and, conversely, not undergoing tests that with more information might have been undergone (Marteau *et al.* 1992b). Having more information about tests before undergoing them might also be of benefit in preparing women for possible adverse outcomes of testing (Weinman and Johnston 1988).

Presenting test results

Negative test results

Informing women of negative test results is recommended practice for bio-chemical screening for Down syndrome (RCOG 1993). The purpose of conveying such a result is to help women to understand that, although the chance of having a child with Down syndrome is below a particular cut-off level deemed high, they still have a residual chance of having an affected child. It is also intended that this information should not cause undue anxiety. Although the impact on parents of false reassurance following a false negative test result is not known, preliminary data suggest that such a misunderstanding may undermine parental adjustment to the birth of a child with Down syndrome (Hall *et al.* 1997). In a recent survey of antenatal clinics in England and Wales, only 29% of 169 programmes made specific arrangements to inform women of negative test results, and in 5% the results were not given at all. In the remainder, the provision of results was dependent on women either attending routine clinics or asking for results (Allanson *et al.* submitted for publication).

The form in which these results were given varied. In 44% of programmes it was presented in the form of a verbal phrase, with one of nine phrases being used: low risk; not at high risk; within normal limits; screen negative; not at increased risk; not needing further action; at reduced risk; very little change; result is fine. The result was presented as a probability figure in 16% of programmes and as both a verbal phrase and a probability figure in 40%. The impact of these different ways of presenting test results has yet to be determined. A trial is underway in which women are being randomly allocated to receive negative test results in one of two ways: as a verbal phrase ('low risk') or as a verbal phrase together with a probability figure (Marteau *et al.* 1996). Preliminary results suggest that understanding of test results is similar in both conditions, but women who receive a probability figure have less positive attitudes towards their pregnancies and, for those at higher levels of risk, are significantly more anxious.

Positive test results

Little is known about the manner in which women are informed of a positive result on screening, for example, how they are informed, by whom, and for how long they must wait before being seen by a specialist midwife or obstetrician. Based on the number and nature of telephone calls to a charity for people with Down syndrome, it has been argued that the needs of distressed users of screening programmes are not being met (Dennis *et al.* 1993).

In a retrospective study of women referred for an amniocentesis following an abnormal result on serum screening for neural tube defects, women reported being encouraged by obstetricians to undergo amniocentesis (Farrant 1985). An observational study of the presentation of amniocentesis to women eligible because of their ages suggests that such encouragement stems from the way that risks are presented by obstetricians (Marteau *et al.* 1993). The word risk was used to denote probability, and often used in conjunction with words such as high or low to denote the obstetricians' own values. Equivalent probabilities were described as low in conjunction with fetal loss following an invasive test and high in conjunction with Down syndrome. Thus information germane to decisions of whether to undergo amniocentesis is frequently presented in ways that encourage undergoing tests rather than fostering informed decision-making.

When presenting amniocentesis either to women eligible because of raised maternal age or because of a positive screening test result, the emphasis is on the chance of the fetus being affected to the neglect of any discussion of Down syndrome. Bekker and Hewison (1996) analysed 22 tape-recorded consultations of one midwife employed in a teaching hospital to counsel women following a positive result on a serum screening test for Down syndrome. Although there was much discussion of the chance that the fetus was affected by Down syndrome and the chance of problems associated with a diagnostic test, there was no discussion of Down syndrome itself in any of the consultations.

Presenting the diagnosis of Down syndrome

To date, there have been no observational studies of obstetricians, midwives or other health professionals informing women of a diagnosis of Down syndrome in their fetuses. Results of several studies suggest that the counselling parents receive will in part depend on the background of the health professional presenting the diagnosis. The great majority of obstetricians in three large surveys in France, the UK and Portugal favour the offer of termination of pregnancies affected by Down syndrome (Julian *et al.* 1989; Geller *et al.* 1993; Michie *et al.* 1995). From a survey of 188 midwives in the UK it would appear that fewer of them than obstetricians feel that termination is justified, with 62% reporting that they felt it was justified (Khalid *et al.* 1994) in contrast with 90% of UK obstetricians (Michie *et al.* 1995). Obstetricians report themselves to take a more directive approach to counselling women after a diagnosis of Down syndrome, placing a greater emphasis on negative aspects of the condition than do clinical geneticists or genetic nurses (Marteau *et al.* 1994). Indirect evidence suggests that the way information about a condition is presented affects the decisions parents make about whether to continue with the affected pregnancy. In two uncontrolled studies, the proportion of women who terminated pregnancies affected by a sex chromosome anomaly was significantly higher among those consulting only an obstetrician, than among women consulting geneticists or paediatricians (Robinson *et al.* 1989; Holmes-Siedle *et al.* 1987). Although the consulting of geneticists or paediatricians may reflect a greater desire to continue with an affected pregnancy, it may also reflect exposure to different information or counselling styles. This is an area of prenatal testing requiring research to determine how information is presented and with what effects as a first step towards training health professionals in optimal ways of counselling.

Summary

The presentation of risk information by health professionals contrasts with the consensus evident in published reports on the importance of decisions about prenatal tests being based on good information.

Optimal methods of providing risk information

Although there is quite good evidence concerning the failure of staff to communicate risk information, relatively little is known about the most effective ways of providing risk information in the context of prenatal screening. Dimensions of the organisation and delivery of care likely to be important are outlined below.

Team approach

Screening programmes need to be organised by teams whose composition reflects the different expertise required to offer a high quality service that meets patient needs. A recent Royal College of Obstetricians and Gynaecologists/British Paediatric Association report recommends the inclusion not only of obstetricians and midwives but also paediatricians, surgeons and general practitioners as well as patient representatives. The inclusion of health professionals with differing knowledge of any one condition may lead to better presentation of information about conditions, a hitherto neglected aspect in communications about prenatal screening.

Training health professionals

Health professionals are rarely given any training before or after qualifying in how to present complex information effectively, or in how to help patients make informed decisions about their care. This is despite recommendations that such training should take place (Drife and Donnai 1991; RCOG 1993). With brief training, modest improvements in the communication about prenatal tests can be made (Smith *et al.* 1995).

Presenting risk

Frequencies

There has been much research in cognitive psychology comparing the impact of frequencies presented in different ways (Brun 1994). This research has largely involved responses to non-personal problems and ones that are not emotionally threatening. One of the findings from such research is that whether frequencies are presented as figures (e.g. 1 in 4) or as verbal phrases (e.g. high risk) makes relatively little difference to subsequent decisions. There is, however, a well-documented phenomenon – the communication mode preference paradox – whereby those faced with decisions prefer to receive frequencies in the form of figures, although their decisions may be uninformed by such precision (Erev and Cohen 1990). Such studies need repeating to determine how applicable they are to the presentation of probabilities of Down syndrome to women undergoing testing.

There is very little research to inform policies on whether frequencies are best presented graphically in contrast to words or numbers, and whether they are best presented relative to some other event or as an absolute frequency.

Down syndrome

Although a full presentation of the risks of Down syndrome requires describing the condition itself, there are few findings from research to guide how this is best done. As has been seen in other areas, health professionals with different clinical experiences perceive the same condition differently (Christensen-Szalanski *et al.* 1983; Marteau and Baum 1984; Britton and Knox 1991; Siperstein *et al.* 1994). Given that the prognosis for any condition is uncertain but tends to be better now than 40 years earlier, the outcome for a child born today cannot be known and therefore can be grounds for much professional disagreement.

Even if agreement could be reached on the prognosis to be conveyed to prospective parents, the optimal ways of doing this are unknown. Possible ways of providing such information include text, pictures and contact with families of affected children. There is limited evidence to suggest that providing pictures or contact with affected children results in more negative attitudes towards the condition and a higher chance of testing and termination (Figueiras *et al.* submitted for publication; Martin Whittle, personal communication). Whether these are better decisions for parents than ones based solely on written descriptions of a condition has yet to be determined. As clinics move towards presenting information about tests using videos and interactive media, women will be presented with more pictorial images of Down syndrome. The effect of this on decision including satisfaction and subsequent adjustment needs to be addressed promptly.

Barriers to implementing good practice in this area

Despite the consensus evident in published guidelines spanning almost 20 years (Black 1979; RCOG/BPA 1996) on the need for women to be given full information about any prenatal screening test, and evidence over the past 10 years that this is frequently not given, there are screening programmes operating that fail to inform women fully about the test. The prevalence of such programmes is unknown. Publication of guidelines is clearly insufficient to effect change in this and indeed other areas of health care (Department of Health 1995). Understanding the barriers to implementation is a first step towards overcoming them. Some of the possible barriers are discussed below.

Resources

In a survey of obstetricians in England and Wales, 46% of 315 obstetricians offering some form of serum screening for Down syndrome said that they did not have sufficient resources to provide adequate counselling (Green 1994). This begs the question of why screening programmes are implemented without sufficient resources for counselling but with sufficient resources for laboratory analyses. This suggests that, contrary to published guidelines, provision of good information is not seen as a core part of screening. Although extra resources may well be necessary, they would not be sufficient to improve communication of risk information given that some midwives and obstetricians lack sufficient information and skills themselves to give the information needed.

Knowledge and communication skills of health professionals

Several surveys of midwives and obstetricians show that they sometimes lack sufficient knowledge to be able to present even basic information about screening, such as false positive or false negative rates (Sanden 1985; Smith *et al.* 1994). In addition to knowledge, health professionals require some basic communication skills to convey sometimes quite complex information effectively. Although relatively brief training can be effective in teaching these skills, in a recent evaluation of such training for midwives and obstetricians only 27% of those eligible participated, and those participating had better skills than those who did not (Smith *et al.* 1995). These results suggest the need for training to be mandatory.

Incentives

Financial incentives seem to operate in the direction of maximising uptake and not in maximising informed decision-making. This is most evident for those providing a commercial service for whom payment is dependent on undergoing a test. Such an incentive may also be operative among NHS providers. Provision of screening services brings laboratory and clinical services such as ultrasound, which are valued outside the screening programme. Providing more information about screening could reduce interest among women in the test and hence reduce the benefits for health professionals of providing such a service.

Another incentive to obstetricians for offering screening in a way that maximises uptake may be the production of birth statistics with a low rate of fetal abnormalities.

Attitudes towards Down syndrome

There have been several critiques of prenatal screening arguing that they are based on a negative attitude towards disability, including Down syndrome (Rose 1995;

Williams 1995). Following a review of genetic textbooks, Lippman and Brunger (1991) reported that Down syndrome, and people with it, were presented in a generally negative light. Although such negative attitudes doubtless reflect the negative attitudes in our society, there is some evidence to suggest that the attitudes of obstetricians towards Down syndrome may be more negative than those of the general public (Drake *et al.* 1996). This may reflect lower expectations among physicians for those with learning disabilities. A comparison of four professional groups in the US showed that physicians had significantly lower expectations and most pessimistic prognoses for children with moderate or severe learning disabilities (Siperstein *et al.* 1994).

Co-ordination between midwives and obstetricians

The provision of prenatal screening requires organisation and skills from two key groups of health professionals: obstetricians and midwives. It would seem that these two groups are not co-ordinating their efforts at a national level to improve the provision of information about prenatal screening. An example of this is the lack of inclusion of midwives on recent working parties, including the current one, to discuss prenatal testing. In part this may stem from differences between the groups in their enthusiasm for prenatal screening, as reviewed above. In addition, these two disciplines in antenatal care do not have a strong history of developing policy together. The implementation of good communication about prenatal testing would be more likely if the lead came from a co-ordinated approach involving obstetricians and midwives as equal partners.

Conclusions

The limited available evidence suggests that, contrary to published guidelines, screening for Down syndrome is not being conducted in ways that facilitate informed decisions about its use. In particular, women's understanding of the test and their results is often poor, in part reflecting a lack of information or ineffectively communicated information. To continue with this situation suggests at best a lack of awareness of how these programmes are failing in one of their core aims and at worst a negative attitude towards disability among those running these programmes. One of the key challenges for those involved in providing antenatal care is to bridge the gap between a policy of screening that embraces the provision of good information and a practice of screening that thus far falls short of this.

Recommendations

1. Implementation of recommendations from previous RCOG reports concerning training of health professionals and provision of good information about screening for Down syndrome. This might involve consideration of a licensing system for screening programmes requiring not only technical quality control but also evidence of effective communication.

2. Research to be conducted on:
   (a) Optimal methods of presenting risk information,
   (b) Barriers to the implementation of guidelines on good communication in the context of prenatal screening.

Acknowledgement. TMM is supported by The Wellcome Trust.

References

Bekker, H. and Hewison, J. (1996) Describing information giving in prenatal testing: a pilot study. Paper presented at the British Psychological Society Special Group in Health Psychology 1996 Annual Conference, 3–5 July, York

Black Report (1979) *Report of the Working Group on the Screening for Neural Tube Defects.* London: Department of Health and Social Security

Boyd, P.A. (1994) Serum screening for Down's syndrome: private patients may receive less counselling. *BMJ* **309**, 1362

Britton, J. and Knox, A.J. (1991) Screening for cystic fibrosis. *Lancet* **338**, 1524

Brun, W. (1994) 'Risk perception: main issues, approaches and findings' in: G. Wright and P. Ayton (Eds) *Subjective Probability,* pp. 295–320. Chichester: Wiley

Burke, B.M. and Kolker, A. (1994) Variations in content in prenatal genetic counselling interviews. *J Genet Counselling* **3**, 23–38

Christensen-Szalanski, I.J.J., Beck, D.E., Christensen-Szalanski, C.M. and Koepsell, T.D. (1983) Effects of expertise and experience on risk judgements. *J Appl Psychol* **68**, 278–84

Dennis, J., Sawtell, M. and Rutter, S. (1993) Counselling needed after screening for Down's syndrome. *BMJ* **307**, 1005

Department of Health (1995) *Methods to Promote the Implementation of Research Findings in the NHS: Priorities for Evaluation.* Report to the NHS Central Research and Development Committee, October 1995

Drake, H., Reid, M. and Marteau, T.M. (1996) Attitudes towards termination for fetal abnormality: comparisons in three European countries. *Clin Genet* **49**, 134–40

Drife, J.O. and Donnai, D. (1991) (Eds) *Antenatal Diagnosis of Fetal Abnormalities.* London: Springer-Verlag

Erev, I. and Cohen, B.L. (1990) Verbal versus numerical probabilities: efficiency, biases, and the preference paradox. *Organizational Behavior and Human Decision Processes* **45**, 1–18

Farrant, W. (1985) 'Who's for amniocentesis? The politics of prenatal screening' in: H. Homans (Ed.) *Sexual Politics of Reproduction,* pp. 96–117. London: Gower

Geller, G., Tambor, E.S., Papiernick, E. (1993) Attitudes toward abortion for fetal anomaly in the second vs third trimester: a survey of Parisian obstetricians. *Prenat Diagn* **13**, 707–22

Green, J. (1994) Serum screening for Down's syndrome: experiences of obstetricians in England and Wales. *BMJ* **309**, 769–72

Hall, S., Bobrow, M. and Marteau, T.M. (1997) Parents' attributions of blame for the birth of a child with Down syndrome: a pilot study. *Psychol Health* (in press)

Holmes-Siedle, M., Ryanen, M. and Lindenbaum, R.H. (1987) Parental decisions regarding termination of pregnancy following prenatal detection of sex chromosome anomalies. *Prenat Diagn* **7**, 239–44

Julian, C., Huard, P., Gouvernet, J., Matteir, J.F. and Aymé, S. (1989) Physicians' acceptability of termination of pregnancy after prenatal diagnosis in Southern France. *Prenat Diagn* **9**, 77–89

Joint Study Group on Fetal Abnormalities (1989) *Arch Dis Child* **64**, 971–6

Khalid, L., Price, S.M. and Barrow, M. (1994) The attitudes of midwives to maternal serum screening for Down's syndrome. *Public Health* **108**, 131–6

Lippman, A. and Brunger, F. (1991) Constructing Down syndrome: texts as informants. *Sante Culture Health* **8**, 109–31

Marteau, T.M. (1995) Towards informed decisions about prenatal testing: a review. *Prenat Diagn* **15**, 1215–26

Marteau, T.M. and Baum, J.D. (1984) Doctors' views on diabetes. *Arch Dis Child* **54**, 566–70

Marteau, T.M., Johnston, M., Kidd, J. *et al.* (1992a) Psychological models in predicting uptake of prenatal screening. *Psychol Health* **6**, 13–22

Marteau, T.M., Slack, J., Kidd, J. and Shaw, R.W. (1992b) Presenting a routine screening test in antenatal care: practice observed. *Public Health* **106**, 131–41

Marteau, T.M., Plenicar, M. and Kidd, J. (1993) Obstetricians presenting amniocentesis to pregnant women: Practice observed. *J Reprod Infant Psychol* **11**, 3–10

Marteau, T.M., Drake, H. and Bobrow, M. (1994) Counselling following diagnosis of a fetal abnormality: the differing approaches of obstetricians, clinical geneticists and genetic nurses. *J Med Genet* **31**, 864–7

Marteau, T.M., Smith, D.K. and Michie, S. (1996) Impact of risk presentation on risk perception. Paper presented at The British Psychological Society Special Group in Health Psychology 1996 Annual Conference, 3–5 July, York

Michie, S., Drake, H., Bobrow, M. and Marteau, T. (1995) A comparison of public and professionals' attitudes towards genetic developments. *Public Understanding of Science* **4**, · 243–53

Robinson, A., Bender, B.G. and Linden, M.G. (1989) Decisions following the intrauterine diagnosis of sex chromosome aneuploidy. *Am J Med Genet* **34**, 552–4

Rose, H. (1995) 'Victorian values in the test-tube: the politics of reproductive science and technology' in M. Stanworth (Ed.) *Reproductive Technologies – Gender, Motherhood and Medicine,* pp.151–73. Cambridge: Polity Press

Round, A. and Hamilton, W. (1993) Prenatal screening for Down's syndrome. *BMJ* **307**, 1211

Royal College of Obstetricians and Gynaecologists (1993) *Report of the RCOG Working Party on Biochemical Markers and the Detection of Down's Syndrome.* London: RCOG Press

Royal College of Obstetricians and Gynaecologists/Royal College of Paediatrics and Child Health (1997) *Fetal Abnormalities: Guidelines for Screening, Diagnosis and Management.* London: RCOG

Sanden, M-L. (1985) Midwives' knowledge of the alphafetoprotein test. *J Psychosom Obstet Gynaecol* **4**, 23–30

Science and Technology Committee of the House of Commons (1995) *Human Genetics: The Science and its Consequences,* vol. I. London: HMSO

Siperstein, G.N., Wolraich, M.L. and Reid, D. (1994) Professionals' prognoses for individuals with mental retardation: search for consensus within interdisciplinary settings. *Am J Mental Retard* **98**, 519–26

Smith, D., Shaw, R.W. and Marteau, T. (1994) Lack of knowledge in health professionals: a barrier to providing information to patients. *Qual Health Care* **3**, 75–8

Smith, D.K., Shaw, R.W., Slack, J. and Marteau, T.M. (1995) Training obstetricians and midwives to present screening tests: evaluation of two brief interventions. *Prenat Diagn* **15**, 317–24

Thornton, J.G., Hewison, J., Lilford, R.J. and Vail, A. (1995) A randomised trial of three methods of giving information about prenatal testing. *BMJ* **311**, 1127–30

Weinman, J. and Johnston, M. (1988) 'Stressful medical procedures: an analysis of the effect of psychological interventions and the stressfulness of the procedures' in S. Maes, C.D. Spielberger, P.B. Defares and I.G. Sarason (Eds) *Topics in Health Psychology,* pp.205–17. Chichester: Wiley

Williams, P. (1995) Should we prevent Down's syndrome? *Br J Learning Disabilities* **23**, 46–50

Counselling the patient: prenatal testing for Down syndrome – the Down's Syndrome Association's perspective

Sarah Rutter[1]

About the Down's Syndrome Association

The Down's Syndrome Association was founded in 1970 by parents who felt the need for support, information and encouragement in bringing up their children with the condition. Their main purpose was to help their children reach their full potential – a potential which had been largely unrecognised by professionals and some parents and carers up to then. The Association has grown and carried on this work and now consists of over 20 branches throughout the UK. Each branch is divided into smaller groups of parents who support each other in whichever way is appropriate. The National Office exists to help administer the work of the branches and also to provide up-to-date information and advice on the condition to parents, carers and the general public. Much of our work involves counselling and supporting new parents.

The work of the Information Officers is to give information and advice on any topic connected with the condition, be it medical, social or educational. Since the advent of prenatal screening tests for Down syndrome, the Information Officers have found that an increasing number of calls come from pregnant women and their partners who are worried about the tests. We now receive an average of three calls per day from people caught up in the testing net. Many of these calls last between 30 and 45 minutes and can be quite complex and distressing. The majority of such calls reveal the inadequacy of the counselling they have received from the health care professionals performing the tests.

The Association feels it cannot refuse to answer such calls despite the fact that time spent in counselling people about prenatal tests is time denied to its members who are parents and carers of people with Down syndrome. The Association has set out its policy as follows:

---

[1] This paper was presented in summary form by Professor Eva Alberman.

The Association does not consider the mere fact of having Down syndrome a reason for having an abortion.

Many people with Down syndrome lead healthy and fulfilled lives, exercising their individual potential; many families have welcomed children with Down syndrome and find great pleasure and delight in them as they do their other children.

The Down's Syndrome Association does however recognise that for some people a child with a disability may not be accepted as readily, particularly if the prevailing attitudes are negative and the availability of support and additional resources is minimal.

The Association's aim is therefore to maintain its present service which is to provide objective and up-to-date information, advice and counselling to people who have had, are about to have or are concerned about the possibility of having a child with Down syndrome, so that they will be equipped with as much information as possible to make their own personal decision for the future.

In order to give accurate and up-to-date information about Down syndrome and prenatal tests in the most efficient way, the Association produced a booklet called *Prenatal Testing for Down's Syndrome* in 1994. This booklet describes what Down syndrome is, what the Association's position is on termination, discusses the different screening and diagnostic tests that are available and the degree of accuracy attributed to each of them. Since it was first published, 15 000 copies of the booklet have been sent out and individual copies are available free of charge from our office. The costs of production, dispatch and staff time which amount to approximately £25 000 over the two and a half years have been borne by the Association, not by those who have developed and marketed the screening tests nor by the Health Service.

We are aware that the following examples of the horror stories we have heard over the telephone are very much anecdotal evidence, but we feel they are none the less a valid reflection of some of the bad practice which is still prevalent among those members of the medical profession who are involved in screening programmes for Down's syndrome.

Example 1

A woman rang our office, extremely upset, requesting information on the genetics of Down syndrome. Through conversation it transpired that she had terminated a pregnancy five weeks before and had not been provided with any information about Down syndrome. She was anxious that she may have another child with Down syndrome and presumed that her two daughters would now be carriers. A health visitor had been to visit her but had not been briefed at all so she could not provide any answers to her many questions. The woman had taken it upon herself to find out more about Down syndrome through books in the library and consequently was beginning to feel that she had made a wrong decision in ending her pregnancy. At no time before the termination had she been provided with any opportunity to discuss any of these concerns.

Example 2

A health visitor rang to request information about testing because one of her pregnant mothers, aged 29, was in distress. She had been given a 1:7500 chance of having a baby with Down syndrome as a result of an AFP test. Her GP received the notification of this while the woman was away on holiday and tried to contact her, saying she must talk to the consultant about it immediately. Her family were worried sick, wanting to bring her back from Tunisia! The health visitor told them not to recall her from holiday, but once the mother returned she saw the consultant who still failed to reassure her – he seemed to think she was wasting his time! The health visitor had tried to explain that 1:7500 was a very low chance, but it was hard to put her mind at ease because of the poor counselling and all the fuss that had been made beforehand.

This woman and her family had been put through days of anxiety, because her GP had not been able to interpret correctly the result of her test. Surely, it would not be unreasonable for GPs to be educated in the issues surrounding prenatal screening, since all GPs must have pregnant women among their patients.

Example 3

A woman who was 32 years old, 19 weeks pregnant in her third pregnancy was told by her midwife that her AFP result was 'borderline'. No explanation was given about what 'borderline' meant, but she was advised to go for an amniocentesis to 'make sure'. The woman had already had a miscarriage and was therefore not keen to undergo any invasive testing. The midwife made her feel ten times worse when she said, 'There's still hope'. The pregnant woman was so upset she could hardly talk when she first telephoned. She told the Information Officer she had not been informed at the start that an AFP test result could turn out to be less than reassuring and she was angry that the midwife could not explain the result properly.

Example 4

A woman rang the Information Office who had spent the three weeks awaiting the results of an amniocentesis reading up about Down syndrome. The amnio had been carried out on the basis of an ultrasound scan, where the radiologist had mentioned the possibility that the baby had Down syndrome. It turned out that the baby had trisomy 13, which was in fact what had been written on the radiologist's notes, yet trisomy 13 had not been mentioned. She could not understand why the radiologist had not even mentioned trisomy 13 when he/she had noted that condition in her notes.

Example 5

In a telephone conversation that lasted about 45 minutes recently, one of our information officers was told by a pregnant woman of over 35 that when she had tested positive on a triple test, she had been told she would have to have an amniocentesis. She was not sure about taking the risk of miscarriage because of her past history and because she saw this as her last chance to have a baby. Her husband was very against the amniocentesis. She was given the impression by the midwives that a baby with Down syndrome was some sort of monster which contradicted her own admittedly limited knowledge of the condition. They tried to persuade her to undergo the amniocentesis by telling her nothing but exaggerated half-truths and, frankly, untruths about children with Down syndrome. Their attitude was that a person with Down syndrome was not really human anyway and so they could not understand why she and her husband were so keen to protect the pregnancy.

Many women have reported that they have been informed of their screening results in such an insensitive way either by their midwife or their GP that they need to phone us to try to make sense of what they have been told. It is really not good enough to tell women over the phone that they have screened positive and that they 'need to go for an amniocentesis' without providing an opportunity for explanation or discussion of the options. Many do not even realise that they can refuse to undergo amniocentesis if they want to. These women feel upset and anxious. They have lost confidence in the very professionals who are meant to be supporting them in their pregnancy.

Quite often women report that they have been told their is no point in them having amniocentesis unless they agree to terminate the pregnancy if the results prove positive. People who have positive amniocentesis results are often made to feel irresponsible if they then decide to go ahead with the pregnancy; they report that the attitude of the hospital staff changes towards them once they have made their decision to continue.

Some women have blood taken without knowing what it is for. They are unaware that they are being screened for Down syndrome. Obviously, these women are given no information about what Down syndrome is, the implications of a positive result or any of the issues that surround the procedure. If they are then telephoned at home with a positive screening result, they are, of course, totally unprepared for the anxiety created.

A large number of women phone us thinking that a positive blood test result means that their baby definitely has Down syndrome. No time has been taken in such cases to make sure the women know the facts about the tests and the difference between a screening test and a diagnostic test.

It is impossible to say how many times we have heard women say that their pregnancy has been blighted by the tests and the anxiety caused by them. It is also not unusual for mothers to say that they wish they had never got involved with what they describe as the 'roller coaster' of testing. Even once their baby has been born without Down syndrome, some mothers find it difficult to believe that their child does not have the condition and continue the anxious search for the characteristics of trisomy 21.

In the light of our experience of counselling people who are already on the 'roller coaster' of screening and testing for Down syndrome, it seems that the basic principle of genetic counselling, that of ensuring that individuals have the facts, presented in an unbiased and clear way, to enable them to make their own decisions, is being flouted every day by those who are performing the tests. The full implications of undergoing screening for Down syndrome should, in our opinion, be made clear to patients before the blood is taken. It would be unthinkable to test someone for HIV or, for example, Huntington's disease, without beforehand discussing the possible consequences of a positive result, so how has it become acceptable to test for Down syndrome without counselling?

The Association is aware that it is impossible to turn the clock back on prenatal screening tests; we know they are likely to be made more widely available, not less. Unless appropriate counselling services are set up alongside the screening programmes, then we shall continue to be called upon to 'fill in the gaps'. At least we can ensure that those women who do contact us are provided with objective and up-to-date information as a result of which some will not be persuaded to terminate their pregnancies out of fear of the unknown.

Chapter 31

Counselling about risk assessment

Discussion

Whittle: A question to Dr Macintosh. I was interested in and to some extent disturbed by your findings about the poor degree of precision between laboratories – the large variation that seems to appear from that. I wonder whether you have information about how many cycles each of those laboratories are processing and whether there is any standardisation there. I remember from our earlier working party that there was a feeling that there might be a critical figure – I don't think we ever arrived at the figure – below which the quality control of an individual laboratory would deteriorate. I think there were 75 laboratories or so. I wonder if you have any feelings about the average or mean or mode of samples processed by each of those laboratories?

Macintosh: There is a huge variation in the number of samples that are going through these various laboratories. Probably one of the biochemists could make a better contribution to the variation, because these reports are sent out by NEQAS to the working laboratories. Would Tim Chard or David Aitken like to comment?

Torgerson: I already have some information on precision which I was going to come up with.

Macintosh: The comment is on the number of tests going through.

Aitken: In Glasgow we might well be one of the largest laboratories in the country and since we started doing AFP hCG screening we average between 27 000 and 28 000 analyses a year. I am sure that all figures below that – and maybe some of them exist in the NEQAS scheme – will be less than a couple of thousand.

Reynolds: In my laboratory we average 3000 samples every year.

Spencer: There are certainly labs doing less than that. Two labs that I know of do no more than 500 samples a year. So there is an incredible variation. The whole process is incredibly variable. You can look at the variability of risk in a variety of ways; it is not just analysing a sample, it is what goes into calculating the risk. Again there is a lot of variability in what people are using, and mathematical packages and a whole host of things have an impact.

Macintosh: This information is available from the questionnaire. I just do not have it with me, but it is about to be published. One other thing I would like to say is that if you contrast the Northern and Yorkshire regions for biochemical screening from the laboratory aspect, the Northern Region is approximately the same size as the Yorkshire region and has 10 or 11 laboratories providing risk estimations, whereas in Yorkshire there are two laboratories. So it is highly variable.

Wald: I have two comments and one question. One comment relates to Dr Macintosh's presentation. As far as risk is concerned, I think the accuracy of risk estimation has been validated. What is less clear is the precision of individual risk. That is vitally important because overall one needs to be confident that one is on target.

My second comment is directed at Professor Marteau's talk. She appropriately pointed out that giving women with a positive screening result an individual risk estimate increases their level of anxiety. She also correctly pointed out that she did not put a value judgement on whether that was good or bad. I just wanted to bring that point out because there is often a presumption that one should just avoid causing anxiety, which certainly Professor Marteau did not say. But many people, and certainly journalists, often make that point. I have seen headlines in the papers saying, 'Test that is designed to relieve anxiety does the opposite'.

Screening is intended to cause anxiety because you identify people with a higher risk of a serious disorder. There is uncertainty and very difficult decisions have to be made, and that always generates anxiety. And anxiety, provided it is appropriately dealt with and is not excessive, is a necessary part of the process. In fact, I would have thought that her particular result there showed that it was appropriate. I would have regarded that as a positive response from the process rather than a negative one, which some people – certainly not Professor Marteau – might have interpreted.

My last point is a question to Professor Alberman. I quite often get stories of mishaps, misinformation and tragedies that have come through screening. What troubles me a little is that I also see – and you will know, Professor Alberman, from our own group that Ann Kennard produced a lot of these – anecdotes of women who have been extremely well handled in the process, who write in on their own accord to say how pleased they were that this was offered, how sensibly the staff dealt with them and how considered it all was. It seems to me that in situations like this it is just as important to bring out the successes as well as the failures. So often one just gets these terrible stories where things went wrong.

My question is this: Don't you think if one were doing this again it would be sensible to show some of the positive responses as well as the negative ones?

Alberman: I am sure you are right. Knowing Ann Kennard and her team, I am not at all surprised that they received positive responses. The very fact that the convenors chose to ask the Down's Syndrome Association for their views made it obvious that they were going to get negative views, because on the whole people do not ring up their information officers to say I've had a wonderful talk with Bart's people and I'm so pleased, they've been very helpful. So you are right.

Having said that, I have enough personal experience to know that with hindsight it may be wonderful; with foresight this is a very anxiety-provoking situation. With hindsight, when all is well, things went well and people were very helpful. With foresight, one's attitude is to look for trouble in a sense. I think everyone knows that giving bad news or even anxiety-provoking news is always problematical. There is plenty of evidence to show that patients forget that they were given helpful advice and only remember the unhelpful parts.

Marteau: May I just clarify part of Professor Wald's comments on the results from the study that I presented. You said that I was presenting the results of how women responded to positive test results. They were negative or low-risk test results. So they were the women's reactions on being given a result where the probability was less than one in 250.

Secondly, the strength of evidence is what we are really talking about. Quite appropriately, the Down's Syndrome Association in their paper have presented cases, because that is what they deal with. They can give us numbers in terms of the number of telephone calls. But this is the tip of an iceberg and the question is, how big is that iceberg? That is part of the exchange that has just gone on between Professor Wald and Professor Alberman. I do not think trading cases is a way of determining how large that iceberg is. We need to be more sophisticated and go in for some of the surveys that Professor Alberman alluded to and, when one does, look at large numbers of women to see what they have understood about the screening tests that have been presented to them. What one sees is fewer than 50% understanding correctly the nature of the screening test that they have been offered and that they are about to undergo.

Nicolaides: What I would like to do now is separate two issues. One is the accuracy and precision of the various tests; the second is the presentation of results, and where we go from here. There is a major confusion among those who give the service and second, the screening aspect. Almost certainly that is a consequence of our lack of precision in the aims of screening.

If the aim of screening is to identify babies who are at risk from DS, preferably 100% uptake of invasive testing, preferably or absolutely desirable termination of all detected DS fetuses with the primary incentive of achieving maximum reduction in the live birth prevalence of DS, then we must make clear recommendation as to how that can be achieved. The RCOG, for example, can write a leaflet on how dreadful a condition Down syndrome is. The Department of Health and Social Security can write another leaflet about the enormous burden to society of having such babies. These leaflets can be very short and quite nasty. Then we can have very short letters to every professor, every clinician, every midwife: our intention by the year 2000, a five-year plan, is to eliminate or do as much as possible to eliminate this dreadful condition and make quite sure that everybody does exactly this.

That would be very easy because there would not be a need for long, serious programmes of counselling and I think that this is a process that could be easily enforced within militaristic societies.

The alternative is that we don't really know what the population wants or we do know that different people want completely different things. They understand different things about DS. One of the biggest problems that I had within my unit was when I asked 10 people last year to produce a one-page leaflet of what Down syndrome is. It was impossible. We wrote it and re-wrote it again and again in order to make it politically correct. At the end the leaflet was so vague that it was not useful at all.

So one of the aspects that you highlight, Professor Marteau and Dr Macintosh, is whether we really know what the intention and the aim of screening is. I raise that issue. Then, if we know, can we make recommendations? Is the failure to make recommendations and the consequences of these horror stories a mere consequence of the fact that we want them to remain horror stories because we are scared of making recommendations. Therefore, the recommendations are so pathetically vague that they are intended to be a political exercise of correctness and they remain vague. Or do you really want to make recommendations?

Let us have discussion about that, and then let's talk about precision values of biochemistry and ultrasound.

Silman: That is something that has been nagging at me all through this meeting, with a private conversation with Dr Macintosh and with what you were actually presented with today when Dr Macintosh was saying that the big difference between the lottery and Down syndrome is that Down syndrome is bad news. You define risk as an adverse event.

I believe that the risk estimation is more accurately defined as a chance estimation or a likelihood estimation. It is a value judgement to say that it is a risk estimation. It goes right to the heart of this confusion about what it is that one is offering. If one is offering a screening programme and one is offering that screening programme non-judgementally to allow a patient to decide whether it is a risk or is not a risk to have a Down's child, should we ever be using the word 'risk' in offering that programme?

I suppose I am taking the extreme politically correct position which is that we should never use the word 'risk assessment'; we should be talking about the 'probability of this outcome'. It is up to the patients to decide whether that is something that concerns them or does not concern them.

A second point, which relates back to your interesting anxiety factor on a screen negative, is that the population that you looked at was obviously dissatisfied at the cut-off point that the statisticians had put there, which was that at one in 250 you need not worry. They went on worrying up to one in 1000. After that they decided OK. Perhaps that cut-off point is more natural for them, and I find that an absolutely beautiful illustration of the distinction between cut-off points put on populations by scientists and the cut-off points that are chosen by individuals.

Cuckle: Down syndrome is a serious medical condition. People have different responses to it and we have to respect those, but it is a serious condition and we are in the business of reducing the birth prevalence of Down syndrome by screening. That is why we are screening. We should not shy away from that. That is not to say that we should be brutal in the information we give: we should give balanced information about the natural history of Down syndrome. We in Leeds show all of our leaflets to the Down's Syndrome Association before we produce them. We give the Down's Syndrome Association helpline in our leaflets and we have made a video recently with the help of the Down's syndrome Association.

However, it seems clear to me that the Down's Syndrome Association does emphasise the positive aspects, and so one has to tread carefully over the eggshells. But we do not need to do so here between us. We can say that this is a serious condition to screen for and in so doing we are being directive. Screening is by its very nature directive. We are saying we want something to be done here. If we had a screening programme and women did not take it up, or they took it up but they did not take up amniocentesis, or they took up amniocentesis and they did not terminate pregnancies – if nobody did we would stop screening. We are not screening simply to inform people about risks; we are screening in order to reduce prevalence: that is the medical aim. We must not shy away from that.

Nicolaides: Can somebody give an opposite view? Have we reached the stage now where that is not a clearly defined aim of screening? Aim – to diagnose, abort, reduce live birth prevalence.

Barry-Kinsella: My experience relates to the Republic of Ireland where there is a constitutional ban on abortion and where the vast majority of patients are Roman Catholics. But that does not preclude from a population interest in screening. When they surveyed all the patients in the National Maternity Hospital they found that 90% of the patients were seeking information if that could be supplied.

In Ireland we do not have population-based screening but we have individual screening and people opt into screening. The purpose of the screening is not necessarily termination; the purpose of the screening is information. That distinction becomes very clear in our population where there is a problem with termination. The ethicality of screening for information only, particularly if it leads to invasive testing, is questionable. But that does not mean it is necessarily questionable to the people involved. People, couples, parents, may seek information without it necessarily leading to termination, and that does not invalidate their request.

Nicolaides: Do you have any information as to whether there is a way of having terminations because it is illegal, or do they seek that information and if the baby is affected they just come across to England to have a termination? Do you have data on that?

Barry-Kinsella: Of all the patients who were screened positive, not only for Down syndrome but for a variety of conditions, half of our patients will seek termination. It is not illegal to travel for termination, we are accommodated very well in that regard. It is not a religious bar; it is more socio-cultural, where a termination is viewed in a different light than in the UK.

This raises another question, which I was going to bring up later. If in the UK there is a 47% take-up of screening in older women, that is a minority. What is happening to the other 53%? We keep talking about what is happening to the minority of women in the UK. Where are all the rest?

Cuckle: They are not being offered screening. Large sections of the population are simply not being offered it because of lack of resources. It concerns me that

Professor Marteau wants to spend lots of money on counselling. I would like to see better counselling, I would like to see better information given. But I know that in Yorkshire one of the reasons why they were not screened is that they say they have not enough money for proper counselling. They may be using it as an excuse, but it is a disincentive.

Many years ago, Dr Macri will remember a meeting in America about spina bifida screening where these arguments were gone through. Twenty years ago I produced a balance and this almost became a symbol of the meeting, that we have to have a balance between what we can afford and what we want to try to do. If you try to do the best, perfect screening programme for any disease you will have fewer resources to do the job. So you have to decide whether you want to have babies with Down syndrome in a society where there are 1000 babies a year with Down syndrome, or whether you want to make an impact on that. But it will cost money and there will be a trade-off between perfect information giving and birth prevalence because of resources.

Nicolaides: That is quite important. You have summarised just that point. But I want more discussion. Do we all agree that the aim of this process is to reduce the birth prevalence of DS? If it is, the amount of money spent on counselling can be reduced, made more effective by biochemical or ultrasonographic screening.

Simpson: I go back to a point I made the other day. I think we are veering off a little bit. In the States, where this really is offered to everybody, we still have only a 50% uptake. And, not coincidentally, that 50% approximates that proportion of the population that do not wish to undergo a pregnancy termination. It is not quite 50%. But the population is probably not as poorly informed as we think they are; I think many are making a conscious decision not to undergo screening and there may be a number – let's say 20% – who are poorly informed. But a lot simply do not want to be screened. So I would support Professor Nicolaides' statement that the purpose of the screening is to offer detection of Down syndrome for that proportion of the population that wishes to have it detected.

Cuckle: It is not 50%, it is 80%. The average uptake in all the prospective studies is 80%.

Nicolaides: But that again can vary as to whether that is a 20% failure for uptake of our screening test or maybe the 30% to make the 50 to 80 who were persuaded to accept.

Cuckle: No doubt there will be some who go in that direction. You see that because some women who have positive screening tests do not have amniocentesis. But there are some in the other direction as well who have not been properly informed, and so we have no real data on a truly, fully properly-informed population – how many of those would really accept screening? We simply do not know. All we can say is that empirically it is 80%.

Nicolaides: We have five minutes and obviously we are not going to deal with the biochemical procedure. There are two options and obviously a lot of interest.

Jauniaux: England has been the leading country in prenatal diagnosis for the last 20 years. The situation in Belgium is now that something published in the *BMJ* or *The Lancet* makes history and is the truth. So the test in Belgium is not being offered to the patient but is imposed on the patient. It is part of the package. When they come to the antenatal clinic between 16 and 20 weeks they have a test. They do not know at all what the test is about, and they get no counselling – except that if the test is positive they get amniocentesis.

Because Belgium is a rich country they were able to offer the test to the whole population. So you are talking about an enormous increase in the numbers of amniocentesis since the triple test was introduced. Is there any quality control for information released from Britain to the other countries in Europe in terms of what counselling is exactly?

Nicolaides: The point Dr Jauniaux is making is that publications in the English scientific literature have tremendous implications for health policies throughout the world, let alone Belgium. That is an important point. Obviously there is no information.

Torgerson: I just want to make a comment about the cost of a counsellor. I was looking at some work on sessions of counselling for the genetic risk of breast cancer, and if you pay the counsellors it is a lot more cost effective than if you pay consultant geneticists plus the senior registrar to counsel the patient for one and a half hours.

Marteau: Your question goes to the very heart of prenatal screening. It is an excellent question and none of us should be allowed to go for coffee until we have had some debate on it. On the table we have Professor Cuckle's suggestion for the objective of prenatal screening programmes, which, as I understand it, is that the aim of the programme is to reduce the birth prevalence of Down syndrome.

If we adopted that – correct me if I am wrong – my understanding would be that that would be the first time that any public body anywhere in the world in the latter part of the 20th century has adopted that as an objective. It could be that until now people have been pussyfooting with political correctness, as you suggested. But I just suggest back to this body that that is the first time we would have that as a stated objective.

Brambati: I don't think there is a problem between mass screening in terms of mothers always being told that it is just to reduce the number of Down syndrome babies. I reject this position because any medical decision should be left to the individual. Screening is a tool just adding to the others in the history of prenatal diagnosis to give women the possibility of deciding about the risk, but the risk should be known. As Professor Cuckle mentioned, the problem of information is very important.

We did an experiment in our clinic, randomly. We evaluated more than 200 patients who had gone to the outpatient service or the clinic in the first part of the second trimester.

Nicolaides: This is an NHS hospital in Milan?

Brambati: Yes. The obstetrician should say only: Do you know that there is a risk during pregnancy of having a baby with some abnormality? Do you know anything about Down syndrome? They asked her and they informed the patient that it was possible to face the problem and that if the patient agreed, she could have counselling. The social class was mainly middle to high, and 100% of the patients agreed to have more counselling about the problem of abnormalities and Down syndrome.

After the first counselling session 96% of the patients decided to undergo screening; 3% refused because they preferred to decide to have an invasive procedure independently of the maternal age; 1% of the patients – two out of 200 – decided not to do anything for religious reasons – 87% of the patients were Roman Catholic, 9% atheist. More than 90% of these patients said that in the case of a Down syndrome fetus they would accept termination of pregnancy. The religious problem was absolutely outside the situation because to decide to have a baby with Down syndrome or other abnormalities is a deep problem; it is not only religious.

We gave a 40-minute questionnaire to the patients and when we asked the patient, 'What do you know about Down syndrome?', for the vast majority the trouble was mental retardation: 85% mental retardation, 10% mentioned abnormalities and a few per cent minor things.

Nicolaides: Professor Brambati's point is that in response to an offer for invasive testing some will always say absolutely not, some will say definitely yes and the majority in the middle will say it depends on the risks. In his study the proportions of women taking these three options were 10%, 3% and 87% respectively. We did a study in a higher risk group and it was 10% at either end. But the real issue is that there are no unselected population-based studies examining this issue.

Marteau: Certainly in the UK – and I think it differs from the US – if we are talking about the proportion of women who would never accept a termination, that is pretty solidly 20% across screening studies in the UK. Those are in large population surveys. That does not mean that 80% would invariably accept a termination for Down syndrome. It is about 20% in the UK and I believe it is about 50% in the US, who would not consider termination. So we are talking about different populations.

Brambati: It depends on the situation when you ask people whether they would like to terminate their pregnancies or not. These women were 87% – you know the situation in Italy about abortion – anyway, they decided to abort when Down syndrome was demonstrated. It depends on the context in which you ask people. If you ask, 'Would you like to abort?' 'No, no, no!' No woman wants to abort, obviously, but in a specific context it is very different.

Wald: It seems to me that an important false dichotomy is emerging and I believe that Professor Cuckle's opinion is being misrepresented. Nobody has said that it should be an aspect of national policy to reduce the birth prevalence of Down syndrome. What has been said – and Professor Cuckle also said it – is that all women should be offered the test, choose whether to have a diagnosis, choose whether to have a termination, and if they wished to, to have it. The ultimate test of whether the screening programme is actually worth doing at all is whether people accept those choices and decide. If they do, it is providing a need; if they do not and no one takes it up, we abandon the screening programme. That is exactly what Professor Cuckle said, and I do believe, Professor Nicolaides, that you have polarised an issue that is not an issue of dissent.

Nicolaides: Cost effectiveness, as we defined it yesterday – before we produce certain tests we must prove their cost effectiveness, and I am trying to understand what these words mean to people other than yourself.

Nørgaard-Pedersen: I want to say that the Down's Syndrome Association has prepared very nice information about prenatal testing and I would certainly recommend that. Also the whole thing about screening is not only for Down syndrome; it is for many other things and this information should be given. It should be about newborns and all other aspects. The overall prescription should be that it is in order to ensure having a healthy baby.

Macintosh: There is no way that we can ever say whether a decision is an informed decision or not; I think we all agree on that. The 47% uptake in the UK maternities does not reflect informed decision making at all. Professor Cuckle's estimate of 80% in all the demonstration projects we know will be an overestimate of what informed consent will involve, because when anything is done in a well-conducted, enthusiastic manner there will be an increase in uptake and testing. Variations in uptakes and studies have varied between under 50% to approximately 90%. There is no correct figure and we do not know what it is.

Finally, I wonder if we did not have this resource problem in the UK whether there would be a dichotomy. I wonder whether we would still express the same objectives of screening if there was absolutely no resource implication whatsoever. I suspect not.

Harper: It is just about why women have the test. Nobody has actually mentioned the fact that perhaps some women have the test simply looking for reassurance; they do not fully understand it and when they get a positive result they are not prepared for it and they have not thought it through. That is why counselling and information needs to be given to women. We could perhaps compare it with the amount of information that has to be given to somebody before they have an HIV test, so perhaps we should be doing a lot more counselling.

Grudzinskas: That is a frightfully important point because you sound like a practising obstetrician and gynaecologist. That is the sort of issue that many of us face. Professor Chard, can you improve on that optimistic note?

Reynolds: Something completely different based on what Dr Macintosh said earlier. A lot of this seems to be whether we take it as a population, one in 250. If we are looking at the patient idea they have to be worked on their own personal risk estimates of what they think risk is. If we are to do that we have to give them an accurate result. The problem with that is that the position of the assays is important. It does not matter if their risk is one in 55 000 or one in 65 000. But around the cut-off zone it is very important, and the more assays you put in – so if you have one analyte you have an 8% CV on a likelihood ratio, two you have 16%, three 24%, which gives you confidence intervals of 16, 32 and 48% as you put more and more assay analytes in. As an example, once you look at the range of likely ratios you get for a patient with a triple test that should be on the cut-off, their risk that they are given can vary from one in 100 to one in 2000.

Grudzinskas: Is this a plea for splendid quality control?

Reynolds: It is pointing out that in fact the more analytes we are putting into screening, the less accurate you are getting in your result, making it more difficult for patients to make a decision. So we are better off keeping the number of analytes low. And that may free up some money.

Davies: Professor Wald, you said that nobody had stated that screening should be introduced because it will reduce the birth prevalence. In 1988 you wrote, 'This test has the potential to reduce the number of Down syndrome births in the UK from 900 to 300.'

Wald: The two statements are not inconsistent.

SECTION 9

PRACTICAL ISSUES OF SCREENING PROGRAMMES

Chapter 32

Cost effectiveness of screening for Down syndrome

David J. Torgerson

Introduction

In 1988 Wald and colleagues demonstrated that by using a combination of α-fetoprotein, unconjugated oestriol and human chorionic gonadotrophin (the triple test), about 61% of Down syndrome affected pregnancies could be detected for a test specificity of 5%, and by using an ultrasound scan the sensitivity of the test could be increased to 67% (Wald *et al.* 1988, 1992a). This represented an advance over previous screening policies for Down syndrome, which based on maternal age could only, at best, detect about 30% of all affected pregnancies (Wald *et al.* 1988). Indeed, between 1991 and 1992 the number of health districts and boards using maternal age screening alone dropped from about 55% to 30%, with increased use of the triple test and other biochemical tests for Down syndrome (Wald and Watt 1994).

There have been a number of cost effectiveness analyses (CEA) of introducing biochemical screening, and all of these evaluations have concluded that such screening is a more cost effective alternative compared with offering diagnostic amniocentesis above a certain maternal age (Sheldon and Simpson 1991; Wald *et al.* 1992b; Shackley *et al.* 1993; RCOG 1993; Piggott *et al.* 1994; Haddow *et al.* 1994; Fletcher *et al.* 1995). However, the introduction of biochemical screening for all pregnant women leads to a general increase in the amount of resources allocated to screening. Whether this increase is economically efficient cannot be completely determined through the use of CEA. Theoretically the only technique suitable to answer the question of whether increasing resources to Down syndrome screening is economically efficient is cost–benefit analysis (Gerard and Mooney 1993; Donaldson and Shackley 1995). Therefore, most published cost effectiveness analyses of biochemical screening may be incorrect when they imply that biochemical based screening is economically efficient.

In this chapter three economic issues relating to biochemical screening for Down syndrome will be discussed. First, the chapter will examine whether biochemical screening is 'cost effective' in the absence of any resource increase. Second, the effect of maternal age on the cost effectiveness of biochemical screening will be examined. Finally, the potential cost effectiveness of future, more effective, markers for Down syndrome will be discussed.

Is biochemical screening cost effective?

The consensus of existing published economic evaluations is that biochemical screening for Down syndrome is 'cost effective'. However, what is meant by cost effectiveness or economic efficiency?

Economic methods

A key idea in economic evaluations is the concept of 'opportunity cost'. Opportunity cost is defined as the benefit or opportunity foregone by using health care resources in a particular manner. For example, paying for biochemical screening means those resources cannot be used to pay for hip replacements, or coronary artery bypass operations or other health care interventions. Hence, biochemical screening for Down syndrome is economically efficient if the lost benefits, be they improved quality of life due to hip replacements or any other alternative use for the resources, is judged to be less than the benefits accruing to the biochemical screening programme. Ideally, this judgement ought to be made through the use of cost–benefit analysis (CBA) whereby all the benefits are expressed in monetary terms and if the benefits of biochemical screening exceed the benefits of any alternative use for the resources then it should be adopted. However, CBA when health benefits are expressed in monetary terms is rarely, if ever, properly undertaken in the health care field for obvious reasons. Therefore, health economists often rely on less powerful evaluative techniques such as cost effectiveness analysis or cost utility analysis.

Cost effectiveness analysis is where all the benefits are summarised in natural units – such as cases of cancer detected or affected pregnancies detected and births avoided. As such it is a useful technique for comparing two different programmes aimed at detecting cases of Down syndrome (obviously, it cannot be used to compare the cost effectiveness of different health care interventions such as breast screening with Down syndrome screening). Usually two or more programmes are compared in terms of their cost effectiveness ratios. A cost effectiveness ratio is calculated simply by dividing the cost of an intervention by its benefit (Torgerson and Spencer 1996). However, there are problems in using cost effectiveness ratios.

Cost effectiveness is a relative term and therefore when it is stated that a health care programme is cost effective this should be in relation to another competing programme. In the context of economic evaluations of biochemical screening it should be explicitly assumed that it is more cost effective than maternal age screening. However, some economic evaluations have made the erroneous implicit assumption that biochemical screening is being implemented where no screening previously existed (for example, Wald et al. 1992a; Piggott et al. 1994). To produce relevant economic results it is important that the incremental costs and benefits of biochemical screening are compared to the existing screening programme that is maternal age screening (Torgerson and Spencer 1996). This applies to future evaluations of better markers of Down syndrome risk. These should be evaluated against existing biochemical markers not against the either do nothing option or maternal age screening. For example, a recent paper has suggested that the addition of dimeric inhibin A to existing biochemical markers will improve screening detection rates (Aitken *et al.* 1996). The appropriate comparison for estimating the extra costs and benefits of this new marker is with, for example the triple test, not maternal age screening.

An alternative to CEA is cost utility analysis (CUA) when the benefits of health care are expressed in utility units such as quality adjusted life years (QALYs). There are obvious difficulties in applying this method to prenatal screening. However, Thornton and Lilford (1995) have proposed that a technique comparing the amount of disutility avoided between different forms of prenatal screening could be useful in clinical decision making. Including this method alongside some estimate of costs could, for example, help decision makers to allocate resources between Down screening or screening for cystic fibrosis. Furthermore, it is argued that, in principle, the technique could be developed such that a comparison could be made between money spent on prenatal screening and other different health care activities. However, to date this has not been attempted.

Previous economic studies

Existing economic evaluations, of Down syndrome screening, have assumed or explicitly shown that biochemical screening produces a lower cost per averted birth or detected pregnancy than the maternal age screening programme it seeks to replace. For example, Shackley *et al.* (1993) showed that for a 26% detection rate maternal age screening resulted in a cost per avoided birth of £24 350. However, replacement of the maternal age screening programme with more expensive biochemical screening produced a cost effectiveness ratio of £20 100 for a 58% detection rate (Shackley *et al.* 1993). It is this type of result that leads health economists and others to the tempting conclusion that biochemical screening is more cost effective than maternal age screening.

Despite biochemical screening sometimes producing a lower cost effectiveness ratio than maternal age screening this does not automatically mean it is more cost effective. Strictly speaking a new health care technology (e.g. biochemical screening) is only more cost effective than the older technology if it produces a better outcome for the same total cost; or it produces the same outcome at lower total cost. If the new technology results in an increase in total costs then it is only cost effective if there is no other better use for the extra resources required to purchase the newer, but more effective, technology.

The problem with existing economic evaluations of biochemical screening is that they mostly show an increase in total costs but with a lower cost effectiveness ratio and this is taken as being 'cost effective'. An increase in total costs but with a reduced cost effectiveness ratio can occur as follows. Let us assume that the existing maternal age screening programme costs £1000 and avoids ten affected births; therefore, this would give a cost effectiveness ratio of £100 per avoided birth (i.e. £1000/10). If biochemical screening is introduced this might increase total costs from £1000 to £1500 but increase the number of avoided births from 10 to 20. This would result in a marginal cost effectiveness ratio of £50 per avoided birth (i.e. the extra cost of £500 divided by the extra benefit of ten) and an average cost effectiveness ratio of £75. Thus, the marginal and average cost effectiveness ratios of £50 and £75 are less than the £100 of the existing programme. This type of result leads the analyst to assume that the newer, more expensive programme is 'cost effective'. However, this judgement depends on what alternative health care programmes could have been funded with the extra £500 which biochemical screening costs. If, for example, the extra resources could have been better used to promote effective smoking cessation for pregnant women, which in turn would reduce the number of low birth weight babies this would have a direct effect of avoiding the birth of a number of mentally and physically handicapped babies (Buck and Godfrey 1994). Therefore, if implementing biochemical screening prevents resources going into a programme that actually could prevent more distress and handicap, then it is not cost effective.

Many existing published economic evaluations of Down syndrome screening fall into the trap of assuming that biochemical screening is more cost effective than maternal age screening because, despite a higher total cost, it produces lower marginal and average cost effectiveness ratios compared with existing programmes (Sheldon and Simpson 1991; Wald *et al.* 1992b; Shackley *et al.* 1993; Piggott *et al.* 1994).

The main reason that biochemical screening leads to a higher total cost than maternal age screening is because it has been assumed that if biochemical screening is to be implemented then it must be given to all pregnant women (with the exceptions of Cuckle 1992; Fletcher *et al.* 1995; Torgerson 1996). It is possible, however, that the extra benefits of offering biochemical screening to all pregnant women may not be worth the extra costs. Fortunately, there are circumstances when biochemical screening is almost certainly cost effective.

Cost effective biochemical screening

Let us consider a screening policy of offering maternal age screening to all women 35 years or older. However, only about 25% of these women accept the offer of an amniocentesis (Piggot *et al.* 1994). Table 32.1 shows the total costs by age group as if such a policy had been in operation for all of England and Wales in 1992. Such a screening programme would have resulted in 25%* of the 51,900 pregnant women 35 and over having an amniocentesis which would have detected 75 affected pregnancies at a total cost of £3 244 000. However, replacing this screening strategy with biochemical screening for all women 35 years and over would have resulted in a reduction of total screening costs by £1 052 000 but increased the number of affected pregnancies detected from 75 to 140 and also reduce the fetal loss rate from 130 to 64. Therefore, it can be safely said in these circumstances that biochemical screening is more cost effective than maternal age screening as not only is there a reduction in total costs but an increase in the numbers of affected pregnancies detected and a certain amount of the disbenefit of amniocentesis, that is losing healthy fetuses, is avoided.

---

* This 25% figure is based on an audit of amniocentesis uptake within a single health district when only maternal age screening was offered (Piggot *et al.* 1994).

Importantly, it should be noted in this example that there is no need to compare the cost effectiveness ratios of maternal age and biochemical screening as a simple comparison of the total costs and benefits is sufficient. However, if the total costs and benefits of the programme are increased then a cost effectiveness ratio might be used to decide whether an increase in total costs is worthwhile.

Extending biochemical screening to younger women

The decision to offer biochemical screening to younger women ought, partly, to depend on whether the resources used to screen these lower risk women have a

Table 32.1. Cost effectiveness analysis of replacing amniocentesis for pregnant women 35 years and over with biochemical screening

Age	Number of pregnant women[a]	Incidence of Down syndrome[b]	Number of affected pregnancies	Age specific detection rate[c]	Age specific false positive rate[c]	Max. number of detectable cases (assuming 100% uptake)	Number of amniocenteses (assuming 100% uptake)
49	50	0.1250	6	0.998	0.938	6	47
48	100	0.0909	9	0.996	0.907	9	92
47	150	0.0667	10	0.994	0.864	10	131
46	200	0.0476	10	0.990	0.812	9	164
45	400	0.0357	14	0.983	0.749	14	303
44	600	0.0270	16	0.972	0.672	16	408
43	800	0.0204	16	0.956	0.597	16	483
42	1000	0.0154	15	0.936	0.519	14	525
41	1500	0.0112	18	0.909	0.442	16	671
40	2100	0.0089	19	0.876	0.368	16	782
39	4000	0.0068	27	0.836	0.300	23	1215
38	5000	0.0053	26	0.792	0.242	21	1225
37	8000	0.0041	33	0.745	0.194	25	1570
36	11 000	0.0033	36	0.699	0.155	25	1724
35	17 000	0.0026	44	0.649	0.122	29	2097
Total	51 900		299			249	11 437

Maternal age screening		Biochemical screening (assumes 75% uptake for screening and 75% for amniocentesis)	
Costs	*Effects*	*Costs*	*Effects*
12 975 amniocenteses @ £250 each=£3 244 000	75 affected pregnancies detected (i.e. 299×0.25); 130 miscarried fetuses.	38 925 biochemical tests @ £15 each=£584 000 and 6433 amniocenteses @ £250 each=£1,608,000.	140 affected pregnancies detected (i.e. 249×0.75 ×0.75); 64 miscarried fetuses.
Total cost=£3 244 000		Total cost=£2 192 000	

[a] Based on age distribution for all pregnant women in England and Wales 1992 (Department of Health 1992)
[b] Based on regression analysis of combined series of Down syndrome births (Cuckle *et al.* 1987).
[c] Taken from Cuckle (1994) and assumes a risk cut-off of 1:250.

Table 32.2. Cost effectiveness analysis of extending biochemical screening to women under the age of 35

Age	Number of pregnant women	Incidence of Down syndrome	Number of affected pregnancies	Age specific detection rate	Age specific false positive rate	Max. number of detectable cases	Number of amniocenteses (assuming 100% uptake)	Cumulative total cost (age specific cost per affected pregnancy detected)[a]
34	20000	0.0021	42	0.600	0.096	25	1941	£589 000 (£42 000)
33	22000	0.0017	38	0.559	0.077	21	1713	£1 158 000 (£47 000)
32	28000	0.0015	41	0.517	0.062	21	1755	£1 802 000 (£54 000)
31	30000	0.0013	38	0.480	0.050	18	1516	£2 423 000 (£61 000)
30	42000	0.0011	46	0.455	0.043	21	1825	£3 238 000 (£69 000)
29	43000	0.0010	42	0.432	0.038	18	1651	£4 031 000 (£77 000)
28	44000	0.0009	39	0.414	0.034	16	1511	£4 810 000 (£85 000)
27	45000	0.0008	37	0.398	0.030	15	1364	£5 572 000 (£91 000)
26	46000	0.0008	36	0.384	0.027	14	1255	£6 324 000 (£97 000)
25	46000	0.0007	34	0.375	0.026	13	1208	£7 068 000 (£104 000)
24	45000	0.0007	32	0.366	0.024	12	1091	£7 779 000 (£108 000)
23	44000	0.0007	30	0.364	0.024	11	1066	£8 474 000 (£112 000)
22	39000	0.0007	26	0.361	0.023	10	906	£9 083 000 (£114 000)
21	28000	0.0007	19	0.357	0.023	7	650	£9 520 000 (£117 000)
20	20000	0.0007	13	0.355	0.022	5	444	£9 828 000 (£118 000)
19	19000	0.0006	12	0.352	0.022	4	422	£10 000 000 (£120 000)
18	17000	0.0006	11	0.350	0.022	4	378	£10 000 000 (£122 000)
17	10000	0.0006	6	0.349	0.021	2	212	£11 000 000 (£122 000)
16	8000	0.0006	5	0.348	0.021	2	170	£11 000 000 (£122 000)
15	3000	0.0006	2	0.348	0.021	<1	64	£11 000 000 (£123 000)

[a] Assumes test cost of £15, amniocentesis cost of £250 and a 75% uptake rate for both.

better alternative use. Ideally, cost–benefit analysis should be used to inform such decision making. Given the difficulty of translating the major benefits of screening – that is 'the avoidance of distress and handicap to the families concerned' (Wald *et al.* 1992) – into monetary values it is often not practical to use cost–benefit analysis. However, screening policy can be usefully informed through the use of cost effectiveness ratios, that is cost per affected pregnancy detected.

A key requirement as to whether we should screen younger women is resource availability. Clearly, in the absence of any resource increase extending screening to younger women will be limited to available resources. However, from the previous analysis we have shown that by implementing biochemical screening for women aged 35 and older results in a resource saving of £1 052 000. Therefore, these saved resources are available to be used to offer screening to some women under the age of 35.

Table 32.2 shows the number of pregnant women under the age of 35 and the number of Down syndrome affected pregnancies by age with the detection and false positive rates for biochemical screening. The final column of the table shows the cumulative cost of extending biochemical screening to younger women and the cost effectiveness ratios for each age band. As Table 32.2 shows, the cost effectiveness ratio increases with the youth of the pregnant population. Assuming we wish to use the £1 052 000 resource savings to screen younger women we can see from the cumulative costs in Table 32.2 that we could just about extend screening to all women aged 33 and over. As argued earlier the decision to use the resource savings to extend screening to younger women should depend on the nature of other health interventions which cannot be purchased by using the resources for biochemical screening. This judgement and the decision as to whether it is worthwhile extending screening to all pregnant women can be informed, in part, by examining the age specific cost effectiveness ratios (Torgerson 1996). These are shown in the last column of Table 32.2. However, there is no accepted cost per affected pregnancy detected threshold for Down syndrome which is generally acknowledged as being cost effective. How much is society willing to pay to detect one affected pregnancy? The implicit values from maternal age screening is £46 000 per affected pregnancy if screening were confined to women over the age of 37 and £97 000 if screening included women aged 35. (This is estimated from Table 32.1 by multiplying all the pregnancies for a given age band by £250 (the amniocentesis cost) and dividing it by the total number of affected pregnancies.) Alternatively, the excess life-time cost of an individual with Down syndrome has been estimated to be in the region of £79 000 (Shackley *et al.* 1993). From Table 32.2, if these figures were used as a measure of benefit, then this would imply offering screening to women aged 32 and older if a benefit estimate of £46 000 were used, women 29 years and older for a benefit estimate of £79 000 and women aged 27 and over if the figure of £97 000 were used. Only if society is willing to pay in excess of £120 000 per affected pregnancy detected is it worthwhile to offer biochemical screening to all women.

Whether biochemical screening should be offered to all or only some women will depend on the relative weights given to cost effectiveness, equity, clinical efficiency and reducing prevalence of Down syndrome. In terms of cost effectiveness whether screening should be offered to all pregnant women depends on the ultimate objective of screening. If the objective is to detect as many affected pregnancies as possible then this can be achieved for least cost by restricting screening to older women and using a lower cut-off point for amniocentesis, say 1:600 rather than 1:250 (Cuckle 1994). This 'two step screen-ing' would also address the issue of reducing Down syndrome prevalence by a given amount. However, such a policy would have the unwanted side-effect of increasing the numbers of miscarried fetuses and has been described as inequit-able (Wald *et al.* 1996). Furthermore, such a policy would conflict with the concept of clinical efficiency whereby for a given total number of amniocenteses the number of affected pregnancies detected is maximised by screening all women with the same risk cut-off.

Future screening evaluations

The current generation of biochemical markers is likely to be superseded or added to in the near future by improved indicators of Down syndrome risk such as dimeric inhibin A (Aitken *et al.* 1996) and urinary markers (Cuckle *et al.* 1995). Whether these newer markers should be used in the future for routine screening should depend to some extent on their relative cost effectiveness compared with existing biochemical markers. It is important for any new technology that it should be evaluated for its cost effectiveness as early as possible given the diffi-culty of withdrawing widely diffused interventions that have been shown later to have dubious effectiveness or cost effectiveness.

With respect to evaluating economically new biochemical markers, a key factor in determining their relative cost effectiveness will be the cost of the new test as other factors such as amniocentesis uptake rates are not likely to differ between the existing screening programme and a future one based on different markers. However, a problem with evaluating many new technologies is that the costs of the new technology in its early stages may not be a good representation of imple-mentation costs. One reason for this is economies of scale. The unit costs of producing small numbers of tests for screening evaluations is likely to be much higher than when large numbers are required for implementation of the new technology. However, even if the cost or price of a new test has not yet been established it is possible to estimate the maximum price differential between the new and the old test for the new test to be relatively cost effective.

As an example, Cuckle *et al.* (1995) have reported the potential effectiveness of using urinary markers of β-core fragment of human chorionic gonadatrophin and total oestrogen as indicators of risk for Down syndrome. Initial results suggest these markers have a better detection rate for a given false positive rate than existing biochemical tests. In Table 32.3 the relative differences in detection rates between the two tests are shown. From knowledge of the existing test costs we can estimate the maximum cost of the new test for it to be certain that it is equally cost effective. This is estimated as follows.

First, let us assume that the new test must have at least the same detection rate as the old test. We can see that both tests have a 69% detection rate when the false positive rate for the triple test is 6% and the false positive rate of the new test is 2%. (Although most current screening programmes operate on a false positive rate of 5%, a 6% was chosen here as this happened to be a published rate of the triple test (Wald *et al.* 1992a) which produced the same detection rate as a 2% false positive rate for urinary markers (Cuckle *et al.* 1995).) If we assume that the current programme screens 100 000 pregnant women then this gives a total test cost of £1 500 000 (assuming a test cost of £15). Given a 6% false positive rate and a 69% detection rate we can estimate that there would be an amniocentesis cost of £1 520 500 (Table 32.3). Thus there is a total programme cost of £3 020 500.

To achieve the same detection rate for the new test implies a false positive rate of 2%, thus this leads to an amniocentesis cost of only £521,750. If this cost is subtracted from the total existing biochemical screening cost (i.e. £3 020 500 – £521 750=£2 498 750) and is divided by the number of screened women the resulting figure of about £25 is the cost that the new test must not exceed for us to be completely certain that it is more cost effective than the older test (even if the new test costs £25 but does not detect more affected pregnancies in this example it is still more cost effective as it has the additional benefit of reducing the miscarriage rate).

Clearly these calculations are affected by the relative cost of the existing biochemical test and amniocentesis costs. If, for example, the cost of an amniocentesis were £350 rather than £250, then this would imply that the new test could cost up to about £29, which is nearly double the cost of the old test and we could still be certain it would be more cost effective.

Although the preceding analysis has demonstrated that, for an existing biochemical test cost of £15 and an amniocentesis cost of £250, urinary markers would be relatively cost effective up to a cost of £25 some purchasers may consider accepting the existing false positive rate and spend more money to achieve a

Table 32.3 Comparison of detection rates for fixed false positive rates between the triple test and urinary markers for 100 000 screened women with a 1.3/1000 incidence of Down syndrome

False positive rate	Triple test detection rate[a]	Urinary markers detection rate[b]	Triple test number of cases detected	Urinary markers number of cases detected	Number of false positive cases
0.01	0.45	0.57	59	74	999
0.02	0.54	**0.69**	70	**90**	1997
0.03	0.59	0.76	77	99	2996
0.04	0.63	0.80	82	104	3995
0.05	0.67	0.82	87	107	4994
0.06	**0.69**	0.84	**90**	109	5992
0.07	0.71	0.86	92	112	6991
0.08	0.73	0.87	95	113	7990
0.09	0.75	0.89	98	116	8988
0.1	0.77	0.90	100	117	9987

Triple test		Urinary markers cost	Unknown
Biochemical test costs	100 000×£15=£1 500 000		
Amniocentesis costs	(5992×£250)+(90×£250)= £1 520 500	Amniocentesis costs	(1997×£250)+(90×250)= £521 750

[a] Taken from Wald et al. (1992b).
[b] Taken from Cuckle et al. (1995).

higher detection rate. As argued previously any screening resource expansion ought to take into consideration any alternative uses for the resources. However, although we do not know the cost of the new test we can undertake some cost effectiveness calculations in order to inform future purchasing decisions.

Fig. 32.1 shows the marginal cost per affected pregnancy detected assuming a 6% false positive rate and a 89% detection rate (Table 32.3). If the test costs £1* over and above the existing test, then the marginal cost per extra pregnancy detected is £5128. Increasing this difference in cost to £10 results in a ten-fold increase in the cost effectiveness ratio to £51 282. Using the information from Fig. 32.1 and the information in Table 32.3 a potential purchaser might consider that if the new test costs £10 extra that it is better to implement the new test and pay for its extra cost from reducing the numbers of amniocentesis. On the other hand if the extra cost were in the region of only £1 or £2 then a purchaser might consider that a policy of maintaining the existing false positive rate is preferable and take advantage of the new test's increased detection rate. Of course, a mixed policy of reducing the false positive rate by a smaller amount than is necessary to cover all the costs of the new test and putting in extra resources to gain an increase in the detection rate, could be implemented.

A further use of the information in Fig. 32.1 could be to inform research into new markers for Down syndrome. For example, if a new marker added £20 to the cost of existing tests then this would result in a marginal cost effectiveness ratio of over £100 000, which might be considered too expensive by the NHS to purchase. In such a scenario, more research effort might be directed into methods of reducing the cost of testing for the new marker before a large expensive clinical trial of a new marker is undertaken.

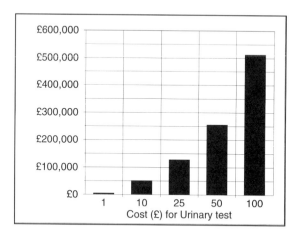

Fig. 32.1. Marginal cost per detected pregnancy

---

* Obviously if the new test is the same or lower cost than the existing test it will be more cost effective as it has a higher detection rate.

Conclusion

This chapter has highlighted a number of important economic issues regarding Down syndrome. Although biochemical screening is certainly an improvement on maternal age screening it is not clear whether extending such screening to very low risk pregnant women is cost effective. There may be more beneficial uses of the health care resources currently being used to screen young pregnant women such as smoking cessation advice to pregnant women (Buck and Godfrey 1994).

There has been a call to develop national guidelines for Down syndrome screening (Wald *et al.* 1996). However, it is important, from an economic perspective, for such guidelines to be sufficiently flexible to allow biochemical screening to be targeted at older women rather than insisting all women should be offered screening.

Finally, it is important for clinical and biomedical researchers to consider the cost implications of their research into newer markers at an early stage. This chapter has demonstrated that it is possible to estimate a reasonable upper cost limit for a new test given some early data on efficacy for it to be relatively cost effective. Should a test have particularly high cost then some research effort might be fruitfully directed at reducing production costs before larger evaluations are undertaken.

References

Aitken, D.A., Wallace, E.M., Crossley, J.A. *et al.* (1996) Dimeric inhibin a as a marker for Down's syndrome in early pregnancy. *N Engl J Med* **334**, 1231–6

Buck, D. and Godfrey, C. (1994) *Helping Smokers Give Up: Guidance for Purchasers on Cost Effectiveness.* London: Health Education Authority

Cuckle, H.S. (1992) Maternal serum screening policy for Down's syndrome. *Lancet* **340**, 799

Cuckle, H.S. (1994) 'Risk estimation in Down's syndrome screening policy and practice' in J.G. Grudzinskas, T. Chard, M. Chapman and M. Cuckle (Eds) *Screening for Down's Syndrome.* Cambridge: Cambridge University Press

Cuckle, H.S., Wald, N.J. and Thompson, S.C. (1987) Estimating a woman's risk of having a pregnancy associated with Down's syndrome using her age and serum APP level. *Br J Obstet Gynaecol* **94**, 387–402

Cuckle, H.S., Iles, R.K., Sehmi, I.K. *et al.* (1995) Urinary multiple marker screening for Down's syndrome. *Prenat Diagn* **15,**745–51

Department of Health (1992) Personal and Social Services Statistics for England and Wales 1992. London: HMSO

Donaldson, C. and Shackley, P. (1995) in R. Detels, W.W. Holland, J. McEwan and G.S. Ommen (Eds) *Economic Studies. Oxford Textbook of Public Health* (3rd edn). Oxford: Oxford University Press

Fletcher, J., Hicks, N.R., Kay, J.D.S. and Boyd, P.A. (1995) Using decision analysis to compare policies for antenatal screening for Down's syndrome. *BMJ* **311**, 351–6

Gerard, K. and Mooney, G. (1993) QALY league tables: handle with care. *Health Econ* **2**, 59–64

Haddow, J.E., Palomaki, G.E., Knight, G.J., Cunningham, G.C., Lustig, L.S. and Boyd, P.A. (1994) Reducing the need for amniocentesis in women 35 years of age or older with serum markers for screening. *N Engl J Med* **330**, 1114–18

Piggott, M., Wilkinson, P. and Bennett, J. (1994) Implementation of an antenatal serum screening programme for Down's syndrome in two districts (Brighton and Eastbourne). *J Med Screening* **1**, 45–9

Royal College of Obstetricians and Gynaecologists (1993) *Report of the RCOG Working Party on Biochemical Markers and the Detection of Down's Syndrome.* London: RCOG Press

Shackley, P., McGuire, A., Boyd, P. *et al.* (1993) An economic appraisal of alternative prenatal screening programmes for Down's syndrome. *J Public Health Med* **15**, 175–84

Sheldon, T.A. and Simpson, J. (1991) Appraisal of a new scheme for prenatal screening for Down's syndrome. *BMJ* **302**, 113–14

Thornton, J.G. and Lilford, R.J. (1995) Decision analysis for medical managers. *BMJ* **310**, 791–4

Torgerson, D.J. (1996) The impact of maternal age on the cost effectiveness of Down's syndrome screening. *Br J Obstet Gynaecol* **103**, 581–3

Torgerson, D.J. and Spencer, A. (1996) Marginal costs and benefits. *BMJ* **312**, 35–6

Wald, N.J. and Watt, H.C. (1994) Choice of serum markers in antenatal screening for Down's syndrome. *J Med Screening* **1**, 117–20

Wald, N.J., Cuckle, H.S., Densem, J.W. *et al.* (1988) Maternal serum screening for Down's syndrome in early pregnancy. *BMJ* **297**, 883–7

Wald, N.J., Cuckle, H.S., Densem, J.W. *et al.* (1992a) Maternal serum screening for Down's syndrome: the effect of routine ultrasound scan determination of gestational age and adjustment for maternal weight. *Br J Obstet Gynaecol* **99**, 144–9

Wald, N.J., Kennard, A., Densen, J.W., Cuckle, H.S., Chard, T. and Butler, L. (1992b) Antenatal maternal serum screening for Down's syndrome: results of a demonstration project. *BMJ* **305**, 391–4

Wald, N.J., Huttly, W., Wald, K. and Kennard, A. (1996) Down's syndrome screening in UK (letter). *Lancet* **347**, 330

Chapter 33

Should screening for Down syndrome be offered?

Nicholas R. Hicks and John Fletcher

Background and introduction

In England and Wales between 1974 and 1987 the birth prevalence of Down syndrome (in the absence of prenatal diagnosis and the induced abortion of affected pregnancies) is estimated to have been about 13/10 000 births or 1:770 births (Cuckle *et al.* 1991). It is the commonest major chromosomal abnormality compatible with life and is a major cause of learning disability. Down syndrome can be diagnosed antenatally by examination of material obtained from amniocentesis and Down births can be avoided by inducing abortion in affected pregnancies. This offers the potential to help women avoid the distress of having a child with Down syndrome. However, amniocentesis is an invasive, relatively expensive investigation that carries a risk of about 1:100 to 1:200 (Tabor *et al.* 1986; Lippman *et al.* 1992) of inducing miscarriage. A decision to undergo amniocentesis should not be taken lightly.

It has long been known that the prevalence of Down syndrome increases markedly with maternal age. This relationship has been used as the basis for screening for Down syndrome. For many years in the UK those at 'high risk', typically women aged 35 years or more (whose risk is quoted at levels from 1:270 (Hook *et al.* 1983) to 1:380 (Dick *et al.* 1996), have been offered amniocentesis. Those revealed as having affected pregnancies, have then been offered termination of pregnancy.

More recently a variety of other easily administered methods for estimating the antenatal risk of Down syndrome have been developed, notably multiple marker serum tests and ultrasound. Wald and colleagues (1988) predicted and subsequently demonstrated (Wald *et al.* 1992) that information derived from measurements of combinations of serum analytes, when interpreted in the knowledge of a pregnant woman's age and the gestational age of her fetus, could predict the risk of Down syndrome better than maternal age alone. Applied to the whole pregnant population these tests offer the opportunity of increasing the proportion of Down pregnancies identified antenatally from about 35% to about 60% without increasing the proportion (about 5%) of pregnant women with normal pregnancies undergoing amniocentesis.

Screening programmes can have multiple consequences and can damage as well as improve health. The benefits of screening for Down syndrome for women include a reduction in the chance of delivering a baby with Down syndrome, the reassurance of a negative result, and better information and greater control over their pregnancies. The main benefit for society is usually seen as a reduction in the number of children with Down syndrome that need caring for. The harms that can be caused by screening include increased anxiety among those with positive results, false reassurance provided to those with false negative results, the further medicalisation of pregnancy, and the loss of healthy pregnancies in amniocentesis induced abortions in women who would not otherwise have undergone amniocentesis. Societal consequences include the loss of alternative benefits that could have been obtained from the resources spent on screening for Down syndrome. It has also been suggested that seeking out and aborting affected pregnancies may further devalue the lives of people with Down syndrome and more generally shift societal values to the disadvantage of people with learning disabilities.

Serum screening for Down syndrome in the UK has been widely adopted. It is an example of rapid translation of research into practice. In 1988 Wald *et al.* predicted the performance characteristics of a serum screening programme. By 1991 51% of UK health authorities and boards offered some form of serum testing. By 1994 this had risen to 76% (Wald *et al.* 1996). However, there was considerable variation in the way in which screening for Down syndrome was undertaken and 31 of 134 (23%) health authorities and boards continued to screen for Down syndrome using maternal age alone. Of the 102 authorities and Health Boards that provided serum screening, only 20 (19.6%) offered serum tests to women over a specified age. The remainder offered serum screening to women of all ages. There was also marked variation in the serum markers that were included in the screening test. This marked variation in the provision of screening for Down syndrome suggested that there was uncertainty about the provision of screening for Down syndrome.

Table 33.1. Wilson and Jungner's screening principles

---

1. The condition sought should be an important health problem.
2. There should be an accepted treatment for patients with recognised disease.
3. Facilities for diagnosis and treatment should be available.
4. There should be a recognisable latent or early symptomatic stage.
5. There should be a suitable test or examination.
6. The test should be acceptable to the population.
7. The natural history of the disease, including latent to declared disease, should be adequately understood.
8. There should be an agreed policy on whom to treat as patients.
9. The cost of case-finding (including diagnosis and treatment of patients diagnosed) should be economically balanced in relation to a possible expenditure on medical care as a whole.
10. Case-finding should be a continuing process and not a 'once for all' project.

There have been reports that both obstetricians (Green 1994) and pregnant women (Statham and Green 1993) are unhappy with the way serum screening programmes for Down syndrome are working. Problems cited by obstetricians include women's anxiety caused by false positive results, and women's lack of understanding of the test and its shortcomings. Women reported that medical staff were unclear about the implications of screening tests and unsure about how to interpret risk. This is consistent with observations that women rarely seem to be given information about the likelihood and implications of possible results before testing (Smith *et al.* 1994) and that psychological consequences of screening for Down syndrome are underestimated (Marteau 1993). Obstetricians also report that the problems with multiple marker screening for Down syndrome are greater than those experienced with alpha fetoprotein screening (Green 1994). For all these reasons, it is important to ask whether the problems are due to imperfect implementation of an otherwise sound screening programme or whether there are more fundamental problems with the screening programme itself.

Deciding whether and how to screen for Down syndrome in Oxfordshire: a case study

The main question that this chapter addresses is whether or not screening for Down syndrome should be offered. The issues are illustrated by describing the way this question was tackled in Oxfordshire. This does not imply that Oxfordshire necessarily made the 'right' decision, but practical experience provides a useful vehicle for raising issues that need to be considered. I would also like to suggest, on the basis of our experience in Oxfordshire, that there may be some additional criteria that could usefully be added to the well established criteria for judging whether a screening programme is worthwhile.

Existing criteria for judging a screening programme

Oxfordshire is a county of about 550 000 people with approximately 7500 births per year. In 1993, in the absence of clear regional and national guidance, Oxfordshire Health Authority had not decided whether to purchase a serum screening programme for Down syndrome. In the same year about a third of women over 35 years of age chose to pay about £50 to have a biochemical test for Down syndrome performed privately. This was widely regarded as unsatisfactory. Both those providing and paying for obstetric services were aware that screening for Down syndrome could cause harm as well as lead to important benefits. We therefore sought a systematic and fair approach to deciding whether and how to screen for Down syndrome.

Wilson and Jungner's screening criteria

We first assessed serum screening for Down syndrome against Wilson and Jungner's old but well-known criteria for judging a screening programme (Wilson and Jungner 1968) (Table 33.1).

Our assessment was that:

- Down syndrome is an important health problem (criterion 1)
- Induced abortion is an accepted treatment for women with an affected fetus (criterion 2)
- Facilities for diagnosis and treatment could be made available (criterion 3)
- There is an antenatal phase in which Down syndrome is recognisable (criterion 4)
- Serum testing and amniocentesis are (arguably) suitable tests (criterion 5)
- Serum testing is acceptable to most of the population (criterion 6)
- The natural history of Down syndrome is understood both antenatally and postnatally (criterion 7)
- People have reached different agreements on whom to treat as patients (criterion 8)
- The cost per case of Down syndrome can be lower using serum testing than using maternal age screening (Shackley et al. 1993) (criterion 9)
- Case-finding could be organised as a continuing process (criterion 10).

Although, on this superficial inquiry, it appeared that serum screening for Down syndrome appeared to meet Wilson's and Jungner's criteria, a number of questions were left unanswered. Particular concerns were that Wilson and Jungner's criteria: (a) did not address the complexity caused by the multiple outcomes of the screening programme, (b) did not help clarify what should be considered 'suitable' tests (criterion 5), (c) did little to help determine if a programme was 'acceptable' to the population (criterion 6), (d) did not provide any basis for comparing different screening policies and (e) did not consider affordability as well as cost effectiveness (see Chapter 32). This last issue was of practical importance to us because even if serum screening for Down syndrome was cost effective (i.e. the cost/case detected with serum screening was lower than with maternal age screening), if a serum screening programme were to cost more than was then being spent on the existing maternal age screening programme it was unlikely to be judged affordable by NHS purchasers.

Table 33.2. Cuckle and Wald's requirements for a worthwhile screening programme

Aspect	Requirement
1. Disorder	Well-defined
2. Prevalence	Known
3. Natural history	Medically important disorder for which there is an effective remedy available
4. Financial	Cost-effective
5. Facilities	Available or easily installed
6. Ethical	Procedures following a positive result are generally agreed and acceptable both to the screening authorities and to the patients
7. Test	Simple and safe
8. Test performance	Distributions of test values in affected and unaffected individuals known, extent of overlap sufficiently small, and suitable cut-off level defined

Cuckle and Wald's criteria

Next we assessed serum screening against Cuckle and Wald's more modern criteria for judging whether a screening programme is worthwhile (Cuckle and Wald 1984; Table 33.2). Our assessment was that:

- Down syndrome is a well-defined disorder (criterion 1)
- The prevalence and incidence of Down syndrome are known (criterion 2)
- Down syndrome is medically [and socially and economically] an important disorder which can be avoided by inducing abortion in women with affected pregnancies (criterion 3)
- Serum screening for Down syndrome can be judged to be cost-effective when compared to maternal age screening for Down syndrome (criterion 4)
- The technical facilities for screening for Down syndrome could be installed easily (criterion 5)
- Inducing abortion in women with a Down syndrome pregnancy is legal and acceptable to all screening authorities but not to all women (criterion 6)
- A blood test is simple and safe to perform but the results may be difficult to convey (criterion 7)
- The distribution of test values in affected and unaffected individuals is known and the extent of overlap is such that a universally accepted cut off level has not been defined (criterion 8).

Again, these criteria, although helpful, did not provide a framework for addressing the questions left unanswered by Wilson and Jungner's criteria. They did, however, reinforce that selection of a suitable cut off for identifying women who should be offered amniocentesis is an important issue. Interestingly, different individuals and institutions were recommending different cut off points (e.g. Barrow *et al.* 1994; Goldie *et al.* 1995), so it was not clear whether and how a 'suitable' cut-off point should be defined. In common with Wilson and Jungner's criteria, Cuckle and Wald's criteria also reminded us of the importance of considering the acceptability and availability of necessary facilities for screening. These should include pre-test arrangements for women who are able to give meaningful informed consent (Smith *et al.* 1994; Vyas 1994).

After applying Wilson and Jungner's and Cuckle and Wald's criteria, two key questions remained, namely:

1. Do the benefits of the programme exceed the harms? If yes,
2. Are the net benefits worth the cost in relation to alternative uses for the same resources?

These questions are very similar to those which form the basis of a new set of screening criteria which are being drafted by a group led by Professor L. Irwig (Irwig, personal communication). Although these are apparently simple and obvious questions, they are not made explicit in well known screening criteria such as those described above. In Oxfordshire I think we took longer than we should have done to agree that these were the key issues. And, although the questions are easy to ask, we have found them difficult to answer. I am not yet sure that we have satisfactory answers.

Using decision analysis to compare policies for antenatal screening for Down syndrome

We wanted to use the large amount of national and local data that was available about biochemical screening for Down syndrome to quantify as many as possible of the likely consequences of different screening options for the population of Oxfordshire. We used the technique of decision analysis, which is a well-documented method for integrating data from a wide variety of sources to explore population policy options (Thornton *et al.* 1992) and to help inform difficult decisions about individuals. The method consists of defining a clinical problem, identifying the components of the decision, arranging the components of the decision as a 'tree' which describes the possible pathways to particular outcomes, and quantifying the probabilities of passing down each branch of the tree (Fig.33.1). This enables the expected consequences of different decisions to be calculated.

We considered six different screening programmes:

1. Offering counselling, ultrasound, biochemical testing, and further counselling to all pregnant women regardless of age, with a 'high risk' result defined as a predicted risk greater than 1 in 250;
2. Offering counselling, ultrasound, biochemical testing, and further counselling to all pregnant women regardless of age, with 'high risk' defined as a predicted risk greater than 1 in 100;
3. Offering pregnant women aged 35 years or more amniocentesis or the option of biochemical testing for Down syndrome paid for by the patient;
4. Offering amniocentesis to pregnant women aged 35 years and above;
5. Offering counselling, ultrasound, biochemical testing, and further counselling to pregnant women aged 30 years and above with 'high risk' defined as a predicted risk greater than 1 in 250; and
6. No screening programme for Down syndrome.

Option 1 was a widely used policy for biochemical screening for Down syndrome in the UK. Options 2 and 5 represented two different approaches to reducing the total numbers of false positive results, by increasing the threshold for labelling a pregnancy 'high risk' (option 2) and by restricting the test to women aged 30 years or more (option 5). Option 3 represented existing practice in Oxfordshire, and option 4 was Oxfordshire's existing policy. The inclusion of option 6 (no screening for Down syndrome) allows the overall population impact of the other policies to be determined.

We constructed a decision tree that described the different policy options and clinical courses of women's pregnancies from the second trimester. At each node or branching of the tree, probabilities or proportions were given to each branch by using published data or, when more appropriate, locally derived data. Once we were satisfied that the tree was a good summary of practice we used it to calculate the expected outcomes of different screening strategies. Where branches are duplicates of others only one full branch has been displayed. A fuller account of this decision analysis has been published (Fletcher *et al.* 1995a).

Seven sets of predicted population outcomes were calculated from the tree for each option: live birth with Down syndrome; live birth without Down syndrome; termination of a fetus with Down syndrome; direct financial costs of the programme to the NHS; and the number of women offered counselling, ultrasound, biochemical testing, and further counselling. Table 33.3 shows the initial assessments used in the decision analysis.

Table 33.4 shows the predicted performance of each of the six screening policies and that different outcomes are optimised with different screening policies; for example, most fetuses with Down syndrome would be detected by

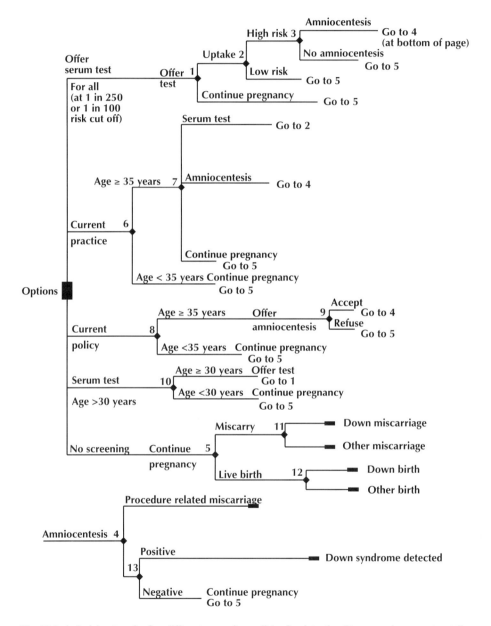

Fig. 33.1. A decision tree for five different screening policies for detecting Down syndrome antenatally. (Reproduced with permission from Fletcher *et al.* 1995b.)

offering counselling, ultrasound, biochemical testing and further counselling to all pregnant women (option 1), but the number of normal births would be greatest with no screening of any sort (option 6). The results also confirm that the numbers of Down syndrome pregnancies detected could be increased and, simultaneously, the number of amniocenteses and associated miscarriages could be reduced, by replacing existing practice with a screening option that includes serum testing.

All the policy options for using a serum test that we considered had important drawbacks: screening women aged >30 years with high risk defined as >1:250 (option 5) would identify fewer Down syndrome pregnancies than screening the whole population with high risk defined as >1:250 and would deny young women the opportunity of improving their chances of detecting a Down pregnancy;

Table 33.3. Starting values used in the decision tree (reproduced with permission from Fletcher *et al.* 1995b)

Variable	Key to Fig.33.1	Value used	Likely range
Prevalence of Down syndrome during second trimester (age standardised to Oxfordshire population)		1.95 per 1000	12–20
Prevalence of Down births in women over 30 years		65/24879	
Number of births per year in Oxfordshire		39/7139	
Prevalence of Down births in women under 30 years		31/47336	
Prevalence of Down births in women under 35 years		57/65094	
Sensitivity of amniocentesis	13	100%	>95%
Specificity of amniocentesis	13	100%	>95%
Sensitivity of screening test (triple test 1 in 250)	2	58%	45%–89%
Specificity of screening test (triple test 1 in 250)	2	95%	89%–96%
Sensitivity of screening test (triple test 1 in 100)	2	44%	
Specificity of screening test (triple test 1 in 100)	2	98.3%	
Probability of miscarriage from second trimester (background)	5,11	1%	0.7%–2%
Probability of miscarriage of a Down fetus from second trimester	5,11	25%	23%–40%
Probability of miscarriage after amniocentesis (added)	4	1%	0.5%–1%
Proportion of pregnancies in women over 30 years	10	40.7%	
Proportion of pregnancies in women over 35 years	6,8	11.6%	
Present chromosomal analysis rate in women over 35 years	7	43%	
Proportion of women over 35 years having biochemical test at present	7	33%	
Uptake of amniocentesis following a positive serum test	3	95%	75%–100%
Uptake of screening test	1	80%	60%–100%
Additional unit cost of CUBC		£13.70	£10–£60
Unit cost of amniocentesis or chorionic villus sampling		£250	£95–£250
Cost of termination		£450	£450–£1000
Number of births per year in Oxfordshire		7533	

Table 33.4. The results of the decision analysis: numbers of predicted events per year in Oxfordshire (reproduced with permission from Fletcher et al. 1995b)

Programme	Unaffected births	Down births	Down mis-carriages	Cases of Down syndrome detected	Amnio-centesis mis-carriages	Number of amnio-centeses	Cost of programme	Programme cost per Down detected 'cost per case'	Amnio-centesis mis-carriages per Down detected 'lost per case'	Number of women offered screening
Serum testing offered to all pregnant women and high risk result defined as risk >1:250	7440	6.2	2.1	6.4	2.9	290	£160k	£25k	0.45	7533
Serum testing offered to all pregnant women and high risk result defined as risk >1:100	7442	7.4	2.4	4.9	1.0	100	£110k	£22k	0.20	7533
Present practice OHA Women over 35 offered amniocentesis on the NHS or private Serum test	7440	7.8	2.6	3.7	3.7	370	£95k	£26k	1.00	874
Current policy OHA Assuming a 75% uptake of amniocentesis by women over 35	7437	7.0	2.3	4.7	6.6	660	£170k	£36k	1.40	874
Offer Serum test for all women over 30 years and high risk result defined as risk >1:250	7442	7.4	2.5	4.7	1.2	120	£70k	£15k	0.25	3066
No screening	7443	11.0	3.7	0	0	0	0	n/a	n/a	None

screening the whole population with high risk defined as >1:250 (option 1) would lead to more miscarriages associated with amniocentesis and more false positive results and would be more expensive than other options; and screening the whole population with high risk defined as >1:100 (option 2) would detect fewer cases of Down syndrome than defining high risk as >1:250 and would be more expensive than what was then present practice.

One advantage of using decision analysis is that the assumptions on which the model is based are explicit. Where there is debate about the numbers that have been used in the calculations it is easy to recalculate the model with the new numbers. Some people have suggested that different numbers should have been used in our analysis (Murray and Tennison 1995; Reynolds 1995; Spencer 1995). However, recalculation does not alter the broad conclusions to be drawn from the analysis (Fletcher *et al.* 1995b).

The importance of having clear aims for a screening programme for Down syndrome

An important conclusion illustrated by this analysis is that the choice of screening programme depends on the overall aim(s) of the screening programme. For example the analysis presented here suggests that if the aim of the programme was to maximise the number of Down cases detected antenatally then, among the options considered in Oxfordshire, option 1 (serum testing offered to all pregnant women with a cut off at 1:250) would be the best option. Alternatively, if the aim was to minimise the financial cost per Down case detected then the best option would be option 5 (serum testing offered to all women over the age of 30 years with a cut off at 1:250). And if the aim was to minimise the number of normal pregnancies lost per case detected then the best option would be option 2 (offering serum testing to all women with a cut off at 1:100). But I submit that none of these population aims are the main reason for screening for Down syndrome: they all ignore the consequences for individual women. The primary reason for (i.e. the aim of) screening for Down syndrome is to optimise the position of each individual woman.

Importance of remembering the individual perspective

Screening for Down syndrome, although often thought of as a population intervention, is also an example of a medical technology delivered to individual women one at a time. The familiar ethics of clinical medicine, with their focus on the individual, cannot be ignored. Indeed there would have to be unequivocal and significant population advantages before contemplating subjugating individuals' needs to those of the population. As well as considering the population outcomes of screening, policy makers and practitioners must therefore consider the consequences of screening for individuals. If this were not the case a screening programme for Down syndrome would conflict strongly with the ethic of respecting individual autonomy. And it is important, that where values vary widely between individuals, well-being should be judged in terms of an individual patient's values because individuals' values cannot reliably be deduced from 'average' population values. One woman may regard losing a normal pregnancy as a greater disaster than having a child with Down syndrome. Another woman may hold quite the opposite views. This has important implications for how antenatal tests for Down syndrome should be used.

Another fundamental ethical principle of medical practice – non-maleficence – is also relevant to the organisation of screening programmes. Its meaning is sometimes summarised in the phrase *primum non nocere:* first do no harm. For all medical interventions, including population interventions such as immunisation and screening, at the moment of intervention both the patient and the professional must believe that the benefits of intervention outweigh the risks for that individual patient. Although this principle is recognised *implicitly* in most population interventions, I believe it is so important that it should be an *explicit* criterion against which screening programmes are judged.

One example of a population intervention in which the principle of beneficence is applied in every day practice is immunisation. The immuniser will seek out those who are most likely to suffer adverse reactions to immunisation and advise against immunising them even though doing so may have adverse consequences for the population (e.g. herd immunity may be more difficult to achieve).

Population benefit and cost effectiveness

The main population benefit of a screening programme for Down syndrome is a reduction in the financial and social costs in caring for people with Down syndrome. Although the cost per case detected for serum screening for Down syndrome is lower than for maternal age screening, Chapter 32 makes it clear that the necessary studies to determine the true cost effectiveness of screening for Down syndrome have not been done. I submit that the population benefits are neither large enough nor certain enough for us to advocate using tests for Down syndrome in ways that make it easy for professionals to ignore the interests of individuals.

Antenatal tests for Down syndrome: individual investigation not mass screening

If it is important to optimise the well-being of individuals and to identify women whose values are such that the risks of screening for Down syndrome outweigh the benefits, then we must change the way in which tests for Down syndrome are currently used. As screening for Down syndrome has multiple consequences and it is likely that women attach different relative values to the consequences of screening, it is impossible that a 'one-size-fits all' mass population screening programme can meet these aims. These aims can only be met by informing individual women of the options available to them and tailoring the selection of investigations and subsequent action to their individual circumstances and values. Existing antenatal tests for Down syndrome should be used as investigations tailored to individual women's needs and not as part of an inflexible mass population screening programme.

Should screening for Down syndrome be offered?

So my answer to the question 'Should screening for Down syndrome be offered?' is : No, an inflexible mass population screening programme should not be offered. However, the relevant investigations should be available to all pregnant women. Women should be told of the options available to them and have the opportunity to discuss these options with an informed attendant. The available tests should then be used and interpreted in such a way that each woman has the maximum chance of optimising her personal position.

Implications for screening programmes with multiple outcomes in populations with variable values

There is a generalisable lesson that emerges from this case-study: inflexible mass population screening should not be undertaken where the proposed screening programme would have multiple outcomes and would be performed on a population made up of individuals who place widely differing values on the various outcomes of the screening programme. Under these circumstances the needs of each individual should be sought, understood, and acted upon accordingly.

The challenge of improving communication

As most screening programmes have multiple outcomes and we are far from certain about the distribution of relative values that people attach to the outcomes of screening programmes, it will be rare to introduce new monolithic screening programmes. The challenge that we face is how we can best organise services so that relevant, valid information is communicated in such a way that patients and staff can together plan appropriate investigation and management for each individual patient. This represents a major challenge for the health professions for the years to come and an area where further research is needed.

Likely benefits of investigating individuals rather than screening populations

Let us return briefly to Down syndrome. If we were to stop thinking about *screening* and instead to think of investigating pregnancies appropriately, it would improve the way in which serum tests for Down syndrome are used. For example, a performance indicator for most screening programmes is the uptake rate. The implication is that a higher uptake rate is better than a lower uptake rate. As the optimal rate of investigation depends on the distribution of individual women's views and values, such an implication would be inappropriate for Down syndrome testing. The concept of screening may be encouraging practitioners to test inappropriately without adequately assessing the balance of risks and benefits in individual women.

Flexible risk cut-off

If we stopped thinking of screening we might also find ourselves asking other questions about the way in which we currently use serum tests for Down syndrome. Why, for example, have we assumed that all women who have had a serum test should have amniocentesis offered to them at the same level of risk? Some might opt for amniocentesis at a risk of 1:50, others at 1:300 or at any other value for that matter. Each value may be appropriate and accurately reflect the views and values of individual women. Obstetricians' instincts tell them that flexibility is desirable but a screening programme makes some feel offering such flexibility is wrong (Goldie *et al.* 1995). If we stopped thinking of testing for Down syndrome as part of a mass population screening programme, most professionals' clinical training would, I believe, mean they would readily tailor interpretation of the tests to women's individual circumstances.

Avoid unnecessary labelling

Why do we distress women with phrases like 'high risk' and 'a positive screening result'? Much of this distress is a direct result of the labels we attach to people which may or may not correspond to what well informed women conceive as high risk for themselves. It would be better for individual women if they were offered the chance to make up their own minds about what constitutes a risk of Down syndrome that is sufficiently high for them to want to go on to amniocentesis. Alternatively, for those women who do not want to make their own decision, their professional attendant should be in a position to base a decision on the woman's values. Again, if we could think of investigating appropriately rather than screening for Down syndrome we would, I believe, reduce the distress presently experienced by too many women.

Other considerations: practicality, affordability and priority

There are two other important considerations that I have not discussed. Is it practical to tailor testing to individual women? And is it affordable? I think the answer to both questions is probably yes. But I do not know. It is therefore important to test the proposals outlined in this chapter thoroughly and assess their consequences. Only a proper evaluation would allow the practicality and costs to be determined. I do not know, for example, how many women would choose serum testing and how many would opt for amniocentesis.

And finally, I have not addressed how the relative priority of investing in tests for Down syndrome compares with the priority afforded to other calls on scarce resources. No one yet has a perfect answer to such questions. Indeed, I do not believe there are any absolute 'right answers'. In my judgement, transparent processes for reaching such decisions that are open to all the relevant stakeholders need to be established. Decisions should be informed by whatever valid and relevant external information is available, which ideally should include cost-effectiveness data. However, even with perfect information about the consequences of medical intervention we will never be able to escape from the value laden nature of resource allocation decisions. So another prerequisite of the decision making process is that it should be underpinned by a clear ethical framework.

Summary

This chapter has addressed the question, 'Should screening for Down syndrome be offered?' by examining how this question was dealt with in Oxfordshire. The main lessons are as follows:

1. The appropriate policy will depend on the aims of the programme.
2. The aim of screening for Down syndrome is to optimise the well being of each individual woman.
3. At the moment of intervention/testing, the benefits should exceed the risks for each individual.
4. The ethical principles of autonomy and non-maleficence should not be ignored for population interventions and screening programmes.
5. Questions that need to be addressed in assessing any potential screening programme should include:
   (a) Do the benefits of the programme exceed the harms for both the population and individuals?
   (b) Are the net benefits worth the costs?

As screening for Down syndrome has multiple consequences and it is likely that different women attach different relative values to the various consequences of screening for Down syndrome, it is impossible to find a one-size-fits-all policy that optimises well-being for each woman. As long as screening for Down syndrome has multiple outcomes and those outcomes are valued differently by different individuals in the population, the concept of mass population screening for Down syndrome should be abandoned and services should be developed which aspire to give appropriate information and provide relevant investigations for all pregnant women.

Acknowledgements. I would like to thank Dr Louise Hicks and Dr Tony Hope for helpful discussions about screening for Down syndrome and for comments on earlier drafts of the manuscript.

References

Barrow, M., Falconer Smith, J. and Stewart, C. (1994) Keeping the concept of risk simple. *BMJ* **309**, 1373

Cuckle, H.S. and Wald, N.J. (1984) *Antenatal and Neonatal Screening.* Oxford: Oxford University Press

Cuckle, H., Nanchanal, K. and Wald, N. (1991) Birth prevalence of Down's syndrome. *Prenat Diagn* **11**, 29–34

Dick, P.T. and Canadian Task Force on the Periodic Health Examination (1996). Periodic health examination, 1996 update: 1. Prenatal screening for and diagnosis of Down syndrome. *Can Med Assoc J* **154**, 465–79

Fletcher, J., Hicks, N.R., Kay, J.D.S. and Boyd, P.A. (1995a) Decision analysis and screening for Down's syndrome. *BMJ* **311**, 1372–3

Fletcher, J., Hicks, N.R., Kay, J.D.S. and Boyd, P.A. (1995b) Using decision analysis to compare policies for antenatal screening for Down's syndrome. *BMJ* **311**, 351–6

Goldie, D.J., Astley, J.P., Beaman, J.M. *et al.* (1995) Screening for Down's syndrome: the first two years experience in Bristol. *J Med Screening* **2**, 207–10

Green, J.M. (1994) Serum screening for Down's syndrome: experiences of obstetricians in England and Wales. *BMJ* **309**, 769–72

Hook, F.B., Cross, P.K. and Schreinemachers, D.M. (1983) Chromosomal abnormality rates at amniocentesis and in live-born infants. *JAMA* **249**, 2034–8

Lippman, A., Tomkins, D.J., Shime, J. *et al.* (1992) Multicentre randomized clinical trial of chorionic villus sampling and amniocentesis. Final report. *Prenat Diagn* **12**, 385–408

Marteau, T.M. (1993) Psychological consequences of screening for Down's syndrome. *BMJ* **307**, 146–7

Murray, D. and Tennison, B. (1995) Estimate of uptake of amniocentesis is overoptimistic. *BMJ* **311**, 1371

Reynolds, T.M. (1995) Costs were overestimated. *BMJ* **311**, 1372

Shackley, P., McGuire, A., Boyd, P.A. *et al.* (1993) An economic appraisal of alternative pre-natal screening programmes for Down's syndrome. *J Public Health Med* **15**, 175–84

Smith, D.K., Shaw, R.W. and Marteau, T.M. (1994) Informed consent to undergo serum screening for Down's syndrome: the gap between policy and practice. *BMJ* **309**, 776

Spencer, K. (1995) Not using age specific values invalidates study. *BMJ* **311**, 1371

Statham, H. and Green, J. (1993). Serum screening for Down syndrome: some women's experiences. *BMJ* **307**, 174–6

Tabor, A., Philip, J., Madsen, M. *et al.* (1986) Randomised controlled trial of genetic amniocentesis in 4606 low-risk women. *Lancet* **i**, 1287–93

Thornton, J.G., Lilford, R.J. and Johnson, N. (1992) Decision analysis in medicine. *BMJ* **298**, 1099–103

Vyas, S. (1994) Screening for Down's syndrome: ignorance abounds. *BMJ* **309**, 753–4

Wald, N.J., Cuckle, H.S., Densem, J.W. *et al.* (1988) Maternal screening for Down's syndrome in early pregnancy. *BMJ* **297**, 883–7

Wald, N.J., Huttly, W., Wald, K. and Kennard, A. (1996) Down's syndrome screening in the UK. *Lancet* **340**, 494

Wald, N.J., Kennard, A., Densem, J.W. *et al.* (1992) Antenatal maternal serum screening for Down's syndrome: results of a demonstration project. *BMJ* **305**, 391–4

Wilson, J.M.G. and Jungner, G. (1968) *Principles and Practice of Screening for Disease.* Geneva: World Health Organisation

Chapter 34

Practical issues of screening programmes

Discussion

Chard: I suggest some slight structure for the discussion of the papers we have just heard. Could we begin with economic and cost effective aspects. Does anyone wish to make any observations or ripostes about that?

Nicolaides: I am always sceptical about these calculations because I am convinced that they are always almost certainly wrong.

Prediction of cost effectiveness has within it the cost of having somebody with DS to care for over the next 60 years. It is incomprehensible to me that you would know the cost of looking after somebody with Alzheimer's disease at the age of 50 in the year 2040 or 2050. So I am dubious about those calculations. I do not know, for example, the cost of needles for amniocentesis in three months from now. That is the first thing.

The second thing is that if all the calculations for cost effectiveness in serum biochemistry are calculated at the cost that is given on the day – add in inhibin or the other test, maybe the quadruple test costs £15, as they said in the advertisement in the *BMJ* a few weeks ago. What is the cost of counselling? What is the cost of the ultrasound scan that is part of the package for dating the pregnancy? Also, all the calculations are part of the subsequent discussions, since I am of the second view – the view that is beginning to be supported by some in this audience – that the aim of screening for DS is mere provision of information and not classification of high and low risk and let them decide whatever they want.

How much of this information can be got from existing provision of care and how much can the existing provision of care be improved by the addition of biochemistry? I am not prejudiced in saying that since antenatal care, to my mind, necessitates an ultrasound scan at 12 weeks for 50 reasons, if part of the package of introducing the ultrasound scan to achieve those 50 reasons has as a side effect that we achieve a certain detection of DS from that, you need to look at the additional cost of adding biochemistry to that to achieve the luxury of giving information to people to let them choose.

Torgerson: First of all, the cost. My calculation of cost of detecting an affected pregnancy is that we should detect the pregnancy and it is up to the individual patient what they want to do about that, whether they want to terminate the pregnancy, carry on or whatever, or just want provision of information.

The second issue is the averted cost issue. None of the studies I quoted included the cost of the averted cost of caring for an individual with Down syndrome, but a paper by Shackley estimated that cost in one analysis which they factored in was £80,000 (Shackley *et al.* 1993). I would agree with you on two issues: first, that the cost of caring for a Down syndrome individual today is very likely to be different from one in 20 years' time. The second, more practical, issue is that you can say to a purchaser that we can do initial microscopic surgery, which would cost a bit more, but we save lots of money on other people's budgets. The purchaser will say so what, that's nothing to do with me, I don't care if you save the social security budget; what I'm worried about is the budget in front of me at the moment.

I personally take the jaundiced view that it is important to calculate the other costs and put them in the equation, but it is also important to present them all separately so that a purchaser is more likely to buy them than to exclude them.

Nicolaides: The other thing is that antenatal care in obstetrics is about other things than DS. This is part of that package of providing for the other things. It is a side effect that you get partial information on DS. You must look at the differential cost effectiveness of adding something else.

Torgerson: Yes, if you are going to evaluate that screening, if you have all the equipment in place anyway whether you are going to do nuchal translucency or not, then you should not take the cost of those overheads into account because they would be there whether you did it or not. What you need to do is factor in an additional cost of extra technician time or extra labour costs, which will be less than starting on a greenfield site essentially.

Nicolaides: Good, it is the other way round. If it is an essential requisite – and I agree with Professor Wald that it is – that you do an ultrasound scan before you have proper second trimester serum biochemistry, i.e. if we did not have serum biochemistry I would for other reasons have to support the introduction of first trimester scanning and therefore on the basis of that work out the cost effectiveness. But if the main reason for introducing first trimester scanning is to do serum biochemistry, it is ridiculous not to include the cost of the first trimester scan in the packet of screening for DS.

Torgerson: Yes.

Nicolaides: But you have not.

Chard: I do not think Mr Torgerson undertook that sort of detailed analysis of all possible scenarios. I don't think you claimed to, did you?

Torgerson: No. I cannot remember but I think that the detection rates I used were reported without the ultrasound scan, so in that sense if I did not use that it is correct, I had reason to do that. If I included figures where you included the use of a dating scan, then that would have needed to be included.

Chard: I am sorry, we must move on and I do not want to focus all the discussion on one point. Could we come to Dr Hicks' paper? If I interpreted the discussion bullet points there, it really comes down to one between mass versus selective screening. I will take any other comments or questions anyone would care to raise.

Wald: The point that Dr Hicks has raised is the critical emerging one. It is not only on this side of the Atlantic, it is emerging in America. I was at a meeting in San Francisco when Dr Goldberg was putting forward the same view. What we really have to consider is whether we are going to give a risk for all and allow people just to decide what they wish to do, and what sort of provision are we going to make for the consequences of that? Those could be substantial – the counselling consequences, amniocentesis, termination of pregnancy. They are likely to be unpredictable, although it is possible that if you did a pilot programme on this you might find that on average you had an estimate and then you could predicate your resources on that.

So we have to ask ourselves what is the reason for having screening, what is the nature of screening? I believe that screening is a legitimate means of limiting the offer of certain tests for treatment to persons who have not sought medical attention for a specific problem.

We then have to ask ourselves, why limit the offer? There are really only two reasons: because the treatment or the subsequent test is harmful or expensive, or both. In both of those elements there is harm, and the individual has to judge the harm in certain situations. But in screening we are offering something that can lead to harm, and I believe there is a professional obligation not to institute a process in a *laissez-faire* manner when you might lead to a situation where, on average, you might well be doing more harm than good.

I recognise that balancing the harm and good is difficult because we are comparing incommensurables. But there is a professional responsibility and I as an individual would feel rather upset if I was leading to something which would result in the death of 50 normal fetuses or babies for one DS detected. If that ratio was more like 4 or 5 to 1 I might find it more acceptable; I am not sure where I draw the line. But as a doctor I have a concern about that risk. I also recognise that the patient will have to balance that. There are basically two parties to a medical transaction: the view of the professional, the doctor, and the view of the patient.

Secondly, there is the expense. If some women with risks of one in 1000 or one in 2000 or one in 4000 say, yes, I'd like an amniocentesis and onward counselling, do we have the resources to give it? I am particularly concerned that if you give a risk to all you will have to counsel every woman, not inform them – we have heard of the difficulties of doing that – and that might be a two-minute or a five-minute exercise. Giving a risk to every woman would be a 45-minute consultation with every woman in the population.

So I believe that that proposition is impractical. It raises ethical concerns to the profession and it is likely to be extremely expensive and may put in threat the whole programme, which already in part is at threat because people say that even with screening we cannot do anything because we do not feel that we can provide the support for counselling and the after care, as Professor Cuckle mentioned earlier.

Hicks: I do not disagree with a word that Professor Wald has said, except that the phrase *laissez-faire* is inappropriate because it is entirely possible to offer individual risks under controlled circumstances, so it is possible to put in a quality control system that maximises both the technical side of the procedure, the biochemical risk estimation, and also, as people have been calling for, whatever the system, whatever the way we choose to use the serum testing. I think we recognise that there is also a need for having a degree of quality control in the way information is given. And those quality control systems will be equally applicable, whichever way we choose to use them. So I would like to get away from the view of *laissez-faire*.

Professor Wald is right. I have no evidence that the model that I am proposing is practical and there are reasons to believe that it may be impractical. But I would suggest that we do not know and that it might be worth finding out.

Reynolds: This actually comes within the recommendations we were asked for at the beginning such as the recommendation for future research. It is quite urgent that we find out what people want. Professor Nicolaides said that doctors and nurses believe somewhere between one in 10 and one in 1000, and they know a lot about it. We need to find out what the population think. We need a model to find out what the effect would be.

Nicolaides: I know in my own patients because I have practised the concept of giving them a number and working out a process of helping them understand what numbers mean. For example, if I tell them the risk of miscarriage is one in 100 and having a DS baby the statistical risk is one in 1000, it means that they feel that they are prepared to have ten miscarriages to avoid the birth of one baby with DS; and the reverse. They have been practising that. If I take a subgroup of women who were over the age of 35, only 30% of a total population actually have an invasive test – a subgroup that would traditionally have had an invasive test. For me there is not a tremendous fear that a policy of offering people a choice will overwhelm the services in terms of invasive tests.

Reynolds: Has anything been published so that we can look at it? We know what the pattern of risk estimate would be and we could then match the risk estimate on that population against what you have as your acceptability range of patients of particular ages. You could get an idea of the effect of this policy quite quickly without being too selective.

Nicolaides: My patients are self-selected patients, but there is a need to address that issue. I do not expect that they will be rushing to have invasive tests.

Macintosh: We have a major problem of decentralisation of our health service. We have great difficulty in initiating this type of study. Professor Wald, would you think it was inappropriate to look at exactly what Dr Hicks has proposed for a region, for example, just offering the test as it is and then observing what the effect was on health professionals in choosing, etc.? I think that that would be quite a rational way forward, but it seems impossible in our decentralised system to be able to organise it at times.

That is addressed to Professor Wald because he said that he felt that we had a duty not to introduce this procedure. Do you really think that? Do you think that it should not be evaluated?

Wald: I gave reasons against the proposition put forward by Dr Hicks. I don't think I would go so far as to say that I would not look at the alternative if a suitable study were to be conducted. We could look at the consequences and quantify them. At the same time, like you, I recognise the difficulties of doing that.

Cuckle: There is a little bit of information on this, which I don't think has been published yet, from Israel, where they have more or less gone over to letting people do what they want. But they have gone completely over the top and vast numbers of women are having inverted prenatal diagnosis. That would be unacceptable here. It is probably acceptable in Israel because they tend to see two or three doctors anyway for every disease that they have and take the average.

This is a semi-private healthcare system and we have to be very careful here, apart from the safety aspects, of wasting public resources. Screening is a kind of rationing; it is a focusing of resources to where they can do the most good for the least cost. It is a kind of *laissez-faire*, what is being proposed. We do not know what the cost will be. It is all right to do a little study of it and it probably would not need to be a massive study, and we would see what happened. But it is a dangerous precedent for screening to be open-ended.

Marteau: I want to endorse the prospect of a properly conducted trial to look at the consequences of offering information about the chance of having a child with Down syndrome without any kind of evaluation added as to whether it is high or low risk. I do not share Professor Cuckle's concern that this would lead to an over-use of resources. The example he gave from Israel – I would want to know how the information was given, how was it framed when it is in a different context. So I would like to see as one of our recommendations for future research some kind of trial where we are able to look at this, and now is the opportunity – and the window of opportunity is fast closing.

Davies: I do not have the dubious pleasure of sitting on the side of the desk which faces the wall but I have been through the process of sitting on the side of the desk which faces the door. When people told my wife and me that we were screened negative or positive, our response to that was, 'How dare you? How dare you presume what we will feel is high risk and low risk?'

The second point is – and it is probably not a popular suggestion – that at the root of all this is money. It is all to do with money. Dr Hicks is concerned, saying you cannot introduce this *laissez-faire*, you cannot tell women they are at risk and let them make a decision. You do women a disservice, if you think that they do not understand this issue. Many of them do, if it is explained properly. So why not accept the fact that resources are limited, and you say OK, you can do what you want; this is your risk, this is what it means. But we are only prepared to pay, we only have enough money to pay, for those at highest risk. If you want CVS and your risk is one in 800 and you are worried, yes, you can have a CVS but we cannot afford to pay for it.

I know that is probably a very unpopular bite-the-bullet scenario, but at least it is truthful and honest.

Chard: It is rather like the French used to do – or maybe still do. They are reimbursed if they have a specific risk factor and not, if they do not.

Brambati: It is what we do in Italy.

Zimmerman: The same in Switzerland.

Jauniaux: The same in Belgium.

Hicks: Two very short points. One is that I can see that screening is one way of limiting how much of a resource gets spent on this activity. But it is also important not to forget that screening also implies there is a population poll and, as Professor Cuckle said earlier on, is it credible to go on minimising the numbers of DS births and maximising the detection rate?

The other point is that it has come through in various forms about the importance of there being some form of quality assurance and quality control. I take great heart from Professor Nicolaides' presentation in demonstrating that it is possible. We may have a decentralised health-care system now, but that does not mean that quality control with hospitals working together is not possible. That is another important message that we ought to push from this meeting.

Reference

Shackley, P., McGuire, A., Boyd, P. *et al.* (1993) An economic appraisal of alternative prenatal screening programmes for Down's syndrome. *J Public Health Med* **15,** 175–84

SECTION 10

RECOMMENDATIONS

Chapter 35

Recommendations arising from the 32nd Study Group: Screening for Down syndrome in the first trimester

The 32nd RCOG Study Group met to discuss new screening methods and the possibility of screening in the first trimester as well as and/or instead of in the second trimester.

The members of the Study Group have attempted to distil the presentations and discussions which took place over a three-day period into a series of recommendations. These recommendations fall into three categories:

1. Recommendations for clinical practice (principally aimed at Fellows and Members of this college) based on research evidence (where available) and on the consensus view of the Group. The clinical practice recommendations have been graded from 'A' to 'C' according to the strength of evidence on which each is based. The scheme for grading of recommendations is based on the system adopted by both the NHS Executive and the Scottish Intercollegiate Guidelines Network.
2. Recommendations for future research in those clinical areas where the Group identified a need for further evidence on which to base practice.
3. Recommendations relating to health education and healthy policy.

In its deliberations, the Study Group noted the recommendations of the RCOG Working Party on Down Syndrome Screening (1993), the report of the Genetics Research Advisory Group (1995) and the draft report of the RCOG and British Paediatric Association Working Party of 1996.

The Group wishes to draw the attention of Fellows and Members of the RCOG to the following recommendations and observations.

1. The Study Group confirms that the objective of screening for Down syndrome is the provision of information for individual(s), on which a decision can be based concerning further care of their pregnancy.

A *Grade C* recommendation based on the consensus view of the Study Group.

2. Although, at present, there appears to be insufficient evidence to recommend routine screening for Down syndrome in the first trimester by biophysical and biochemical markers, the Study Group wishes to state:

   2.1. *Nuchal translucency:* there are sufficient data to consider screening for Down syndrome by the measurement of nuchal translucency at 10–14 weeks' gestation an acceptable procedure. Preliminary reports indicate that the detection rate for a given false positive rate can be at least similar if not superior to serum screening with multiple markers at 15–22 weeks' gestation.

   A *Grade B* recommendation based on experimental data.

   Nuchal translucency screening should only be conducted where:

   2.1.1. The centre has staff with the high level of ultrasound competence and experience required which has been certified by an external agency and subject to external quality control procedures.

   2.1.2. Centres have in place high standard precision equipment, clinical protocols and external systems of quality assurance and ongoing audit.

   Grade C recommendations based on the consensus view of the Study Group.

   Attention is drawn to the view of the Study Group that randomised controlled trials (grade A evidence) in this field were considered to be inappropriate.

   2.2. There are sufficient data to consider that specific serum markers for Down syndrome at 9–13 weeks' gestation (notably pregnancy associated plasma protein-A and the free β subunit of hCG) may be as effective as those serum markers in established use at 15–22 weeks' gestation. There may be additional serum markers which will become applicable in the first trimester.

   A *Grade B* recommendation based on experimental data.

   The introduction of serum markers in first trimester screening for Down syndrome should only be considered when:

   2.2.1. Robust assay kits, which meet international standards, are available.

   2.2.2. Centres can demonstrate that their staff has expertise and experience in the use of these tests.

   2.2.3. The centre has clinical protocols and systems of quality assurance and ongoing audit.

   Grade C recommendations based on the consensus view of the Study Group.

   2.3. The combined use of screening with nuchal translucency and serum markers in the first trimester (9–13 weeks' gestation) might have a detection rate for Down syndrome superior to either serum markers or nuchal translucency used in isolation.

3. Recommendations for future research
3.1. Research into improved methods of rapid genetic diagnostic tests.
3.2. Research into the optimal way of provision of test results to clinicians and pregnant women (qualitative, e.g. screen positive, i.e. >1:300 versus quantitative, e.g. risk is 1:670 or 1:85).

Grade B **recommendations based on experimental data.**

4. Recommendations relating to health education and policy
As screening for Down syndrome in the first trimester with serum and ultrasound markers will require the active participation of the health professions in the community as well as institutions, the following issues will need to be addressed:

4.1. Education and training of health professions such as family doctors, midwives, obstetricians and health visitors.

4.2. Increased provision of information to health professionals and pregnant women.

4.3. Expansion of counselling services.

4.4. Expansion of expertise and regularly performed diagnostic tests such as chorionic villus sampling and early amniocentesis. This may require a policy of centralisation of these services until the safety of these techniques is demonstrated by clinicians intending to provide these interventions. Recommendation of minimum numbers of cases to be performed is important.

4.5. A revision in the provision of therapeutic abortion services.

4.6. Central quality assurance of a continuing audit of counselling, information and education as well as biochemical and biophysical tests.

4.7. A recommendation regarding the advisability of nationwide screening for Down syndrome.

4.8. Evaluation of the cost implications of the introduction of a national policy of screening for Down syndrome.

Grade C **recommendations based on the consensus view of the Study Group.**

Dissenting opinion from Professor Eva Alberman, Professor Theresa Marteau and Professor Nicholas Wald

We believe that some of the above recommendations do not accurately reflect a consensus of the 32nd RCOG Study Group. In particular we draw attention to the following. It has not been shown that nuchal translucency measurement is a better screening test than second trimester screening using four serum markers (see 2.1). Nuchal translucency measurement requires quality control but we do not agree that a case has been made to limit nuchal translucency measurement to centres certified by an external agency (see 2.1.1). First trimester serum screening is, on current evidence, not as effective as second trimester screening using four markers (see 2.2). Since the results of first trimester serum and ultrasound testing are not materially correlated, their combination must be more effective than either alone although the precise method of combining these two tests is still in development (see 2.3). We are of the opinion that further research is needed to compare the performance of first and second trimester screening to determine which should be recommended for use in routine screening practice.

Index